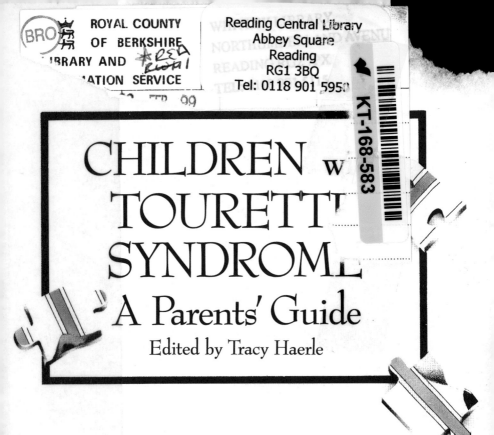

CHILDREN with
TOURETTE
SYNDROME

A Parents' Guide

Edited by Tracy Haerle

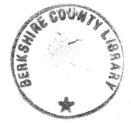

WOODBINE HOUSE • 1992

For information regarding sales of this book please contact:
Woodbine House, 5615 Fishers Lane,
Rockville, MD 20852, 800/843-7323.

Cover illustration & design: Lili Robins

Library of Congress Cataloging-in-Publication-Data

Children with Tourette syndrome : a parents' guide / Tracy Haerle, editor
   p. cm.
   Includes bibliographical references and index.
   ISBN 0-933149-44-1 (pbk.) : $14.95
  1. Tourette syndrome in children—Popular works. I. Haerle, Tracy.
RJ496.T68C45   1992   90–50766
618.92'83—dc20   CIP

Manufactured in the United States of America

4 5 6 7 8 9 10

TABLE OF CONTENTS

i

WEST GRID STAMP

NN		RR		WW	
NT		RT		WO	
NC		RC		WL	
NH		RB		WM	
NL		RP		WT	
NV		RS		WA	
NM		RW	10|96	WR	
NB		RV		WS	
NE					
NP					

ACKNOWLEDGEMENTS

Many people were more than generous with their time, their expertise, and their support in the development of this book. I owe a special thanks to all the parents and to the children and adults with Tourette syndrome who shared their lives with us in this book.

I want to thank the folks at the Tourette Syndrome Association—especially Sue Levy, Dave Spiler, Alan Levitt, Phyliss Levine, and Stephanie George—for all their support in the preparation of this book.

I am especially indebted to the chapter authors, all of whom were so patient and generous with their time—all for the purpose of increasing public awareness, education, and providing support to families affected by TS. A special thanks to Jim Eisenreich for his support.

Thanks goes to Susan Stokes for all her hard work, and to Irv Shapell and the rest of the Woodbine House staff for being interested in this project and making it a reality.

Finally, and most important, I want to thank my family—especially my son, Jeff. Because he has opened me up to the world of Tourette syndrome, I have been able to expand my sensitivity, my understanding, and my wonder at the complexity of the human mind. It is my fondest hope that in the future we all will have learned enough about Tourette syndrome—its cause and its treatments—that a book like this may no longer be necessary.

FOREWORD

JIM EISENREICH*

A few years ago, my dream of playing professional baseball almost came to an end. I didn't know it then, but I had Tourette syndrome. I was bounced from one doctor to another and was treated for problems that I didn't have. It was a nightmare.

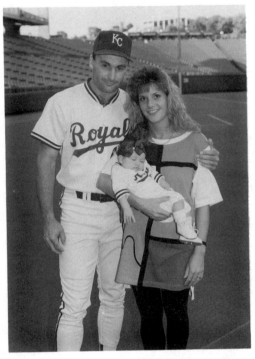

Fortunately, I was eventually diagnosed correctly, and proper treatment now allows me to lead a normal life. My baseball career is back on track, and best of all, my wife and I have a lovely new daughter.

When I first realized that there was a name for what was wrong with me, I felt relieved . . . I wasn't alone. And I found that help was available. When you have Tourette syndrome, one of the most important things you can do is educate yourself and others about the disorder. This book provides a great deal of useful

---

* Jim Eisenreich has been an outfielder with the Kansas City Royals since 1987. Previously, he played for the Minnesota Twins. He is active in public awareness and fundraising efforts for the national Tourette Syndrome Association.

information and does so in understandable terms. It also depicts the very broad range of Tourette syndrome, from almost unnoticeable symptoms to those that are quite visible and severe. Most cases are in the mild range, and when necessary, medications can usually help control symptoms.

In the last few years, great progress has been made in research and treatment for Tourette syndrome, and the future looks bright. Having Tourette syndrome didn't stop me from pursuing my dreams, and it shouldn't stop anyone else, either.

INTRODUCTION

TRACY HAERLE

The first time that either my husband or I heard the words "Tourette syndrome" was the day our seven-year-old son was diagnosed. And yet, we had both studied child psychology in college, and I had been a professional social worker and therapist. In addition, we had been scouring libraries and consulting an endless stream of physicians since our son first began showing symptoms at age two and a half.

Once we had the diagnosis, we assumed that information would be easier to come by. We immediately began searching for facts on Tourette syndrome (TS), but the libraries had no books on the subject, and the schools knew nothing about it.

By this time, our son was having social and academic problems at school, our health insurance was refusing to pay his medical bills on the erroneous grounds that TS was a mental illness, neighbors were calling our son terrible names such as "retard" and "spaz," and our extended family was blaming our son's behavior on our parenting skills—even though they praised those same parenting skills when they looked at our daughter. Then followed horrendous medication trials, which had our son "on the ceiling" one day, and "out to lunch" the next. We felt overwhelmed and alone.

Finally, we stumbled on the Tourette Syndrome Association (TSA) and began to receive some of the support and information we needed to cope with our son's TS. Now, four years later, our son's school is more responsive to his needs, his medications are stable, he has good friends, and we have a great doctor and family support system. Our life is back on an even keel.

It is my hope that this book can make the introduction into the world of Tourette syndrome less stressful for your family than it was for mine. By providing basic facts about how TS can affect all areas of a child's life, this book should better prepare your family for the challenges ahead. Chapters cover medical, educational, legal, family life, daily care, and emotional issues, and also provide a look at what can be expected in the future. You'll notice that I've used the personal pronouns "he" and "she" alternately by chapter. Although more boys than girls have TS, I didn't want to imply that all children with TS are boys, and it can be cumbersome to constantly use "he or she" to refer to a child.

The Parent Statements at the end of each chapter are a highlight. In these statements, parents share their feelings, thoughts, and experiences in raising a child with Tourette syndrome. Many statements contain nuggets of practical advice; others, I think, will help you realize that you're not in this alone. I've also included a glossary at the back of the book to help you decipher medical and educational jargon you may come across.

I do not intend this book to be the final authority on Tourette syndrome. All the scientific facts about TS are not in yet; much research is currently going on. But we who live with TS on a daily basis cannot wait until the final word is in about causes and treatments of TS. We need help *now*—with whatever resources are presently available. This book will, I hope, provide the beginning point in your journey, but it is just a beginning. The future holds much more knowledge and understanding of this complex disorder. Please use the Reading List at the end of the book for suggestions of other useful publications, and contact the Tourette Syndrome Association to find out about newly discovered information. The Resource Guide in the back of the book has the address for the TSA, as well as many other helpful national and local organizations.

Studies show that the severity of a child's Tourette syndrome is not what determines how successful he is in life. More important are high self-esteem and the acquisition of skills that enable him to cope with TS in a society that does not understand neurological disorders. My dream is that this book will help families get started in that all-important task of preparing their child with Tourette syndrome for adult life. My ultimate goal is that every person with TS will be accurately diagnosed and treated, and that they will be given every opportunity to reach their highest potential.

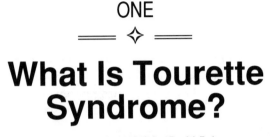

ONE

What Is Tourette Syndrome?

CARL R. HANSEN, JR., M.D.*

Introduction

Tourette syndrome (TS) is a baffling disorder. It may sneak up on you so gradually that for years, you may only have a vague suspicion that your child is "different." Perhaps he seems unusually hyperactive, impulsive, or quick to anger, but when you discuss your concerns with physicians, they say it is nothing to worry about. Tourette syndome may also appear with little or no warning. Years after you have begun to feel as if you really know your child, he may suddenly start making peculiar sounds or movements. At first, you may think that your child's actions are deliberate, but eventually you realize that they are out of his control.

While your child's strange movements and sounds gradually increase in number and frequency, you may spend months or years searching for the reason behind them. You may take your child to an eye doctor if he seems unable to control his blinking. He may have his tonsils removed if he continually clears his throat, or be diagnosed as having allergies if he constantly twitches his nose. Even when parents get an explanation for their child's behavior right away, the diagnosis often means little to them. Most people have never heard of Tourette syndrome, and if they have, they

---

* Dr. Carl R. Hansen is a child, adolescent, and adult psychiatrist at the Hansen McLeod Neuropsychiatric Clinic in Golden Valley, Minnesota.

probably know only of extreme cases which cause people to "bark" or "swear."

Because of the difficulty getting a diagnosis, parents sometimes conclude that there are no answers or solutions to their child's problems. Not true. There are medical treatments that can help many children control their symptoms, and educational strategies that can help them around the learning problems sometimes associated with TS. There are also plenty of up-to-date facts about the nature and causes of Tourette syndrome that can help children and their families cope with the disorder, as well as to dispel public misconceptions.

Because Tourette syndrome *is* such a vastly misunderstood and misdiagnosed disorder, you need current, accurate information at your fingertips to ensure that your child receives the treatment and education he needs. This chapter is designed to give you the basic understanding of Tourette syndrome—its symptoms, causes, treatment, diagnosis, and prognosis—you need to get started.

What Is Tourette Syndrome?

Tourette syndrome is a physical disorder of the brain which causes involuntary movements (motor tics) and involuntary vocalizations (vocal tics). Motor tics can occur in any part of the body, and include eye blinking, facial grimacing, shoulder shrugging, head jerking, and hand movements. Common vocal tics include throat clearing, sniffing, making loud sounds, grunting, or saying words. Both motor and vocal tics may occur many times a minute, or only a few times a day. They may be so mild as to be barely noticeable, or so severe as to be highly distracting, if not disabling. Tics begin before the age of twenty-one, most often around the age of seven. Over the course of time, tics may change in location, frequency, and severity, but they usually last a lifetime. Symptoms must be present for at least a year for a diagnosis of Tourette syndrome to be made.

Like other "syndromes," Tourette syndrome is so called because it is diagnosed on the basis of the symptoms it produces, not with a specific diagnostic test. Both motor and vocal tics *must* be present for the diagnosis of Tourette syndrome to be made, but there are also a variety of other symptoms that *may* be present. The following section reviews both the types of symptoms that all children with TS have, as well as those that only some children have.

The Symptoms of Tourette Syndrome

Tics

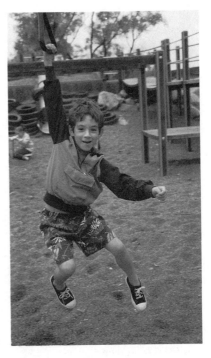

As explained above, all children with Tourette syndrome have tics—sudden, repetitive, and uncontrollable movements of muscles in the body. Tics in the muscles that control speech cause involuntary sounds such as coughing, hissing, snorting, or outbursts of words or phrases. Tics in other muscles of the body produce involuntary movements such as eye-blinking, grimacing, and leg-jerking.

Medical professionals sometimes classify tics as *simple* or *complex*, depending on how many parts of the body are involved. Brief, isolated movements of only one part of the body (head twitching, eye blinking, or shoulder shrugging) are considered simple motor tics. Likewise, simple noises—produced by air or sound moving through the vocal cords, throat, or nose (throat-clearing, sniffing, coughing, spitting)—are considered simple vocal tics. Complex tics involve more complicated, seemingly purposeful movements or sounds, and include hitting, pinching, poking, smelling objects, complex touching movements, and saying recognizable words or phrases.

Here are some examples of common motor and vocal tics:

Motor Tics	Vocal Tics
Simple	*Simple*
blinking eyes	throat-clearing
jerking neck	sniffing
shrugging shoulders	coughing
grimacing	grunting
flipping head	spitting
kicking	yelling
tensing muscles	belching
sticking tongue out	
finger movements	*Complex*
	animal sounds
Complex	repeating words or phrases out of
	context ("Oh boy," "I don't
facial gestures (eye rolling)	know," or words from advertising
grooming behaviors (smoothing hair)	jingles on TV)
smelling things	coprolalia (using obscene or other
touching	socially inappropriate words)
jumping	palilalia (repeating one's own words
hitting	or sounds—"Do my work,
biting	work, work")
echopraxia (imitating others' actions)	echolalia (repeating the last sound,
copropraxia (obscene gestures—	word, or phrase spoken by
giving the finger)	another person—saying "Come
self-injurious behaviors (picking	over here" after mother has just
scabs, rubbing sores raw, mouth	said, "Come over here")
biting, hitting self)	

More than half of all children with Tourette syndrome develop an eye tic first. In other children, the first symptom may be other facial tics, involuntary vocal sounds such as throat clearing, or vocal and motor tics together. Other tics usually develop in the weeks or months after the first tic. Common examples of early motor tics are grimaces, head jerks, or hand-to-face movements. The first vocal tics are often throat-clearing, grunting, sniffing, or snorting. Tics usually develop in upper extremeties first, then move down the body. Tics involving the trunk or legs usually occur fairly late in the course of the syndrome, as does coprolalia.

To receive the diagnosis of Tourette syndrome, children must have at least two motor tics and one vocal tic. (There are other types of tic disorders in which children may only have motor *or* vocal tics.) Children with Tourette syndrome may have any combination of vocal and motor tics. In addition, their symptoms usually change over time as new ones appear, replacing or adding to old ones. Bear in mind, however, that no child develops all, or even most, of these tics. For example, although television dramas may give the impression that everyone with Tourette syndrome has coprolalia, in reality, only about 30 percent do.

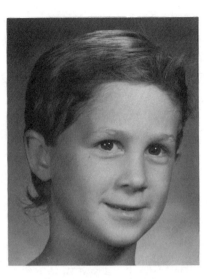

Likewise, only a small percentage of people with Tourette syndrome develop self-injurious behavior such as hitting themselves, mouth biting, or violent motor tics which may injure muscles.

Your child's tics may be mild, moderate, or severe, depending on their frequency and the degree to which they disrupt day-to-day activities. For example, they may range from a mild, easily disguised nose-wrinkling tic to loud, violent, disruptive full body movements. Symptoms will also wax and wane—or vary in intensity—from hour to hour, day to day, and year to year. There may be times when there are no tics, and then times when many tics occur, many times a day.

Often the intensity of tics increases during early adolescence (ages twelve to fifteen). To add to the difficulties, teenagers with TS may become increasingly self-conscious about their disorder, and less tolerant of their own differences. Fortunately, tics often diminish significantly around the ages of sixteen to eighteen, as adolescents move toward adulthood. No matter how severe tics were in childhood, there is usually at least some improvement in adulthood, although improvement is not as notable in the more extreme cases.

Although scientists do not understand exactly what causes Tourette syndrome, they do have a good idea about what causes the tics that accompany the condition. Presently, researchers believe that tics are caused, at least in part, by an excess of, or oversensitivity to, the brain chemical *dopamine*. (Dopamine is a chemical which ordinarily helps transmit signals involving control of motor movements from one nerve cell in the brain to the next.) Clearly, tics are involuntary. Your child is not deliberately making movements or sounds to draw attention to himself, to annoy others, or for any other conscious reason. He may be able to suppress or hold back tics for short periods of time, but eventually the need to give in to them will be irresistible. Many people with TS report that this "need" is felt as a conscious awareness of tension building up within themselves, sometimes in the part of the body where the tic occurs. They may "hear" a word or sound coming into their mind, and feel that they "have" to say it. A discharge of tension occurs when the tic is performed. (See Chapter 9 for more information about what it feels like to have tics.)

Some environmental factors can increase or decrease the intensity of tics. For example, tics occur less frequently during sleep or activities that absorb a child's concentration. But they can occur *more* frequently during a bout with hay fever, allergies, or viral illnesses. Caffeine may increase symptoms in some children with Tourette syndrome, as may stimulant medications such as methylphenidate, amphetamine, and cylert used to treat attention deficit hyperactivity disorder (ADHD), or allergy medications such as pseudoephedrine. Under intense emotions such as anxiety, fear, frustration, or anger, tics may also increase. Stress, too, can make tics worse. For this reason, never ask your child to try to suppress a tic, as this only puts increased stress on him and may cause his tics to become even more pronounced.

If increased stress makes tics worse, it stands to reason that you can help control your child's tics by reducing stress as much as possible. Ignoring tics, helping your child manage his time, providing clear expectations for behavior, and working with teachers to develop an educational plan that gives your child the best chance at success are just some of the ways you can make the environment less stressful. Chapter 4 details these and other strategies for reducing stress. As Chapter 3 explains, there are also a variety of medications that can often provide some relief from vocal and motor tics.

Obsessive-Compulsive Behavior

In addition to having tics, at least 50 percent of children with Tourette syndrome have obsessive-compulsive (OC) symptoms. Examples of OC behavior include insisting on wearing clothing that is a certain color or made from a certain type of fabric; repeatedly checking that doors are locked or the stove and lights are off; always having to be first in line or to sit in the same place; or erasing a sentence over and over until the paper tears in an effort to get the letters "perfect."

To understand what is behind these actions, it is essential to understand what medical professionals mean by the terms "obsession" and "compulsion." An obsession is a thought, idea, impulse, or image that, at first, seems intrusive or senseless to the person experiencing it. For example, a child may continually repeat words or thoughts in his mind, mentally count or group objects, or think about forbidden actions such as touching strangers or standing on a desk. Young children with TS and OC symptoms often think again and again about having a certain toy or going to a certain store or other destination. These obsessions are experienced as a product of the person's mind. That is, someone with OC symptoms does not think he is hearing voices, or that he is getting the obsession from some other outside influence. A compulsion is a repetitive behavior (thought or action) designed to stop the obsession, reduce anxiety, keep a dreaded event from occurring, or prevent discomfort. Examples include placing objects just right, smelling hands, touching things three times, or turning the lights off and on many times.

Adolescents and adults with OC behaviors are usually aware of the bizarre nature of their obsessions and compulsions. They may try to stop or ignore their obsessions and compulsions, but because this causes extreme anxiety, they cannot succeed in stopping the OC behavior. Young children with OC symptoms, on the other hand, may not realize that their behavior is inappropriate. They may not be able to verbalize what their obsession or compulsion is, and may therefore see it as normal. For example, they may not realize that their behavior is unusual if they feel an overwhelming need to buy a certain toy or to ride down a road over and over again.

Obsessions and compulsions can greatly disrupt daily life. To begin with, they are often time-consuming. This means other activities that a child needs or wants to do frequently fall by the wayside. For example, if a child feels a need to turn a circle after each step, he may be late for class. They can also impair school or work performance. A child may check and recheck his work so often that he is unable to complete it in the allotted time, or he may lose his concentration if he is constantly counting the dots on his teacher's tie. In addition, OC behaviors are distressing to the child, family members, and others. The child himself may feel weird and out of control, while parents and siblings may be at a loss to understand and deal with the behaviors.

When obsessions and compulsions significantly interfere with someone's abilities to perform his schoolwork, job, or other aspects of daily life, he is said to have obsessive-compulsive disorder (OCD). As Chapter 3 discusses, medications can often help control OC behaviors. There are also daily care strategies, explained in Chapter 4, that can help reduce OC behaviors, or, at least, reduce their impact on your child's life.

Attention Deficit Disorders

An attention deficit disorder is a neurological condition that makes it more difficult for a child to focus his attention, control his impulses, and behave appropriately. As is the case with tics, these problems are caused by a chemical imbalance in the brain. About half of all children with Tourette syndrome have attention deficit disorders.

Symptoms of attention disorders can include:

1. fidgeting with hands or feet, squirming in the seat, or, as a teenager, having a feeling of restlessness;
2. not being able to remain seated when appropriate;
3. being distracted by sights, sounds, smells, etc., in the environment—often by stimuli such as the ticking of a clock that someone without ADHD wouldn't notice;
4. having difficulty waiting turns in games or groups;
5. blurting out answers before questions have been completed;
6. having difficulty following instructions as to how to do a chore, school assignment, or other task, despite the willingness to cooperate and ability to comprehend the instructions;
7. having trouble sustaining attention in work or play activities;

8. often shifting from one uncompleted activity to another activity;
9. having difficulty playing quietly;
10. talking excessively;
11. interrupting or intruding on others;
12. appearing not to listen when spoken to;
13. losing things needed for activities at home, school, or work;
14. taking physically dangerous risks without thinking of consequences or consciously seeking thrills.

To be diagnosed as having an attention deficit disorder, your child must have at least eight of these symptoms. Symptoms must be present for at least six months, and begin before your child is seven years old. If one of your child's symptoms is hyperactivity, his condition will be called "attention deficit hyperactivity disorder (ADHD); otherwise, it will simply be called attention deficit disorder (ADD).

To determine whether your child does indeed have an attention deficit disorder, the doctor will not only evaluate how well your child is able to concentrate and control his impulses, but also how your child's abilities compare with other children's of the same age. For example, just because your two-year-old has trouble waiting his turn does not mean this is a symptom of an attention deficit disorder. *Most* two-year-olds have trouble waiting their turn. If, however, your child has problems taking turns when he is eight, his difficulty could very well be due to an attention disorder.

In children with Tourette syndrome, symptoms of attention disorders often appear before motor or vocal tics do. Studies show that ADHD symptoms are usually noticeable by age four or five. As a result,

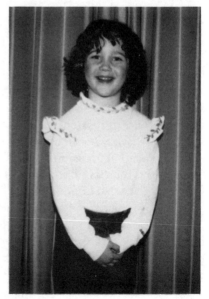

doctors may begin by treating attention deficit disorders as they would in any other children—by prescribing stimulant medications intended to make it easier to concentrate and control impulses. But in children with Tourette syndrome, these medications can actually make tics worse or hasten their appearance. Fortunately, there *are* medications that can reduce attention deficit symptoms without worsening TS symptoms. Chapter 3 describes these appropriate medical treatments for children with Tourette syndrome and attention deficit disorders. In addition, Chapter 4 offers some guidance in handling ADHD on a day-to-day basis within the family, and Chapter 7 gives practical help for dealing with ADHD or ADD in school.

Aggression

For about 25 to 35 percent of children with Tourette syndrome, controlling tantrums and aggressive behavior is a problem. They may appear to have a "short temper" and get into fights for little or no reason. They may attack other people or destroy property without provocation, or turn their aggression on themselves, perhaps by impulsively punching a wall. Often, the target of their aggression is a parent or someone not likely to harm them in any way. Usually, children who have problems with aggression greatly regret their explosive outbursts. Between outbursts they are reasonable, and feel guilty about their behavior.

Aggression occurs more frequently in children with TS who also have hyperactivity, impulsivity, and other attention difficulties. In addition, aggression can increase when tics increase. Often, but not always, children with more severe tics have greater difficulty controlling their aggression.

Exactly what connection there is between Tourette syndrome and increased aggression is still being studied. It may be partly to do with the increased pressure of dealing with TS on a daily basis. But scientists also believe that there may be an underlying biological problem that makes it more difficult to regulate aggression.

As with attention deficit disorders, tantrums and aggressive behavior may arise in toddlers with Tourette syndrome *before* any tics develop. This type of behavior can also develop months or years *after* tics appear. Often, a child's aggressive behavior is worse in some settings than others. For example, a child may be able to control his aggression at home or in the classroom, but have difficulty in the neighborhood or on the playground.

Treatment involves first helping the child learn that fighting and destructive behavior are not acceptable, and then helping him learn to control his impulses. Sometimes a psychologist or other mental health professional can help the child learn to recognize when he is about to lose control by keeping track of physical signs such as a faster heart rate. He can then avoid an impending conflict. Through role-playing and assertiveness training, a psychologist might also help the child develop better skills in conflict resolution. Social skills groups, too, can help children learn better ways of dealing with others and increase their success in relationships. Yet another option is relaxation therapy biofeedback—a technique through which the child is trained to relax his muscles. In addition, medications are sometimes helpful in reducing aggression. Chapter 3 discusses the medical treatment of aggressive behavior in more detail.

Sensory Integration Problems

The term "sensory integration" refers to the process by which our brains organize and process information received from the senses of sight, hearing, smell, touch, movement, and balance. Some children with TS have sensory integration dysfunction. This means that their brain has difficulty processing incoming sensory information or stimuli. They may be over- or under-sensitive to input from one or more of their senses, or be unable to use sensory information efficiently. For example, they may over-react to touch (tactile defensiveness), and consequently be distressed by the feel of certain fabrics on their skin or the texture of certain foods in their mouth. Or they may have difficulty telling where parts of their body are in space, and therefore appear clumsy. Sensory integration problems can also contribute to problems with speech, muscle development, hyperactivity, aggressiveness, and learning problems.

Sensory integration dysfunction is best treated by an occupational therapist with expertise in S.I. therapy. An occupational therapist is skilled in using special exercises and activities to help children overcome problems in development that interfere with their activities of daily living. Chapter 6 goes into sensory integration in more detail.

Learning Problems

Tourette syndrome has no effect on intelligence. Some children with Tourette syndrome have mental retardation and some score in the "gifted" range on IQ tests, but most have about average intelligence. This is as it is in the population as a whole.

Even though most children with Tourette syndrome have average or above average intelligence, they *are* more likely to have learning problems. In fact, about one-third have specific learning disabilities—delays or difficulties in learning one or more specific types of information. (This is in contrast to mental retardation, which causes delays in *all* areas of learning.) Children with learning disabilities may, for example, have greater than usual difficulty with reading, handwriting, or mathematics. They may also have problems with auditory processing—taking in information through the sense of hearing and reacting appropriately—for example, by following spoken instructions. Children with learning disabilities do more poorly in an area than expected, given their level of intelligence. By definition, learning disabilities are not the result of other causes such as mental retardation or hearing and vision problems.

Tics, distractibility, or obsessive-compulsive symptoms can also contribute to learning problems in children with Tourette syndrome. For example, eye blinking or head jerking can impede reading; hand jerking can make writing impossible. Likewise, if a child has a compulsion to count mentally, concentration can be reduced. Medications used to control tics can also interfere with learning or memory, or make children too sleepy to pay attention in class.

Learning problems most often become apparent when a child enters school and has difficulty reading or understanding math concepts. At this point, a thorough professional assessment of the type discussed in Chapter 7 can help determine the best way to deal with the learning problems. For example, if a reading problem is found to be related to head jerking tics, reducing or eliminating the tics through medication would likely be the simplest strategy. But if the reading problem is not related to any TS symptoms, then the child might benefit from special educational strategies. In any case, if you are aware of your child's specific learning disabilities, you and his teachers can plan ways to help him overcome these problems. Chapter 7 explains how you can work to discover how your child learns best and incorporate that knowledge into his educational program.

What Causes Tourette Syndrome?

For many years, Tourette syndrome was believed to be the result of underlying psychological problems. And unfairly enough, parents were sometimes blamed for causing the mental conflicts that led to these problems. Today, however, researchers have proven that this simply is not true. Nothing you did caused your child's tics, obsessive-compulsive behavior, or other symptoms, nor does he have a mental illness. Although the precise cause of Tourette syndrome has yet to be pinpointed, studies suggest that it is due to chemical abnormalities in the brain.

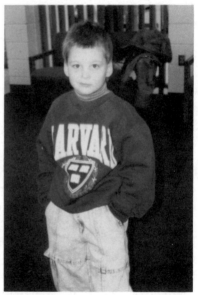

The first clue that Tourette syndrome is caused by biological factors came in the early 1960s. Researchers found that tics could sometimes be reduced by using Haldol™ (scientific name: Haloperidol), a medication which blocks or diminishes the brain chemical dopamine. As mentioned earlier, dopamine is a chemical that acts as a *neurotransmitter* or messenger between brain cells, and is involved in some way in the control of motor movements. There are many other neurotransmitters, and studies are currently underway to discover whether abnormalities in any of these chemicals might also play a part in Tourette syndrome. In addition, researchers are investigating specific parts of the brain to determine what, if any, role they play in TS. The Tourette Syndrome Association (TSA) supports this ongoing research into the specific cause of TS, in hopes that determining the cause will lead to a cure.

In the late 1970s, researchers discovered that Tourette syndrome is, in fact, a genetic disorder. In other words, it is caused by an alteration in the normal make-up of the genes or chromosomes. (Genes are the bits of material in every cell of the body which determine all of a person's traits—from eye and hair color, to foot size and special talents. Chromosomes are the microscopic, rod-shaped bodies which contain the genes.) Just as your child's genes determine whether he will be tall or short, musically gifted or tone deaf, they also determine whether or not he will have tics or obsessive-compulsive symptoms.

As with other genetic disorders, the predisposition to develop Tourette syndrome is usually passed on within families, from one generation to the next. (Geneticists call this predisposition "vulnerability.") Mothers and fathers who are themselves vulnerable to Tourette syndrome can pass the tendency on to their sons or daughters. When one parent has the Tourette syndrome gene, each child he or she has will have a 50 percent chance of inheriting the vulnerability for Tourette syndrome.

All children who inherit the Tourette syndrome gene do *not* go on to develop Tourette syndrome. For reasons that are not fully understood, about 30 percent of girls who inherit the gene do not have any symptoms at all, whereas the figure for boys is only 1 percent.

When the Tourette syndrome gene *does* cause symptoms, these symptoms can vary greatly from person to person. For instance, some children have both OCD and the vocal and motor tics associated with Tourette syndrome. Others have just one condition or the other. This is because genetic research indicates that the same gene that causes the tics of TS may also cause OC behaviors. Some children, too, may have one of the other tic disorders described below in the section on "Getting a Diagnosis." In general, boys are more likely to have tics, and girls are more likely to have obsessive-compulsive symptoms. Both boys and girls, however, can have any of the symptoms of Tourette syndrome, in any combination, and in any degree of severity.

Although Tourette syndrome is usually due entirely to genetic causes, sometimes it may be caused by other factors. For example, brain damage resulting from viruses, lack of oxygen at birth, or other prenatal problems may also be involved in causing TS.

How Many People Have Tourette Syndrome?

Tourette syndrome is more common than once believed. Estimates are that it affects about 1 in 2,500 people in the United States today. Some studies show that in boys, the figure may be as high as 1 in 1,000. Up to three times as many people may have some, but not all, the symptoms of Tourette syndrome. For example, they may have motor tics, but not vocal tics, or have obsessive-compulsive symptoms alone. According to some studies, transient tics (tics lasting less than twelve months) occur in 5.4 to 18 percent of boys and in 2.9 to 11 percent of girls.

Because boys who inherit the Tourette syndrome gene are more likely to have symptoms than girls are, more boys are diagnosed than girls. Presently, boys with TS outnumber girls by about 3 to 1.

Having Other Children

If you already have one child with Tourette syndrome, any other children you have will have a fifty-fifty chance of inheriting the Tourette syndrome gene. And, as explained above, any daughters that inherit the gene will have a 70 percent chance of developing symptoms; any sons, a 99 percent chance.

At present, there are no pre-natal tests to determine whether a baby will carry the gene or develop symptoms. There are also no tests to determine which parent passed on the gene or whether a younger sibling also inherited the gene or will develop symptoms. Currently, however, researchers are trying to discover which one of the forty-six chromosomes in each cell harbors the gene for Tourette syndrome. Once its location is discovered, not only will genetic testing for Tourette syndrome be possible, but better treatments and perhaps a cure can eventually be developed.

In the meantime, it is important to remember that symptoms of Tourette syndrome can vary widely from child to child. If your other children *do* inherit Tourette syndrome, their symptoms may be much milder *or* more severe than either their sibling's or their parent's. A genetic counselor can explain your chances of having additional children with Tourette syndrome and the possible range of symptoms. He or she can also help you cope with your feelings about embarking on another pregnancy that may produce a child with Tourette syndrome. You may also find it helpful to talk to other parents who have chosen to have additional children and then wound up with more than one child with TS. The final decision, of course, is up to you.

Getting a Diagnosis

Getting a firm diagnosis of Tourette syndrome can be difficult for several reasons. First, because of the tendency of tics to wax and wane and change over time, it may take a while before your child's doctor gets a complete picture of his symptoms. Second, children often suppress their symptoms when they are around strangers, including doctors. And third, there are a variety of other conditions with similar symptoms that can sometimes be confused with Tourette syndrome. Provided your child sees a specialist or specialists with training and experience in tic disorders, however, the diagnosis process should be fairly straightforward.

To reach a diagnosis, the doctor follows guidelines in a book called the *Diagnostic and Statistical Manual of Mental Disorders,* third edition, revised (DSM-III-R). This book, published by the American Psychiatric Association, outlines the "official" criteria for identifying most mental and emotional disorders. The DSM-III-R lists the following criteria for diagnosing Tourette syndrome:

1. both multiple motor *and* one or more vocal tics have occurred at some time, but not necessarily at the same time;
2. tics occur many times a day, nearly every day, or intermittently throughout a period of more than a year; tics usually occur in bouts (groups);
3. the anatomic location, number, frequency, complexity, and severity of the tics change over time;
4. the tics begin before age twenty-one;
5. tics do not occur only during drug or alcohol intoxication, and are not the result of a known nervous system disease such as Parkinson's disease.

In addition to checking your child's symptoms against these criteria, the doctor will also perform a *differential diagnosis.* A differential diagnosis involves comparing your child's behavior with the behavior of children with other disorders that might produce the same symptoms. In other words, it is a way of ruling out what disorders your child does not have, and determining what disorder he does have.

In making a differential diagnosis of Tourette syndrome, several similar tic disorders, as well as other conditions, must be ruled out. The tic disorders include:

1. chronic motor tic disorder;
2. chronic vocal tic disorder;
3. transient tic disorder; and
4. tic disorder not otherwise specified.

In contrast to Tourette syndrome, chronic motor and chronic vocal tic disorder cause only motor *or* vocal tics, not both. Transient tic disorder may cause both one or more motor tics *and* one or more vocal tics, but the condition lasts less than twelve consecutive months. Tic disorder not otherwise specified is a catchall diagnosis for all other types of tic disorders. For example, the name may refer to a disorder that causes both motor and vocal tics but begins *after* age twenty-one. Or it may refer to a disorder that causes vocal tics and just one motor tic, in contrast to the multiple motor tics in Tourette syndrome. Most researchers believe that these tic disorders are milder variations of TS, possibly due to the same cause, but this has not yet been proven.

Other conditions with symptoms similar to Tourette syndrome that must be ruled out include: duchenne muscular dystrophy, head trauma, brain tumors, epilepsy, and autistic disorders. The doctor must also make sure that tics and other symptoms are not due to over-exertion or drug use.

The Diagnosis Process

Observation plays a large role in the diagnosis of Tourette syndrome. Medical professionals will need to look not only at the type of tics your child has, but also at their severity, frequency, and the extent to which they disrupt your child's daily activities. Because your child may suppress his tics or have fewer than usual in the doctor's office, the doctor will also question you about your child's behavior in the past. You can help a great deal if you prepare

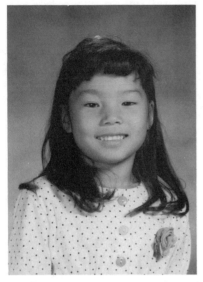

a list of all your child's past tics or OC behaviors ahead of time. You may also want to document your child's tics by taking home videos. In addition, you might suggest that the doctor follow your child into the waiting room or a restroom if your child suppresses his tics in the office. Determining what factors make your child's symptoms worse or better is especially important. In addition, the doctor should question you about your family's history of tics, obsessive-compulsive behavior, hyperactivity, or other related symptoms.

Before your child receives the diagnosis of Tourette syndrome, he will probably see a variety of specialists with differing expertise. Ideally, these specialists will consult with one another and share their observations about your child with one another in order to arrive at the best possible understanding of your child's disorder. When specialists from different disciplines work together in this manner, they are known as an interdisciplinary or multidisciplinary team. Multidisciplinary teams are often involved in diagnosing children with mental retardation, autism, cerebral palsy, and other developmental disorders. Unfortunately, the concept of using multidisciplinary teams to diagnose TS has not yet really caught on in most areas. If a team with expertise in TS is not available in your area, it will be up to you to coordinate the efforts of each specialist, making sure each knows about test results and conclusions reached by other other specialists. Specialists with expertise in diagnosing Tourette syndrome include:

Pediatric Neurologist. A pediatric neurologist is a medical doctor specializing in diagnosing and treating neurological disorders in children. Neurological disorders—disorders of the brain, spinal cord, or nerves—include epilepsy, cerebral palsy, and Parkinson's disease. In diagnosing TS, the neurologist will do a number of tests to rule out these other neurological disorders and to look for specific neurological impairments or weaknesses. Tests may include blood tests and perhaps an electroencephalogram (EEG)—a test that measures the electrical activity of the brain and helps identify seizure activity. The neurologist will also talk to you to get a picture of your child's medical history.

Neuro-Psychiatrist. A neuro-psychiatrist is a medical doctor with expertise in diagnosing and treating mental disorders of neurological orgin, including OCD, depression, bi-polar disorders (manic-depression), and neurological dsorders such as ADHD with behavioral symptoms. Like the neurologist, the neuro-psychiatrist may do an EEG or blood tests to test for abnormalities such as lead poisoning. He or she may also do a CAT (computerized tomography) scan, a test that uses a series of X-rays to form a computerized picture of the brain at different levels. Although both the neuro-psychiatrist and pediatric neurologist are qualified to diagnose TS, the neuro-psychiatrist is generally more familiar with medications used to treat associated difficulties such as OC behaviors or ADHD.

Psychologist. A psychologist is not a medical doctor, but a professional trained in understanding human behavior, emotions, and how the mind works. Psychologists cannot diagnose Tourette syndrome, but can help your family cope with the diagnosis and help your child with self-esteem or emotional issues related to living with TS.

Occupational Therapist. An occupational therapist specializes in helping people with neurological impairments or other movement problems improve the motor skills needed to carry out their daily activities. During the diagnosis process, they perform tests to find specific motor problems which may relate to a neurological impairment.

If you are lucky enough to be able to work with a multidisciplinary team, after each member of the team has completed his evaluation, you will be given a summary of the team's findings, together with their treatment recommendations. If a team is not involved with your child, you should work with the professional you consider to be your child's primary physician to discuss the different findings and develop a treatment plan.

The History of Tourette Syndrome

For most of history, Tourette syndrome has been grossly misunderstood. Centuries ago, people with Tourette syndrome were thought to be possessed. Often, they were kept isolated from others; sometimes they underwent extreme "treatments" such as flogging, lobotomies, or even being burned at the stake. Later, medical professionals theorized that the condition was due to mental or emotional problems arising within the child himself, or triggered by "bad parents." People with TS were sometimes committed to insane asylums, or went through psychoanalysis to work through the past emotional traumas they were believed to have suffered. And as recently as the 1970s, Tourette syndrome was frequently misdiagnosed as schizophrenia, obsessive-compulsive disorder, epilepsy, or just plain "nervous habits."

These misconceptions persisted even though the idea that Tourette syndrome was a genetic disorder had been around since at least 1885. In that year, Georges Gilles de la Tourette, a French neurologist, first identified Tourette syndrome as a distinct syndrome and suggested that the disorder was hereditary.

Since that time, medical researchers have written many reports and made many systematic studies. Today, although the cause of Tourette syndrome is still somewhat of a mystery, much progress has been made in understanding the condition, as well as in developing effective treatment strategies. As mentioned earlier, there is a very real hope that researchers will eventually be able to pinpoint the exact cause of TS, and that a cure will not be far behind.

Your Child's Future

Many of the barriers that previously prevented people with Tourette syndrome from reaching their full potential have now fallen. Federal and state regulations and laws guarantee your child the right to a public education tailor-made to his unique learning needs. By prohibiting discrimination against people with disabilities, state and federal laws also ensure your child's right to work and participate in community activities. And, although misunderstanding and prejudice may still be encountered, growing awareness and public understanding of the disorder is helping to reduce negative attitudes. The Tourette Syndrome Association, in particular, has taken a leading role in combating misconceptions, as well as in providing essential support services and advocacy for people with Tourette syndrome.

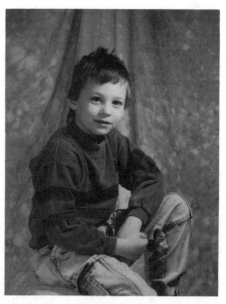

How well your child will eventually flourish in this new climate of acceptance and opportunity depends on many factors. Some of these factors are out of your control. For example, the severity of your child's tics, the presence of associated symptoms such as attention deficit disorder or obsessive-compulsive disorder, and his intelligence can all affect his ability to adjust. Continued difficulties with mood, aggression, or handling frustration can also contribute to problems in adulthood.

But other factors vital to your child's adjustment *are* under your control. Your child's level of maturity as an adult and his ability to cope with the stress of having Tourette syndrome are perhaps *the* most important factors in determining how happy and fulfilling his life will be. These are things that you, as a parent, can help nurture with a steady diet of support and encouragement. You can learn to foster your child's independence and mastery without neglecting his special needs. Your child's school program, too, can play a large part in helping him achieve the successes he needs in order to feel good about himself and his abilities. In fact, no matter how severe your child's symptoms are, his future should be as bright as any other child's, so long as he has the right attitude and effective coping skills.

Most children with Tourette syndrome go on to lead normal, independent adult lives. As with other children, how far they can go in school is limited only by their intellectual abilities and drive. Many graduate from high school; others go on to complete college and graduate school. People with Tourette syndrome are equally successful on the job—provided personal strengths and preferences are taken into account in choosing a career. Someone with loud coprolalia, for example, probably shouldn't choose a job in a library, any more than someone who has claustrophobia should choose to work in a coal mine. As long as he has a healthy acceptance of both his strengths and weaknesses, however, your child will find his place in society.

Conclusion

There is no denying that Tourette syndrome is a disability. It is a chronic condition that can have a major impact on your child's psychological development and relationships with others. Depending on the severity and the presence of associated disorders, it may also make it harder for your child to develop skills in certain areas. But unlike many other disabilities, which often place very definite limits on what a child is able to learn and achieve, Tourette syndrome in itself rarely prevents children from reaching their potential. Many highly successful people have had Tourette syndrome, including Dr. Samuel Johnson, one of the greatest English writers of the eighteenth century.

In short, remember that Tourette syndrome is only one small part of your child. And although it is a part that cannot—and should not—be ignored, it is also a part that both your child and your family can learn to work around. Like every child, your child with Tourette syndrome deserves to be given the chance to make the most of his life. With proper medical treatment, appropriate education, and support from your family, he should be well on his way to reaching that goal.

Parent Statements

When Billy was four, he had this sniffing thing which lasted for four months. Then it went away. He then started to blink his eyes, and after a couple of months he started clearing his throat. It's been like that ever since—one thing starts and then goes away, and then another starts. Sometimes he has three or four tics at once.

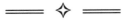

When she was seven, Joan's tics were causing her lots of problems. She had this cough—she did it fifty or a hundred times a day. She would also squint her eyes and jerk her shoulder. This was enough of a problem, but on top of that, she had this hand-washing routine. I couldn't count how many times a day she washed her hands. She had to have a clean towel each time and she was wild over germs. She thought everything had germs; we had to cover the plates before each meal, and if someone coughed or sneezed in the kitchen or at the table, she wouldn't eat.

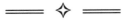

My son has had every diagnosis possible.

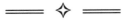

Often doctors—especially psychologists—say your kid has conduct disorder, plain and simple.

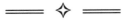

The pediatrician put her on medication for ADHD. When I reported to him that she was making noises, he said, "It's just a nervous tic; it will go away." Two months later, we were at the neurologist to get her medication dose and schedule finely tuned, but the neurologist said, "She must go off medication immediately—she has TS."

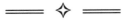

After three years of being treated for Tourette syndrome with ADD, the child neuro-psychiatrist changed the diagnosis to Tourette syndrome and seizure disorder. He said that although Michelle had ADD symptoms, she didn't really have ADD.

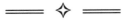

All kids with TS aren't the same. Each one needs an individualized approach. My friends' kids have similar problems to Ken's, but they are also unique.

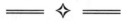

We knew there was something wrong with our daughter. Our pediatrician said she was just nervous, and refused to refer us to a neurologist. After asking three times, he finally gave in. The neurologist immediately diagnosed TS.

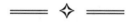

I knew he was "hyper" from the time he was a toddler. From six in the morning until eleven at night, he was like a motor you wind up. It was go, go, go.

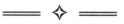

We don't want her labeled a "bad" kid. She has enough to deal with without putting that label on her.

I wish I could bottle and sell some of Dave's energy.

Allen is creative, bright, loving, caring, and affectionate. He has many facial, hand-to-face, and vocal tics. He exhibits SIB [self-injurious behavior] and aggressive behavior much of the time.

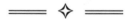

We knew about TS, the lip smacking and the way he flipped his head like he was trying to get the hair out of his eyes, but we didn't know about the echoing. He started repeating the last two or three words of each sentence. At first it was a whisper and then out loud. We had four very tough months before someone told us that the repeating (by this time he would repeat things we said out loud) was also a part of the TS. He got in so much trouble at school because of this, and we weren't able to help him at home because we didn't know.

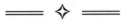

I'm always amazed at how interesting Sharon's obsessions can be. She is able to transfer her unusual thoughts into very creative art, games, and puzzles.

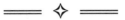

My son only swears when he's angry or under stress, so people don't believe it's coprolalia. We know it is. My greatest fear is that the coprolalia will get worse.

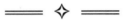

His symptoms began around age five with prolonged sniffing, which we thought was a habit. If we told him to stop, he would then start clearing his throat. The throat-clearing lasted for months and then he began repetitious movements—head to shoulder, hand to nose, eye, and ear. That's when we brought him to the doctor.

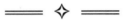

TWO

$\diamondsuit$

Adjusting to Your Child's Diagnosis

TRACY HAERLE*

There is really no such thing as a "typical" case of Tourette syndrome. In addition to mild to severe tics, your child may have hyperactivity, obsessive-compulsive behaviors, or attention deficits, in any ·combination of symptoms and in any degree of severity. Her symptoms may have unfolded overnight or developed so gradually that you were scarcely aware of their arrival. They may have appeared as early as late infancy or as late as early adolescence.

But despite the countless forms Tourette syndrome can take, most parents' experiences shortly before and after their child's diagnosis are quite similar. Often parents spend months or years desperately seeking an explanation for their child's puzzling behavior. They get conflicting advice from family, friends, and doctors. Many parents are blamed for the very behavior they would do anything to understand. And depending on how their child is doing and what the latest doctor says, they may be alternately buoyed up by hopefulness or paralyzed by dread. Then, when their child finally receives a diagnosis of Tourette syndrome, they are flooded by a fresh torrent of emotions and experiences.

Our family's story may sound very familiar to you. Our son, Jeffrey, was born in August, 1981. An active, happy baby, he walked

---

* Tracy Haerle is the mother of two children, one of whom has Tourette syndrome. She holds a B.S. in social work and has experience in adolescent counseling. A past president of TSA Minnesota, she currently works as a parent advocate and educator.

early and was soon into everything. He seemed to be very excited about the world and needed to touch and experience everything. In marked contrast to his older sister, he kept me very busy chasing after him, trying to keep him out of danger. I began asking our pediatrician about Jeff's activity level before he was two. The doctor said that Jeff was "all boy," and gave me the impression that he thought I was just a nervous mom. I thought maybe he was right.

By the time Jeff was three, my concerns had deepened. He just couldn't seem to control his behavior as other three-year-olds could. For example, no matter how many times we warned him not to, he would impulsively run into the street or hit other children and grab their toys. He did not seem to be able to read others' reactions to his behavior. For example, whenever he hit other children, he always seemed very surprised by their angry reaction. He was also very rigid about changes. Once he got an idea in his head, he could not be swayed. He would only wear green clothes, demanded that certain routines be carried out, and insisted on playing with particular toys. In addition, he was impossible to discipline. He just could not seem to understand that his behavior was inappropriate no matter how many times he was corrected. Jeff needed constant supervision, and we could not take him into malls, restaurants, or many other public places without him running wild.

Frustrated and exhausted, we turned to a local psychologist. During a one-hour session, the psychologist focused only on our parenting skills. He told us that Jeff had probably picked up hostility from something in our home. Although my husband and I were convinced that Jeff acted this way not out of hostility, but because there was something wrong in his brain, we still felt guilty. The psychologist did not tell us he was not qualified to do neurological testing and offered no suggestions. With no idea what to do next, we felt helpless and powerless. It seemed no one would listen to us or take our situation seriously.

When Jeff was four, we took him to the public school for pre-school screening. Jeff ran around the room from one activity to another and could not pay attention to the testing. Although his behavior was embarrassing to me, it qualified Jeff for special education.

The school referred my son to a pediatric neurologist, who diagnosed Jeff with attention-deficit hyperactivity disorder

(ADHD). Jeff had a slightly abnormal electroencephalogram (EEG), and therefore could not take medications usually prescribed for ADHD. The doctor suggested that we try behavior modification and special education.

For the next two years, we worked hard to understand our son's needs and to help him learn to behave in more socially acceptable ways. We learned that a calm, relaxed environment helped Jeff to be more in control. He still had no friends, however, and because we could not get a babysitter, my husband and I had no social life, either.

At times we believed that Jeff would "grow out" of his hyperactivity. At other times we were overwhelmed and depressed. We tried special diets and explored allergy theories. We were desperate for solutions.

Jeff's first-grade year began with problems. He couldn't get along with the other children, and he had trouble following the teacher's directions. On the bus and at the bus stop, Jeff did impulsive, inappropriate things, and the older kids began making fun of him. The behavior modification program the teacher and I tried didn't work. As a result of all these failures, Jeff's self-esteem was sinking fast. He also seemed to be developing "nervous habits"—clearing his throat, blinking, pushing hair out of his face, and making meaningless noises. All year long, whenever the phone rang, I feared it would be one of Jeff's teachers venting their frustration on me.

Near the end of first grade, the school psychologist observed Jeff in class. I will never forget his phone call. He said that he suspected a neurological problem and did not think Jeff was acting this way on purpose. A breakthrough at last! We returned to the pediatric neurologist, who diagnosed Jeff with Tourette syndrome. I had never heard of Tourette syndrome, but was very relieved to have a doctor validate what we had felt for so many years. And when the doctor told me that medication could be used, I felt very optimistic.

The News Sinks In

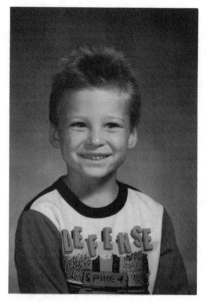

If your child had moderate to severe TS symptoms, including hyperactivity, obsessive-compulsive symptoms, or behavior problems, you probably felt as relieved as I did to hear that there is a medical name for the condition. But the relief fades fast as the realities of living with TS hit you. Medications may help somewhat, but eventually you realize that there is no cure for Tourette syndrome. You learn that it is lifelong, and that things will probably get worse before they get better. And teachers, neighbors, and other children *still* do not understand you and your child. Like your child's TS symptoms, your worry, frustration, and sorrow wax and wane, at times almost overwhelming you.

Your situation may be somewhat different if your child's Tourette syndrome came on suddenly and you were fortunate enough to get an immediate diagnosis. Instead of relief, your initial reaction may have been shock, denial, or anger. If so, the emotional fallout from your child's diagnosis may hit you even harder and sooner than it would have if you had had the opportunity to adjust to the news more gradually.

If your child has mild TS symptoms, coping will probably be easier. Your child and your family will generally have fewer problems inside and outside the home, and you may not even think of your child as having a disability. But then again, there may be times when the reality of your child's neurological impairment and the changes that it brings seem very difficult to face.

No matter how and when you get the news of your child's TS, you could face a long, complicated adjustment process. This is because you, like most parents, probably had idealized expectations for your child's life. When your baby was born, you had hopes and dreams that she would be happy and successful. But once your child is diagnosed with Tourette syndrome, you may fear that you will have to let go of some of those hopes and dreams. Instead of hoping that your child will one day become a doctor, athlete, or lawyer, you may now wonder (rightly or wrongly) how she will make it through high school. These feelings are part of the mourning process for the "perfect" child that will never be. Often it awakens intensely painful emotions in every member of the family.

No two families handle the adjustment process in quite the same way. But it is easier to handle if you are prepared for some of the emotions you may have and understand why you feel the way you do. This chapter is designed to give you that understanding, as well as to suggest some strategies to help you get on with your life.

Your Emotions

In coming to terms with your child's diagnosis, it is normal to be besieged by a variety of emotions: shock, helplessness, guilt, anger, grief, and resentment, to name a few. You may feel a number of these emotions simultaneously, or may move in stages from one to another. Occasionally you may seem to get "stuck" in one emotion for a while. Even after you think you have conquered one emotion, something may happen to set it off again. For example, whenever Jeff's symptoms begin to worsen, I re-experience the grief and helplessness I felt right after his diagnosis. Or when I see a young boy shopping cooperatively with his mother, I grieve over the many years I've lost struggling with Jeff in stores.

Regaining your equilibrium can be tough. There are no foolproof coping methods, and sometimes it can seem as though you take three steps back for every two forward. But with time, most parents learn to master their emotions and enjoy the good things their child and their life have to offer. To help you sort out what you might be feeling, the sections below describe some of the most powerful emotions parents typically have en route to acceptance.

Shock and Denial

Many parents react to the diagnosis of Tourette syndrome with shock. This reaction is especially common if your child's TS came on abruptly and you had no clue it was anything serious. But even if you have been searching for answers for years, hearing the words

"Tourette syndrome" is shocking. Most people have never heard of TS before this moment, and to learn suddenly that something is wrong inside your child's brain is a tremendous jolt. You may go numb, and might not feel or think anything other than "this is not really happening to me."

Shock, in fact, serves a useful purpose. It helps insulate us from the total blow of a painful experience. It gives us a grace period before we must face reality and begin to actively deal with our problems. If you get stuck in this phase too long, however, you may have trouble accepting the reality of TS in your family. Because of the waxing and waning of symptoms or their subtlety, you may easily fool yourself into thinking that the tics are just "bad habits" and fall into the trap of long-term denial. This could make it harder for you to recognize and do something about your child's needs. In this situation, it may help to talk to other parents of children with Tourette syndrome and see that many otherwise "normal" families are in your situation.

Helplessness

As the shock wears off, a feeling of overwhelming helplessness may set in. Your child's problems may seem so numerous or complicated that you don't know how to begin helping her. Especially if teachers and other professionals have previously tried and failed to improve her symptoms, you may wonder if there are any real answers. And just the thought of dealing with the platoons of doctors, never-ending problems at school and in the neighborhood, medication side effects, and daily care of your child may make you want to run away. Worst of all, when you think about the future, you see no end to the constant drain on your time and energy.

When I first realized the extent of Jeff's needs, I cried for three days. I felt unequipped to handle the present problems, and looking into the future brought overwhelming worry. Advice from well-meaning friends who didn't understand what I was going through only made matters worse. In trying to make me feel better, some denied Jeff's TS or tried to minimize my pain. My feelings of powerlessness did not begin to lift until other parents of children with Tourette syndrome showed me that it really could be done. It was especially helpful to talk to parents of older children and to adults with TS and hear their success stories.

Guilt

Guilt is another emotion that can really run you through the emotional ringer. After you learn that TS is genetically transmitted, you may scour through family histories, looking for other family members who may have had Tourette syndrome. You then may blame yourself or your spouse for not knowing that TS runs in the family. Whether or not a genetic link is found, you may feel terribly guilty for somehow "causing" your child to suffer so much. If one parent has TS and knows the child inherited it from him, he may feel an added burden of guilt, knowing first-hand what problems their child will likely endure.

Often parents fault themselves for their treatment of their child before diagnosis. They may feel guilty for punishing their child for tics and other behaviors that were out of her control. My husband and I, for example, felt guilty about the behavior modification we had used to try to stop Jeff's tics. We had had him wear a rubberband on his wrist and snap the rubberband whenever he had a tic. Although this method stopped one tic, two new tics appeared to take its place. We also felt guilty about our frustration over his behavior, once we learned that he definitely could not control it. Sometimes parents think back to the many times people made fun of their child's tics and feel guilty about not intervening. And then there is the lingering guilt about being a "bad" parent, even though you know in your heart you didn't cause your child's TS. For example, any time a professional, friend, or relative suggests that something might be my fault, I feel angry and guilty at the same time.

Remorseful as you may feel, it is important to realize that you are not to blame for your child's troubles. Tourette syndrome may be genetic, but there are no pre-natal tests that could have predicted that your child would have the condition. You are also not to blame for failing to realize that your child's symptoms were out of her control—even the best specialists sometimes have difficulty recognizing Tourette syndrome. Your energies are far better spent in helping your child today, than in blaming yourself or your spouse for what happened yesterday.

Anger

There is a lot to be angry about in dealing with Tourette syndrome. We are angry at all the doctors and professionals who misdiagnosed or minimized our child's Tourette syndrome, and angry that they can't make our child "better." We are angry with all the people who blamed us as parents for the TS symptoms. We are angry with the schools, churches, and social organizations for the way they may have misunderstood and mishandled our child. Often we are angry at God for allowing this to happen, and at our families and friends for minimizing our situation or for not giving us support.

For my part, I was outraged at the ignorance of people who constantly misunderstood our son and judged him mercilessly. My husband and I were also furious at the medical insurance system when they refused to pay Jeff's medical bills, claiming that TS was a mental illness, not a neurological impairment.

Anger is a powerful emotion. If you can channel it in the right directions, it can be a great impetus for needed change. My anger over the public's ignorance about TS motivated me to become involved with my local TSA as a parent advocate. I now try to educate people about TS whenever possible. And our anger about the insurance issue propelled us to take the insurance company to an appeal board. We won the appeal, and they had to pay our claims. But when your fury is out of control or you become "stuck" in your anger, it can lead to roadblocks in communication with school staff, doctors, and others who could help you with your child. You may enter a conversation with a hostile, defensive attitude, which impedes open communication and makes it difficult for you to understand what people are saying. Getting mired in anger can also make you sick or depressed. In these situations, it's essential to vent your anger with others—your spouse, the parents in a support group—who understand what you're going through.

Grief

Grief is the deep sense of loss we feel when we lose something or someone dear to us. It is a lonely, empty, painful feeling that seeps into your very being like a poisonous gas, altering your whole outlook on life. In the early days, your grief can be all-encompassing when you think of the idealized child—the perfect family life—that will never be. As my husband and I did, you may grieve about losing years of your life to constant stress and struggle. Later, grief can intrude on you when you least expect it, rekindled by everyday experiences that remind you that your family is different than average. Watching two girls amiably playing together in the park, for instance, you may suddenly be overcome with sadness that TS will always set your child apart from other children. My husband and I still have trouble accepting that typical vacations and many normal family activities are not feasible for our family.

Although it is almost inevitable that you will feel some sense of loss when your child is diagnosed with Tourette syndrome, grief does lessen with time. At first when you look at your child, the TS may be all you are able to see. As you learn more about your child and about Tourette syndrome, however, your main focus will shift away from TS. Like all parents, you find out what your child is capable of and adjust your expectations. Your idea of the perfect child is replaced by a more realistic view. And although you may still feel occasional twinges of grief, you recognize them for what they are: expressions of your love and concern for your child and of your desire that she have the opportunity to live the best possible life.

Resentment

Everything can seem so *unfair* when you have a child with Tourette syndrome. Other families can go out to eat or to a movie and melt right into the crowd; you and your child may immediately become a magnet for stares if you venture outside. Other parents can just assume that their child will adapt to her teacher and the classroom; you may have to trudge to the school for meeting after meeting to work out your child's educational problems. Other children have sleep-overs and go on outings with friends; your child may not be able to handle these situations. Thinking about how much harder your family has it then other families can naturally lead to strong feelings of resentment.

Often, your resentment doesn't stop with people who take normal family life so much for granted. For example, you can also resent people who say insensitive things about your child. I sometimes resent society in general for being so narrow and intolerant as to look at people who are different as freaks. And even though you know that your child cannot control her tics and other symptoms, you may even resent her for making your life more difficult. I find that if I spend too much time caring for my son by myself, I am much more apt to feel resentful toward him for his disability. I lose my perspective, get tired, and my resolve is worn down by constant demands and interventions. I have had to learn that I need a break now and then from the stress of raising a child with Tourette syndrome. I *need* support from others—husband, friends, and family. And then sometimes I resent being different from other families and needing help.

Although all these types of resentment are normal and understandable, it is important not to let it rule your life. Dwelling on your resentment can come between you and your child, lead to self-pity, and drive away the very people you need for support. To keep from getting stuck in resentment, it helps to be aware of these feelings, and to remind yourself of the good things in your life. I find that reading inspirational books such as *When Bad Things Happen to Good People*, which is included in the Reading List, helps me put my feelings in perspective. This may seem like small consolation at the moment, but most people have felt at one time or another that their lives, too, are unfair.

How to Adjust

Acknowledge Your Feelings

When you're hurting, it's senseless to pretend that you're not. You cannot make rational decisions when your mind is a jumble of painful and conflicting emotions. Nor can you see things as they really are when your thoughts are colored by despair, anger, or guilt. Getting the support you need from other people can also be more difficult if your feelings short-circuit open communication.

Obviously, you must first come to terms with your own emotions if you are to be effective in meeting the needs of your child and the rest of your family. This means you must first honestly own up to everything you are feeling. In the beginning, this can be difficult: you may have so many emotions at once that you aren't sure *what* you're feeling. You may also feel ashamed of certain feelings you are having, and worry that you must be an awful person to be having such "bad" feelings. For example, I thought that feeling resentful was a selfish thing to do, and that feeling helpless was "weak." It can help to remember that any feeling you're having has probably been shared by thousands of parents before you. Your feelings are a normal reaction to hearing devastating news, and are neither good nor bad.

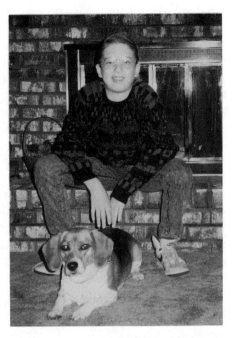

Everyone has their own way of coping with difficult emotions. Some find it helpful to work out their frustrations through exercising or concentrating on a hobby. Others cry, talk to a friend, or seek help from professional counselors. My husband and I cope by talking things over many times. A friend of mine copes by swimming laps every day. Do whatever seems right to you. Remember, you have a right to have whatever emotions you are feeling *and* to express them.

Take Your Time

Following your child's diagnosis, you may feel as if you should rush right out and try to solve all her problems immediately. You don't want to waste a moment discovering the medication that will best control her tics or devising the educational strategies that will best help her learn. In fact, my husband and I began experimenting with medications and trying to set up a special education program for Jeff right away. But coming on top of everything else you are feeling, the very thought of everything that needs to be done may be overwhelming.

Take your time. If you don't feel emotionally ready to handle major decisions yet, then by all means, put them off until you do. Just like broken bones, emotional wounds take time to heal. You cannot rush or force the adjustment process. But if you're good to yourself, you *can* make things easier on yourself. Make whatever changes to your lifestyle you can to make this time less stressful. For example, simplify things or cut back on stress-producing family activities or social events. Look at your short- and long-term goals for your family, and set priorities. For instance, is it more important to sell pies at the PTA fund raiser or to spend relaxed time at home with your family? Is it more important to attend family social gatherings, or to find less stimulating activities for your child that won't send her behavior out of control?

It *is* important for your child to receive the right medical treatment and educational program and to become an accepted part of the community. But it is also important that you be emotionally ready to give your child the support she needs to make the most of her opportunities. I would suggest taking it easy before you plunge into a whirl of activities. Later on, when you and your child with TS have developed better coping skills, there will be time to make decisions and to take part in activities. (See Chapter 4 for practical methods of coping with community activities.) Remember, you can be your child's most powerful ally—if you allow yourself time to grow stronger.

Get the Facts

When it comes to Tourette syndrome, there are no stupid questions. People with TS have been misunderstood and mistreated for so long that there are all kinds of erroneous bits of information floating around out there. Then, too, because Tourette syndrome is such a complex disorder, you will probably have many questions even if you have access to the most accurate and up-to-date information.

Becoming informed about Tourette syndrome is the best way to put needless worries to rest. It helped my family immensely to learn about the expected outcome of TS. We could mentally prepare ourselves for coping with the next six to eight years of worsening symptoms. And we could prepare for the changes as a family. Information is also essential to being able to deal effectively with school staff and doctors. In addition, knowledge about TS can boost your confidence in your abilities as a parent because you will be better able to interpret your child's behavior and needs. You also need the facts about TS so you can help your child understand and deal with her symptoms.

To gather information about your child's symptoms in particular, it is essential to find a doctor who is not only knowledgeable about TS, but also accessible to parents. As problems arise, you may need to contact your doctor for immediate advice.

For information about TS in general, contact the national Tourette Syndrome Association (TSA) at the address in the back of the book for information about their many helpful pamphlets, booklets, and videos. Your local TSA should also be a great source of information. In addition, it may be helpful to contact the Obsessive-Compulsive Foundation, learning disabilities organizations, or ADHD associations, which are listed in the Resource Guide. The Reading List also suggests useful books and journals that may be available through your library. Finally, you may want to attend one of the conferences on TS held throughout the U.S. and Canada. My husband and I have found these conferences to be a great way to learn the latest TS findings, and meeting other parents and hearing their experiences is enriching. Information on conferences can be obtained through your local TSA.

Seek Support

Meeting other parents of children with Tourette syndrome can be a lifeline for exhausted and bewildered parents. Better than anyone else, other parents are equipped to tell you about what lies ahead and how to deal with it. They can help you out with everything from inside information about your school system, to practical strategies for dealing with specific problems at home or in public. Best of all, they can offer an understanding ear when something is troubling you.

My husband and I felt nervous at our first support group meeting. But people were so understanding and accepting that we soon felt comfortable. In fact, we found that talking about our family was therapeutic. Who better to tell your story to than people who are going through, or have been through, the same experience?

Your local TSA chapter most likely sponsors a TS support group. To make contact, call the national Tourette Syndrome Association or the nearest local chapter. These phone numbers are in the Resource Guide at the back of this book.

Besides sponsoring support groups, most state TSA chapters put on social events for families of children with Tourette syndrome. Not only do these social events allow you to meet and swap information with other parents, but they also allow you to truly relax without worrying that someone will criticize your child's behavior.

If your family takes part in your local TSA activities, your child can meet older role models with TS, as well as children their own age. It has helped Jeff to realize there are others in the same boat as he is and to accept his TS. "Normal" siblings are also welcome at TSA activities. They can vent their frustrations about their brothers and sisters (and they do!). Our daughter has become good friends with several other siblings of children with TS, and the whole experience has helped our family immensely. Everyone in the family now realizes that they are not alone with their feelings and frustrations about Tourette syndrome.

Telling Your Child

As the person most directly affected by TS, your child deserves to know why she has tics and other behaviors. Just like you, she has probably agonized over why she cannot seem to control certain sounds and movements no matter how hard she tries.

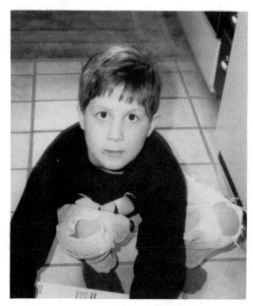

How you break the news to your child will depend somewhat on her age. It was pretty easy telling our seven-year-old that he had TS, because he was well aware of his "hyper" behavior and problems with friends. We explained to him that there was a problem in his brain that made it harder for him to control his behavior and calm down. If your child is somewhat older, she may want more factual information on the neurology of TS. For help explaining your child's diagnosis, you can contact the national TSA. They offer video tapes and pamphlets which explain TS to all age groups, from very young children to adults. Several useful children's books about TS and ADHD are also available. These can be found in the Reading List at the back of this book.

Whatever your child's age, you don't want to overload your child with more information than she is ready for at this time. But it is often helpful to reassure her that as she grows older, she will probably be more in control of her Tourette syndrome, and chances are good that symptoms will improve. It is also imperative to give honest answers to your child's questions about TS. Many young children want to know if they will die from TS or whether it is contagious. When specific symptoms occur, your child may wonder, "Is this TS, or am I crazy?" If you don't know the answers to questions, talk to other children or adults with TS, as well as their parents. You might also urge your child to make a list of questions for the doctor to encourage her to begin taking responsibility for her own care.

In our family, we felt that merely learning *facts* about TS was not enough. We thought it was also important to learn how it *feels* to have TS by getting to know adults with TS. This knowledge pays off every day. I cannot tell you how many times my son has complained of feeling "different" or "weird" only to discover that his feeling is a typical TS symptom. One day, for example, Jeff was concerned about how "grossed out" he was at the feel of the gooey glue they were using in school, when the other kids seemed to enjoy it. Because of my knowledge of TS symptoms, I recognized that Jeff's disgust was caused by tactile defensiveness—a type of sensory problem which causes a strong, adverse reaction to the sense of touch. I was able to allay Jeff's fears and explain that people with TS often have this reaction. He felt much better.

Once you break the news to your child, you can expect that she will go through the same grieving process that you experienced. When we first told Jeff about his diagnosis, he crawled under a blanket and said he didn't want to hear about it. We watched him slowly progress through each phase until he, too, reached acceptance. Now he even tells TS jokes and talks openly about his latest tics or compulsions. If your child is somewhat older when you get the diagnosis, she may have more difficulty coping. During the early adolescent ages of eleven to fifteen, children all want to be exactly alike, and peer pressure is exceptionally strong. Because of your child's "difference," she may feel overwhelming denial and anger at first.

In addition to her feelings about the diagnosis, your child will also have to cope with feelings resulting from years of being misunderstood. Because your child was probably blamed, shamed, and humiliated because of her symptoms, her self-esteem may be very low by this time. She may have little trust in adults or teachers because no one would believe her or help her. You must reassure her that her symptoms are not her fault, and that people who make fun of them are wrong. You will also need to educate everyone in your child's world—at school, around the neighborhood—so that teasing or punishing is stopped. Family counseling, too, may help your child develop higher self-esteem, as well as cope with feelings such as anger and frustration that have built up over years of being misunderstood. Chapter 4 provides more information on boosting your child's self-esteem.

Your Family and Friends

It is not enough for you to love and accept your child. If she is to grow up feeling like a valued member of society, others around her must also treat her with caring and understanding. The logical source of this added emotional support is your family members and friends.

Most family members and friends gladly rally to the support of a child with Tourette syndrome. But before they are able to do so, they usually must go through their own process of adjusting to the diagnosis. Like you, they will have many questions and concerns and will have to work through their feelings in their own way. Often, however, they will follow your lead. For this reason, the following sections offer some suggestions for gently guiding others toward acceptance.

Brothers and Sisters

If your older children are old enough to ask "Why?" they have probably noticed at least some differences in their sibling with Tourette syndrome. Whether or not they've actually articulated their questions, you can be sure an explanation about TS would be welcome. In our family, Jeff's nine-year-old sister had stored up a lot of anger about how he treated her. Jeff could not seem to lose a game graciously and often hit or kicked her. In addition, his behavior at school often embarrassed her. Understanding that he didn't do these things on purpose helped her cope.

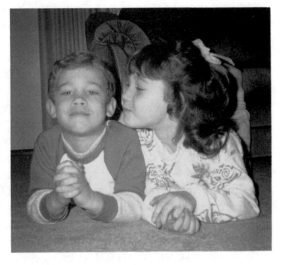

In explaining Tourette syndrome to brothers and sisters, there are several basic points to cover. First, you must help them understand that their sibling cannot control certain sounds and movements even though most people can. It may help if you compare having tics to having hiccups or sneezes or to having your knee tapped with a mallet by the doctor. Second, you should tell your other children that their sibling's tics increase if she is stared at, so they should ignore the symptoms whenever possible. Most children are very good at ignoring tics once they have this understanding.

If your child has more than simple tics and noises, explaining TS will be more complicated. Some obsessive-compulsive rituals or aggressive or impulsive behavior may appear purposeful, especially in the eyes of a child. For example, your child with TS might insist that her siblings follow a bedtime ritual or might have a compulsion to spit at family members. Telling siblings that their brother or sister with TS "can't help" behavior like this brings up many concerns about fairness and what to expect from siblings. At first, you may have to explain TS as each puzzling incident occurs. Counseling by a psychologist experienced in working with TS can also be a great help in coping with these family issues. Chapter 3 provides more information on psychological counseling.

After your other children have absorbed the information about your child's TS, they will probably go through many of the same stages you did in adjusting to the diagnosis. They may be angry and resentful because you seem to spend more time with their brother or sister. Or they may worry that they somehow caused their sibling to get Tourette syndrome. Like your child, they will need to be reassured that people do not die from TS and it is not contagious. Of course, if your other children are still quite young, there is a possibility that they, too, may develop TS, because of its genetic nature. It is probably *not* a good idea to bring this possibility up, as young children would not be able to understand genetics and there is no sense awakening needless worries.

Try to give your other children what they need—whether it is information about how TS will affect their sibling, or someone to talk to about their worries. Especially at first when you are busy with doctor appointments, school meetings, or TS support groups, take care that their emotional needs don't fall by the wayside. We fell into this trap when Jeff was first diagnosed. Our daughter—who is usually pretty independent—let us know in so many words that she resented the neglect. Be sure you set aside some special time to spend with your other children doing activities they enjoy. And by all means, arrange for your children to get to know other siblings of children with Tourette syndrome.

Grandparents and Other Relatives

How grandparents, aunts, uncles, and other relatives initially react to your child's diagnosis will likely depend on how aware they were of your earlier concerns. If relatives have been involved with your family and are aware of your concerns about your child, they may feel relief at having an explanation. If they were not previously aware of any problems, they may react with shock or disbelief. We experienced both of these reactions by relatives. Some had been concerned about Jeff for years, as we had. These relatives were relieved when we finally had a name for Jeff's problems. Others, who had had less contact with Jeff, denied and minimized the diagnosis, and again hinted that our parenting (or lack of discipline) must be the problem.

After the news has sunk in, your relatives are sure to have similar emotions to yours—perhaps with a new twist. Grandparents, for example, may blame themselves for passing on "defective" genes to your child. Aunts and uncles may worry that they, too, may have inherited the TS gene and will pass it on to their own children. This is a legitimate concern, and they need to know the facts: that there is a fifty-fifty chance that they have the gene. Your relatives may blame your spouse for giving your child Tourette syndrome, and your spouse's relatives may blame you. Everyone—especially grandparents—will probably grieve. Grandparents may grieve not only about the loss of their "perfect" grandchild, but also about the pain that you are going through.

You can help relatives adjust by reassuring them that their feelings are normal. Realize that this is a difficult time for them, too, and try not to be upset by questions and comments that seem insensitive or off the wall. Instead, volunteer information you think will help them and encourage them to ask questions. Try to allow for individual coping styles; don't expect them to come to terms with Tourette syndrome overnight. Let them know how important their understanding and acceptance is in reassuring your child that she is a welcome member of the family and of the human race. Also tell them how much *you* value their support. Chances are, you will find, as we have, that the relatives who take the time to really know your child will become great allies in her life.

Friends

Finding out that your child has Tourette syndrome can permanently or temporarily disrupt old friendships. Some friends may feel genuinely uncomfortable around your child. Others may stay away for fear of doing or saying the wrong thing. Then again, friends may think that you have your hands full just caring for your child and that they would be in the way.

On the other side of the coin, you may send your friends subtle or not-so-subtle messages that you wish to be left alone. For example, you may think that your friends cannot possibly understand what you are going through, and therefore avoid them. Or you may stop attending parties and other social events because you feel you must devote yourself totally to your child. In our family, we cut back on socializing because Jeff became overly excited whenever we had company. I also sometimes found it very hard to be around my friends because I resented their normal lives. They would talk about their children's sports activities or family social events, and seemed insensitive to the way our lifestyle would have to change because of Jeff's TS.

Obviously, there is much room for misunderstanding. You may think your friends are "deserting" you, at the same time they think that you are shutting them out of your life. The best solution is usually for everyone to be honest with one another about how they feel and what they have been going through. With enough background information, many of your friends will probably adapt well and be eager to help out however they can.

Often, parents discover new friends through Tourette Syndrome Association activities or through special education. As mentioned earlier, other parents of children with Tourette syndrome can offer you unparalleled understanding. I don't know if I could have survived the first year after Jeff's diagnosis without the support of friends I made through TSA.

Your Marriage

The first few months after your child's diagnosis can really be taxing. In addition to coping with your emotions, you may need to try out new medications and monitor their side effects, work on setting up an educational plan for your child, learn how to manage your child's behavior, and deal with medical insurance problems. Through teamwork, however, most parents find that the physical and emotional drain becomes more manageable.

In our case, it took some time to work out a smooth-running system. At first I was overwhelmed with all the new responsibilities and all I needed to learn. My husband, Clyde, had to take a great deal of time off from work to help me at home and to meet with school personnel and doctors. Eventually, we each settled into doing what we did best and started working as a team. Clyde's strong point turned out to be organizing household jobs and activities. I handled daily care, school meetings, and doctor appointments. Because I spent so much time with Jeff during the day, Clyde took over at night to give me free time to go out with friends. When Jeff's needs were more intense, meal preparation and household duties often took a back seat, and we both became more flexible in our roles around the house.

While you and your spouse are working out ways to handle the practical aspects of raising your child, do not neglect each others' emotional needs. No one understands you as well as your spouse does, and no one can help you cope with your feelings quite so well. It is important to remember, however, that everyone copes in a different way, at a different rate. Your spouse may be feeling guilty the day you are feeling angry, or may seem to skip right over an emotion that engulfed you for weeks. The important point is to listen to your spouse without judging and to acknowledge that he or she has a right to feel that way.

Finally, try not to let your marriage revolve around Tourette syndrome. It *is* necessary and important for you and your spouse to discuss your concerns about your child, but this should not be your sole topic of conversation. Nor should all your activities be related in some way to TS. After all, your child with Tourette syndrome is not the only one in the family with special needs and interests. To recharge your batteries, you and your spouse must occasionally take a break and do something *you* enjoy. Although it is difficult to find a sitter for Jeff, my husband and I make a point of setting aside time to be alone. Just as "normal" couples do, we enjoy going out to shop, eat, or watch a movie. All parents need to learn to balance their time and energies between family and self, and you are no exception.

Keeping Your Perspective

Having a child with Tourette syndrome is certainly no laughing matter. TS can complicate almost every aspect of your child's life and challenge your family's coping abilities to the utmost. But believe it or not, developing a sense of humor about TS can be an integral part of coping. Almost every adult with TS I know says that their ability to laugh at themselves and others with TS has been a lifesaver. They often tell the funniest stories about tics (especially vocal tics) and people's reactions to them. One person with TS told me, for example, about a TS conference in which a speaker was talking about the Statue of Liberty. Suddenly, an audience member with TS let loose a hilariously appropriate vocal tic: "BIG MAMA!" The audience greeted this tic with a hearty laugh, which is actually the best way to cope with funny vocal tics. I don't mean that you should laugh *at* someone for having TS, but you may want to laugh along with her. A friendly laugh can sometimes do more than anything else to ease a potentially awkward situation.

For me, remaining open to the genuine humor in everyday situations is only part of the sometimes difficult task of keeping my perspective. It is also important to remember that TS, in and of itself, is not going to rob your child of her potential to succeed in life. As long as she develops effective coping strategies, there is no reason to believe your child will not achieve her personal, academic, or career goals. Today there are adults with TS pursuing successful careers in almost every profession you could mention, from doctor and lawyer, to professional athlete and musician. Samuel Johnson, the great eighteenth-century British writer and compiler of the first English language dictionary, is believed to have had Tourette syndrome with OCD. And two of the chapter authors of this book—successful professionals in their own right—also happen to have TS.

Conclusion

Right now, your child's diagnosis of Tourette syndrome may seem to hover overhead like a monstrous thunder cloud. It overshadows everything else in your life and makes the years ahead look long, dark, and hopeless. Even when a ray of sunshine manages to pierce the gloom, it only seems to spotlight your child's latest tics and behaviors. Maybe you feel that you will never be happy and carefree again. This is how I felt when my son was diagnosed.

It has now been four years since we found out about Jeff's Tourette syndrome. And I want you to know that there *is* life after Tourette syndrome! The clouds disperse and everyone in the family gets on with their lives. True, the life you have after the diagnosis will likely be different than the life you knew before. But do not assume that these differences will be for the worse. In our case, we moved from a relatively expensive house into a more affordable one, enabling me to quit my job. This meant we had to give up some of our material goals—to let go of the American Dream of enviable prosperity and success. But because the smaller house required less upkeep, it also meant we both had more energy to devote to our children. And because we had moved into a school district known for the highest quality education, we had more assurance that Jeff would have his special needs met at school.

Through our experiences with TS, we have been stretched, as people, in so many ways. I have learned, for example, never to look askance at a child who is acting up in a restaurant or mall. (And, because not everyone is so enlightened about behavior problems, I've learned to be tough skinned about criticism when my family is on the receiving end.) Along the way, I think I've developed a heightened sensitivity for all people who are being judged in ignorance. In addition, as my gut feelings and instincts about my son have proven correct time after time, my trust of my own instincts has been reinforced. My husband, too, feels he has learned to trust his instincts, and that the experts are not always the people with a Ph.D. behind their name. My daughter, I believe, accepts differences in others with a tolerance rare for her age, and Jeff has learned that people love him and understand him just the way he is. Together, we have faced up to the fact that we will never be a perfect family. We have loosened up and accepted that we will always be different than the norm. And as TS has pulled our family closer together as a team, we have also discovered our own private brand of happiness.

Eventually, your family, too, will adjust to Tourette syndrome. You will learn to appreciate the "waning" times, and to cope with the "waxing" times. And as your love and acceptance grow, you will realize that what your child *does* is not nearly as important as who she *is*. One day you will see that whatever tics, rituals, attention deficits, or other symptoms she has are just part of the total package that makes her the unique and special child that she is. You will see her not as your child with Tourette syndrome, but simply as *your* child.

Parent Statements

We have gone through many emotional stages since our son was diagnosed with TS two years ago. Counseling has helped us to sort through our feelings. Although we still feel great sadness that our son has a disability that will affect him all his life, we are coming to understand that he can have a good, fulfilling life despite having TS.

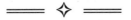

There are many paths to happiness, and our daughter will find hers.

═══ ✧ ═══

It is devastating to have family, friends, and neighbors—not to mention doctors, counselors, and teachers—accuse you of bad parenting. I went it alone—in anguish—until I went to my first TSA meeting. The problems and stories told by the other members were so totally similar to my experience I could hardly believe my ears.

═══ ✧ ═══

If it hadn't been for the support and affiliation of other parents (and TS camp), I don't know what would have happened to me.

═══ ✧ ═══

Sometimes the condemnation of so-called "well-meaning" others is so hurtful it's impossible to convey in words.

═══ ✧ ═══

After years of looking for a diagnosis, we finally found a child neurologist who said my daughter had Tourette syndrome. I was shocked and grief-stricken. Yet at the same time, this doctor and his very sensitive nurse were the first to assure me that I was in no way responsible for her symptoms.

═══ ✧ ═══

I'm still learning to adjust to the fatigue that hits me when Robby's going through a trying phase. I try to forget the outside world's expectations of me. If I don't feel I can have relatives over or go to social events, I don't.

═══ ✧ ═══

Going to TS summer camp was very enlightening. Seeing all these loving parents with their children, it was obvious that these parents were not causing the problem behaviors.

═══ ✧ ═══

No one understands like other parents of kids with TS do. Not even the very best of "TS doctors" in our area understands to the fullest. I wish he did, though.

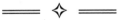

As a parent, I got to the point where what I needed more than anything was understanding. Everyone blamed me for Jim's TS, ADHD, and OCD behaviors until his diagnosis.

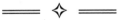

The TS support group people don't doubt my observations or experiences. They *know* there is no hidden agenda. TS parents are the true professionals when it comes to this disorder.

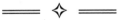

And then there are the people who accept that your child's behavior is due to neurological problems. Those people want to know if you drank or did cocaine during the pregnancy. Explaining to friends and neighbors that NO, he has TS, seems to fall on deaf ears.

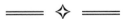

People thought I was wrong to deal with the hyperactivity. They said I should punish it. You get a lot of so-called well-meaning criticism. I'm so glad I followed my own instincts.

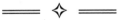

I have three college degrees in the helping professions. Having a child with Tourette syndrome brought me out of Ivory Tower ignorance and into the wisdom of the trenches.

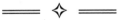

After she'd watched the tapes on Tourette syndrome, my son's grandmother was overheard saying, "I still wonder if he could have caught it from the dog."

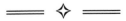

When I told my parents about our daughter's TS, they said, "It couldn't have come from our side of the family, by God!"

==== ✧ ====

It was a long journey, but when we found out, it was as if somebody had opened a window. Everything Brad did made sense.

==== ✧ ====

When Cindy was diagnosed, the first thing I did was join the TSA support group. What they were saying fit Cindy to a tee. It seemed like they were all talking about my child.

==== ✧ ====

I will never forget the day he was diagnosed. I felt relieved and sick to my stomach at the same time; also guilty. My heart began to break. These feelings are still with me.

==== ✧ ====

Developing a sense of humor will go a long way in helping you to live with Tourette syndrome.

==== ✧ ====

THREE

$\diamond$

Medical Treatments and Professionals

ORRIN PALMER, M.D.*

As yet, there is no "cure" for Tourette syndrome. But there *are* medical treatments that can help reduce the effects of the condition on your child's life. Medications can not only help control motor and vocal tics, but can also help control obsessive-compulsive disorder (OCD) and attention deficit hyperactivity disorder (ADHD) behaviors that often accompany Tourette syndrome.

Whether your child will benefit from these treatments depends on the severity of his symptoms. Children whose symptoms do not interfere with daily life generally do not need medical treatment for their TS. Their symptoms can often be controlled through strategies such as reducing stresses which increase symptoms, making classroom modifications, and educating people in their life about Tourette syndrome. On the other hand, children whose symptoms do interfere with daily life need a carefully monitored medical treatment plan.

If medication is prescribed for your child, you will be closely involved in his treatment. Depending on your child's age, you may need to make sure he takes his medications on schedule, and your observations will be invaluable in helping your child's physician

---

* Dr. Palmer is a graduate of New York Medical College. He completed his internship at Yale University and his residency and fellowship training at Mount Sinai Hospital and Medical Center in New York. He is currently Medical Director of Psychiatry at Frederick Memorial Hospital in Frederick, Maryland, and also has a private practice in neuro-psychiatry.

judge the effectiveness of medications. To help you know what to expect, this chapter reviews the most commonly used medications, as well as their benefits and side effects. To help you ensure that your child receives optimal care, it also offers some tips on selecting and working with medical professionals.

The Medical Treatment of Tourette Syndrome

The treatment of choice for Tourette syndrome is medication—it can be the quickest and easiest way of reducing or eliminating tics and other symptoms of TS. Many different medications are used to treat TS, and each has its own unique combination of desired, beneficial effects and unwanted effects, or *side effects*. In choosing a medication or group of medications, your child's physician should attempt to maximize desired effects, at the same time minimizing side effects. Ideally, your child will be given the drug or group of drugs with the fewest side effects and the lowest possible dose.

The medications children with TS may be prescribed fall into three broad categories: 1) anti-tic drugs; 2) anti-OCD drugs; and 3) anti-ADHD drugs. Each of these types of medications reduce symptoms by interacting with different brain chemicals *(neurotransmitters)* that transmit nerve signals from one nerve cell to the next. Anti-tic medications work by blocking the activity of the neurotransmitter *dopamine*. This is because tics are believed to be caused by too much dopamine or by a heightened sensitivity to dopamine. Anti-OCD medications help to restore the proper balance of the brain chemical *serotonin*, which is involved in mood stabilization and obsessive compulsive behavior. And because ADHD is caused by too little of the brain chemical *norepinephrine* (and possibly dopamine) in parts of the brain, anti-ADHD medications increase the flow of these chemicals to the brain. The sections below discuss the types of these medications most often used in the treatment of Tourette syndrome.

Anti-Tic Medications

Anti-tic medications are often effective in improving both motor and vocal tics in children with TS. Occasionally, they eliminate tics completely, but more often they reduce the frequency or severity of tics. For unknown reasons, some children with TS show no improvement of symptoms at all when taking these drugs. There is no way of predicting how effective anti-tic medications will be for any given child. For example, there is no proven relationship between the severity of a child's tics and how readily they respond to medication. The only way to find out whether anti-tic medications will help control your child's tics is to try them.

To control motor and vocal tics, the medications that are traditionally tried first (first-line drugs) are known as *neuroleptics*. The two neuroleptics that have been found to be most useful in treating TS are Haldol™ (scientific name: haloperidol) and Orap™ (pimozide). Haldol is generally given in a dosage ranging from 0.25 mg to 5.0 mg (child to adult dose) per day in divided doses. In doses above 5.0 mg (and in some people, well below 5.0 mg), the drug produces disturbing side effects which worsen as the dosage is increased. These side effects may include: 1) cognitive dulling (short-term memory loss, slowed thinking); 2) restlessness (known medically as *akathisia*); 3) sedation or drowsiness; 4) decreased coordination; 5) dry mouth, blurred vision, and constipation; 6) weight gain; 7) depression; and 8) difficulties leaving home or one's parents, or going to school (school phobia). The lower the dosage, the less likely these side effects are to appear.

These same side effects typically also occur with Orap at higher dosages. The dosage range for Orap is roughly 0.5 mg to 8.0 mg.

A rare complication of neuroleptic therapy should be mentioned. Occasionally, another movement disorder, called *Tardive Dyskinesia*, will develop in people taking neuroleptic medication, usually after long-term usage. This disorder produces involuntary movements, most often of the tongue and of the muscles around the mouth. It may or may not go away upon discontinuation of the neuroleptic.

Catapres™ (clonidine) is an alternative first-line drug. In most people, it seems to produce fewer side effects than neuroleptics do, and does not, as far as we know, pose any possible long-term risks such as Tardive Dyskinesia. It does not work well on everyone, but can be more effective than the neuroleptics in controlling complex tics. Unfortunately, Catapres may lose its effectiveness with time in some people. Typical dosages range from 0.05 mg to 0.3 mg per day. Side effects may include sedation and dry mouth, both of which lessen considerably with time. Like the neuroleptics, Catapres may also cause cognitive dulling, but usually to a lesser degree, and it usually improves over time. Because Catapres is used to treat high blood pressure (hypertension), your child's blood pressure may drop on this drug. Therefore, his blood pressure may need to be periodically monitored if he is prescribed this drug.

Neuroleptics and clonidine are generally most effective in treating the involuntary movements and vocalizations of Tourette syndrome. If your child's TS is complicated by OCD or ADHD, or both, additional medications may be necessary.

Anti-ADHD Medications

Anti-ADHD medications can often help control symptoms of attention-deficit hyperactivity disorder. They may reduce or eliminate symptoms such as impulsivity, poor attention, or fidgetiness. As with anti-tic medications, however, their effectiveness varies widely from child to child. In some children, anti-ADHD drugs may improve all symptoms of ADHD; in other children, they may only improve some symptoms; and in still others, anti-ADHD drugs may not be effective at all.

For most children with ADHD, the treatment of choice is Ritalin™ (methylphenidate). Unfortunately, Ritalin often, but not always, makes the symptoms of TS worsen. This is because Ritalin is a stimulant drug, and stimulants increase the flow of the brain chemicals norepinephrine and dopamine. Since children with TS already have too much dopamine in parts of their brain, stimulants exacerbate tics. If your child with TS has great difficulty sitting still and concentrating, and is easily distracted, a trial of Ritalin *may* be warranted. If his tics get worse on Ritalin, it should probably be discontinued.

Typical dosages of Ritalin range from 5 mg to 30 mg per day. Side effects may include initial sedation, reduced appetite, nervousness, and insomnia. If your child is prescribed Ritalin, his physician may recommend occasional drug holidays, preferably during summer break, because some studies show it can cause stunting of physical growth if taken on a continual basis. This stunting of growth does not occur, however, if the drug is not taken for approximately four weeks out of the year.

An alternative to Ritalin in the treatment of ADHD is a group of medications known as tricyclic antidepressants. These drugs are less likely than Ritalin to make TS symptoms worse. Probably the two best to use in children with Tourette syndrome are Norpramin™ (desipramine) and Anafranil™ (clomipramine). 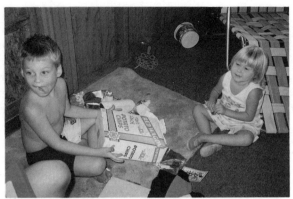 These drugs are used together with other first-line TS medications such as Haldol, Orap, or Catapres.

For Norpramin, dosages should be started at 10 mg per day; for Anafranil, at 25 mg per day. Maintenance dosages for Norpramin should be between 10 mg and 100 mg per day; for Anafranil, between 25 mg and 100 mg per day. (The maintenance dosage is the level at which optimum control is achieved with the fewest side effects.) Possible side effects include sedation, dry mouth, mild blurred vision, constipation, lightheadedness upon standing, and mild memory impairment. Because these side effects are worse when the drug is first taken, it's probably best to take both of these medications at bedtime. Anafranil seems to cause more side effects than Norpramin, but if your child also has OCD, it is probably the better drug. As explained below, this is because Anafranil can also control OCD behaviors. Before your child begins treatment with either of these medications, he should be given an electrocardiogram (EKG), as people with certain types of heart disease cannot take them. However, these problems are rare, especially in children.

Anti-OCD Medications

Anti-OCD medications can sometimes completely eliminate a child's obsessive-compulsive symptoms. More often, however, the main benefit of these drugs is in reducing the frequency of unwanted, intrusive, disturbing thoughts. Because children on these medications often have fewer OC behaviors than they would otherwise, they are better able to concentrate on schoolwork and daily activities.

OCD in children with Tourette syndrome is treated with either Anafranil or Prozac™ (fluoxetine). Higher dosages of Anafranil are needed to treat OCD than to treat ADHD and side effects are therefore increased. Prozac does not cause the same or as many side effects as Anafranil or Norpramin. Although people frequently experience an "energizing" effect or nervousness upon beginning treatment with Prozac, this is short-lived, lasting three to four weeks at most. Other side effects, which may or may not disappear, are nausea, diarrhea, heartburn, headaches, and insomnia.

Prozac comes in only one size, a 20 mg capsule. But people with TS are particularly prone to the initial "energizing" effects of Prozac when treatment is begun at 20 mg per day. One way of reducing the severity of this side effect is to spill out the contents of the 20 mg capsule into eight ounces of juice. Mix the solution vigorously, as Prozac does not dissolve well. Then immediately have your child drink two ounces, equivalent to a 5 mg dose of Prozac. Store the remaining solution in the refrigerator in a glass covered with plastic wrap. On the next day, again mix vigorously and give your child another two ounces, thereby dispensing another 5 mg. I recommend gradually increasing the dosage by 5 mg every four to five days as tolerated using this procedure.

To treat OCD associated with TS, your child's dosage of Prozac will probably eventually be increased to 10–40 mg per day. (Adults with TS require higher dosages of approximately 60–80 mg a day.) To minimize insomnia as a side effect, Prozac should be taken in the morning.

Other TS Medications

For no known reason, the first-line drugs described above some-times do not produce the desired improvement of symptoms. When the drugs traditionally used to treat TS do not work, several other medications may be used.

To reduce motor and vocal tics, Inderal™ (propranolol) is some-times prescribed. This drug is traditionally used to treat high blood pressure. In TS, low dosages are used, ranging between 10 mg to 100 mg per day. Side effects may include sedation, dizziness or lightheadedness, and rarely depression. Inderal should not be used by people with asthma. Its usage in the treatment of TS is still somewhat experimental. Once it has accumulated a longer track record, it may be prescribed more often for tics.

Buspar™ (buspirone), a drug that is marketed as an anti-anxiety drug, is sometimes useful in treating the OCD component of TS. Like the more traditional anti-OCD medications, it can decrease OCD behaviors. Side effects are rare, but may involve a feeling of lightheadedness or of a "rush" thirty minutes after taking the medication. Maintenance dosages range from 40–60 mg per day in adults and usually between 15–30 mg per day in children in divided dosages. Buspar is only used in addition to first-line TS drugs.

A final drug that may be used in conjunction with other first-line TS drugs is Klonopin™ (clonazepam). Klonopin is classified as a minor tranquilizer and is useful in treating certain types of epilepsy. For people with Tourette syndrome, Klonopin may be prescribed to treat OCD symptoms. It is also sometimes useful in reducing symptoms of anxiety. Dosages for children usually range from 0.25 mg to 1.0–2.0 mg per day. Side effects may include sedation and mild memory impairment. Unfortunately, a small number of individuals taking Klonopin may become dependent on it and develop some *tolerance*. That is, they need increasing dosages to achieve the same effect.

Treatment of Aggressiveness

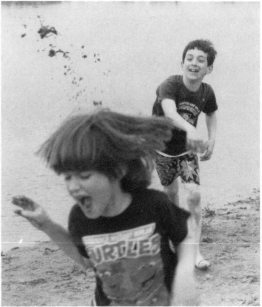

Some children and adults with TS have difficulty controlling their aggression. They may hit, or threaten to hit, other family members, throw objects across the room, or become verbally abusive. (Medical professionals sometimes refer to this problem as "behavioral discontrol.") If your child has uncontrolled aggressive urges and explosive emotions, there are two drugs that may help decrease these symptoms. The first drug that is usually tried is Tegretol™ (carbamazepine). Lithium carbonate is also sometimes used. If your child is prescribed either drug, you and your child must work closely with your doctor. Rare, but serious side effects are associated with these drugs, and your child will need to be closely monitored.

The "Right" Dosage and Medication

In prescribing medications for your child, your doctor will try to produce the maximum improvement in symptoms with the minimum of side effects. Striking this delicate balance can be difficult, however, since no two children respond in quite the same way to medications or have quite the same combination of symptoms. Generally, your doctor will begin by giving your child the lowest dosage that is often effective, gradually increasing the dosage to see how your child responds. He or she will closely monitor your child—with your help—to see whether the benefits achieved outweigh the side effects. For example, a moderate dosage of Haldol might significantly reduce your child's tics, but might not be the best choice if it causes a great deal of cognitive dulling and makes it harder for your child to keep up with his class.

If one medication is not effective in controlling a child's TS, OCD, or ADHD symptoms, a combination of drugs may be tried. Using a combination of drugs may also make it possible to reduce or avoid undesirable side effects. Rather than taking a relatively high dosage of one drug, your child might take lower dosages of two or more drugs and receive the same or better benefits with fewer side effects. For instance, if a high dosage of Haldol reduces your child's tics but causes depression, the depression might be reduced by decreasing the dosage of Haldol and adding Prozac.

Over the course of your child's life, the type of medications as well as dosages prescribed may occasionally need to be changed. For example, as your child's body weight increases, it may be necessary to increase the dosage of medications—but only if your child's symptoms worsen. Likewise, if symptoms become temporarily or permanently milder, dosages will be decreased. A change of medications might also be in order if the nature of a child's symptoms change. For example, in elementary school a child might have relatively innocuous OCD symptoms that do not need to be treated with medication. But when the child reaches adolescence, his symptoms might become more sexually oriented and disruptive so that it is advisable for him to begin taking anti-OCD medication.

Some people with TS continue to take medications all their lives. But in about 75 percent of people with TS, tics begin to decrease between the ages of sixteen and eighteen. About 50 percent of adults with TS eventually decide to stop taking TS medication altogether—either because their tics become mild enough that no medication is needed or be-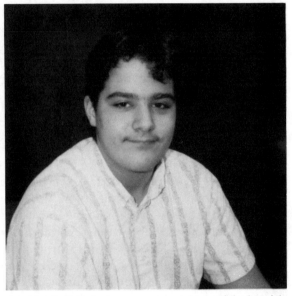cause they would rather deal with their symptoms than with the side effects of medication.

No matter why your child's medications are being decreased or changed, they should never be stopped abruptly. If stopped too quickly, many of these drugs can produce a "rebound effect"—a temporary worsening of symptoms or run-down, tired feelings similar to those produced by the flu or viral infections. Never allow your child to stop taking a medication without consulting a physician. Your child's dosage should be gradually tapered off according to your doctor's directions.

Over-the-Counter Drugs

Always consult your doctor before giving your child with TS any over-the-counter medications. There may be potentially harmful drug interactions you should be aware of. For example, if your child is on Anafranil, taking decongestants may make his symptoms much worse. In fact, many nonprescription drugs sold for cold, flu, and allergy symptoms can worsen the symptoms of TS, whether or not your child is currently taking prescription drugs for his TS, OCD, or ADHD. Antihistamines and decongestants are especially to be avoided. Remember, too, that alcohol is a drug. As your child approaches adolescence, make sure he understands that it is never a good idea to drink alcohol while on medications.

Controversial Treatments

From time to time, you may hear or read of "miracle treatments" for Tourette syndrome. Muscle relaxants, electric shock, and hypnosis have all been touted at one time or another as effective methods for reducing or eliminating the symptoms of TS. But the truth is, there is no evidence that these controversial treatments are useful in treating TS. The only safe, proven ways of controlling TS symptoms are through use of the medications described in this chapter and the types of behavior management strategies discussed in Chapters 4 and 7. Be wary of any doctor who suggests any other kind of treatment. Do not waste valuable time and money chasing after miracle cures.

Medical Professionals

Over the course of his life, your child will see many kinds of medical professionals. Some may prescribe and monitor the drugs described above, or help your child learn to cope with the emotional aspects of having Tourette syndrome. Others will see your child for general check-ups and for treatment or preventative care of conditions that are unrelated to his TS. To help you ensure that your child receives the best possible medical care, the following section reviews the types of professionals children with TS commonly encounter and offers some tips on how to choose them.

Neurologists and Neuro-Psychiatrists

Neurologists and neuro-psychiatrists are the physicians best trained to treat Tourette syndrome. Neurologists are medical doctors who specialize in medical problems associated with the brain and spinal cord. They can diagnose TS and prescribe medications that control tics. Neuro-psychiatrists are psychiatrists with special training in behavioral and emotional conditions which have a neurological cause. If your child has OCD, ADHD, or aggressiveness in addition to TS, a neuro-psychiatrist is therefore recommended. The anti-depressants, anti-anxiety drugs, and other newer drugs used in treating these conditions need to be prescribed by a specialist in neuro-psychiatric drugs.

Ideally, you will be able to find a neurologist or neuro-psychiatrist with first-hand experience in working with children with Tourette syndrome. If you can't, look for a physician who has had experience working with children with other special needs or one who expresses an interest in learning more about TS. Because researchers are constantly looking for more and better ways of treating TS, it is essential that your child's neurologist or neuro-psychiatrist keep up with current developments by reading medical journals and attending conferences on TS.

Before you choose a neurologist, meet with several you are considering, if possible. Consider the way each doctor interacts with you and your child before making your choice. Look for a physician who tries to make your child comfortable. For example, does the doctor let your child wait in an examining room rather than the waiting room if he finds waiting stressful? It is also crucial to find a physician who pays attention to *your* concerns and treats you as an expert on your child and his symptoms.

For help locating a physician with experience working with children with TS, contact either the national TSA or your local chapter. Both have physician referral lists. Other parents of children with TS are also excellent sources of recommendations. *Keep searching* until you are satisfied that you have found a doctor who listens, believes, and helps.

Pediatricians

Children with TS are just as likely to enjoy good health as other children are. That is, Tourette syndrome is not associated with any illnesses or conditions that will adversely affect your child's health. Consequently, your child should see a pediatrician only for the reasons that other children do—for routine checkups, immunizations, and treatment of childhood illnesses. Do not consult a pediatrician for treatment of Tourette syndrome. Most pediatricians are not trained in neurological conditions and can sometimes be sources of misinformation about TS. For questions and concerns about TS, always consult your child's neurologist or neuro-psychiatrist. Your child's pediatrician, however, should be kept informed about the TS medications your child is using so he can take any drug interactions into account.

Although you should not rely on a pediatrician for treatment of your child's TS, it still helps to find one who is experienced in working with children with special needs. A doctor who will go the extra mile to understand your child's special needs is much more likely to keep stress to a minimum. An experienced doctor will be better prepared to help your child cope with potentially traumatic procedures such as shots or blood tests. He or she will also know that as a parent, you can provide valuable information that will make your child's medical care go more smoothly. Once again, the best way to locate a pediatrician who is good with children with TS is to talk with other parents in your area.

Psychologists

Psychologists are professionals who are trained in understanding human behavior and learning. In contrast to psychiatrists, they are not medical doctors and therefore cannot diagnose neurological conditions such as Tourette syndrome. They also cannot prescribe medications to control TS symptoms. Instead, they use counseling and discussion to help identify and resolve problems in cognitive, behavioral, and social-emotional development. They can teach coping strategies, help sort out emotional issues, and build self-esteem. Thus, although a psychologist could not help your child control his tics, he or she *could* help your child learn to accept his tics and feel better about himself as a person.

Psychological counseling is often helpful for children with Tourette syndrome and their families. A well-informed psychologist might, for example, be able to help a family through a crisis that arises because the parents do not understand their child's

TS symptoms or because siblings resent the special treatment their brother or sister with TS gets. A psychologist could also help a child with TS cope with the anxiety he feels because of rejection by school peers or help him learn to handle teasing more effectively. In addition, psychological counseling can help children with TS deal with feelings of depression related to negotiating the world with a disability.

It is imperative to find a psychologist with experience in working with families with a child with TS. Otherwise, the psychologist might misinterpret your child's TS behaviors as *psychogenic*—caused by emotional problems in the family. Too often, families waste years of their lives and thousands of dollars seeing a psychologist who cannot help them because he is not trained in TS. The best bet is to get a referral from your neuro-psychiatrist or neurologist, or to contact the state or national TSA. TSA operates an information bank on local professionals with expertise in Tourette syndrome.

Dentists

Children with Tourette syndrome can pose special challenges for dentists. For example, a child's tics may prevent him from sitting still long enough to have his teeth x-rayed. Or vocal tics and sudden head jerks may make filling cavities more difficult. Obviously, you will want to find a dentist who will understand these special needs and be willing to work around them. Especially if your child's tics are severe, you should look for a dentist who specializes in treating children with special needs. Some major hospitals and medical centers operate dental clinics for people with physical or mental handicaps. You can also contact the National Foundation of Dentistry for the Handicapped, listed in the Resource Guide, for names of qualified dentists in your area. In addition, the TSA information bank can help you locate a dentist. If there are no dentists in your area experienced in working with children with special needs, look for a pediatric dentist who is willing to learn about TS, is patient and understanding, and is willing to allow your child to release his symptoms when necessary.

Becoming Part of the Team

As a parent, you need to take an active role in your child's medical treatment. Although it is up to your child's neurologist or neuro-psychiatrist to prescribe the best medications in the proper dosages, he or she cannot do this without your input. At least while your child is young, you must keep the doctor informed about symptoms your child has outside of the doctor's office, as well as about the side effects and benefits of medications prescribed. You must also make sure your child takes his TS medications properly. Because the level of medication in the blood needs to be kept constant, it is very important for your child to take his medications on time (sometimes four times a day) and not to miss a dose. Because children are often forgetful, you may need to monitor his use of medications until the age of sixteen or even longer. And because many children are not aware of problems with medications or are unable to talk about them until the age of eleven to thirteen, you will need to carefully monitor side effects.

Although your child may not be able to take complete responsibility for his medications until he is a teenager, he should be included as much as possible in decisions about his medical care. He needs to develop a relationship with his physician so that he feels comfortable asking questions about his TS. He must be informed about possible side effects of medications so he can recognize them if they occur. As he grows older, he should be encouraged to take on more and more responsibility for medical decisions, until he is eventually able to take over.

Most physicians recognize the crucial role parents and children with TS play in ensuring the best possible medical treatment. They use a team approach, routinely including parents and their child with TS in medical decisions. To help you become an effective team player, here are some guidelines:

Be a Careful Observer. The physician will often rely on you for information about your child's symptoms outside of his office and the effectiveness of medications. This means you should monitor your child carefully. Keep a notebook in which you record your observations about your child's tics, obsessions, and compulsions: their nature, when they begin, situations that appear to make them increase. Also record observations about your child's waxing and waning cycles: how long are tics at their severest and how long are they at their mildest? Finally, keep a record of any side effects your child's medications cause. For example, lower grades on your child's report card may be a sign that neuroleptics prescribed for tics are causing cognitive dulling. Be sure also to talk regularly to the school nurse and your child's teachers to find out what symptoms and side effects your child has at school.

Be Informed. It pays to be an informed consumer, whether you're purchasing a new car or medical care for your child. Read all you can about TS, and keep abreast of the most current developments. The Reading List at the back of the book is a good starting point; you will also want to get on the mailing list for the TSA newsletter and request some of TSA's pamphlets. Find out what members of your parent support group know about TS and how their child's symptoms are being treated. If you hear or read about a treatment that sounds like it might work for your child, by all means, ask your physician about it. In fact, do not hesitate to ask the physician questions about any aspect of your child's Tourette syndrome and his treatment. Unless you understand your child's medical needs and problems, you won't be able to make informed decisions about his medical care.

Get to Know the Doctor. For medical treatment to be effective, both you and your child need to feel comfortable with the doctor. Your child needs to have an open, trusting relationship with his doctor so that he will be able to talk freely about his tics and compulsions. And you need to feel that you can contact the doctor any time about immediate concerns and problems. If your doctor does not seem willing to take the time to put you and your child at your ease, consider switching doctors.

Conclusion

Medical treatment can help most children with Tourette syndrome control tics, attention problems, and OCD behaviors. This treatment can be a mixed blessing, however, bringing a variety of beneficial effects as well as an assortment of unwanted side effects. Determining which medication or combination of medications will best help your child may therefore take some time. But if you, your child, and your child's physician work together to develop the most effective treatment plan, eventually your child should achieve optimal control of his symptoms.

Parent Statements

We thought Robby's restlessness and pacing might be a side effect of medication. But then again, it could be because his ADHD is waxing. Last fall he started having more anxiety attacks, phobias, and OCD. We are seeing more physical expressions, so we can't be sure if it's the TS or side effects of medication.

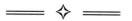

I've found that doctors diagnose according to their specialty. Dr. X always says the mother is too involved and the father is too distant. Dr. Y always says the child has ADD, but no TS. And Dr. Z always diagnoses TS with OCD.

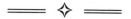

I think even the best and most eclectic doctors have biases that affect their diagnoses and treatments. Once parents understand this, they can take what fits their kid and leave the rest.

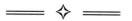

Some doctors are much better than others, so parents must educate themselves to enable them to recognize the difference.

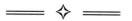

After years of useless behavior modification and talk therapy, we finally got the diagnosis of Tourette syndrome and then some helpful medication.

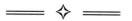

It helps to understand that very, very few professionals understand TS or its complications *and* that professionals don't admit this. Instead they refer you on to someone else.

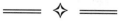

He started having temper tantrums at the end of fourth grade. His neurologist said he did not deal with problems like that and referred me to a neuro-psychiatrist. The new doctor took Ken off one drug and put him on another. His tantrums stopped immediately.

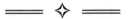

The medication hasn't ended Sally's behavior problems. Although she is able to concentrate longer, she's still hyperactive and displays obsessive compulsive behavior about anything from water to candy bars. She also has temper tantrums during which she is unable to regain control.

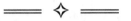

Medication wipes Brad out. He gets so tired, and as soon as his body changes a little, the medication needs to be changed, too. Then we start all over again.

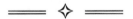

It was a real blessing to have TS diagnosed with one referral and one visit. I know families that go from doctor to doctor not knowing what is wrong.

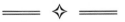

Right now, medication controls about 60 percent of the tics. We don't go for total control because of the possible side effects.

═ ✧ ═

Kids with TS need counseling as they approach adolescence. An eleven- or twelve-year-old wants to be just like his peers, and having TS sets him apart. Lots of anger and frustration build up. They ask questions like "Why did this happen to me?" "Will girls ever like me?" "Will I be able to get a job when I grow up?" Counseling gives them an outlet to express all of their feelings and it helps to build up self-esteem and eventual acceptance of themselves.

═ ✧ ═

Jim wants to take Ritalin so he can pay better attention at school. He says he'd rather suffer with the tics than be called on while "off task."

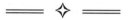

I'm hopeful that with early diagnosis we'll be ready in case things change. As Julie grows older, I know we will have to make some medication adjustments.

Remember the "Three M's" of Tourette syndrome. 1) Medication: If you keep on trying, you'll eventually find the right medication and method of dosage that will help to lessen the TS symptoms. 2) Maturation: As your child matures, usually by his late teens, there's a good chance that the chemical imbalance of TS will "self-correct" and his ability to control his symptoms and emotions will increase. 3) Motivation: With maturity comes eventual awareness and desire to control the most disruptive behaviors of TS for inner reasons of self-worth—inner motivation rather than punishment from outside of himself.

FOUR

$$\Longleftarrow \diamond \Longrightarrow$$

Daily Life with Your Child

MARILYNN KAPLAN*

For most parents, good advice on child care is easy to come by. When they have questions about discipline or mealtimes, for example, they have only to consult their own parents, their neighbors, or their child's pediatrician for suggestions. But when you have a child with TS, you may find that what works for other parents does not always work for you.

It is not that your child's daily care needs are any different from any other child's. It is just that her TS, together with any related conditions such as ADHD, OCD, sensory integration problems, or developmental delays, sometimes make daily care more challenging. For example, children with TS and ADHD have trouble keeping their attention focused on one activity, so they may need more reminders or supervision when they are cleaning their room, setting the table, or completing some other chore. Children who also have OC symptoms may have rituals or routines that interfere with their family's daily routine. For example, if a child has a compulsion to wash her hands repeatedly before breakfast, her parents might have trouble getting her dressed and ready for school in time to catch the bus. In addition, the need to keep your child's tics to a minimum by reducing stress can dictate the way the whole family's life is run.

---

* Marilynn Kaplan is the parent of a ten-year-old with severe Tourette syndrome and associated neuro-behavioral difficulties. She serves on the board of directors of the Minnesota TSA and PACER (Parent Advocacy Coalition on Educational Rights), as well as on the governor's Ombudsman's Committee on Mental Health and Retardation for Minnesota. She also conducts inservice training on TS for educators.

Each day, you may have to follow a set routine so that no unexpected events increase the stress your child feels. To add to your problems, your child's symptoms of TS wax and wane and frequently change. This means you must constantly re-evaluate your child's needs and develop new strategies to meet them.

In the end, how you adapt your daily care routine to your child will depend on her personality, symptoms, and developmental abilities. Because children's personalities and TS symptoms vary so widely, there are no magic formulas and no absolute right and wrong answers. With attention, planning, and nurturing, however, you can learn what works with your child. And although your role as a parent may sometimes be more challenging, you can help ensure that your child develops the independence and self-esteem she needs to succeed as an adult. This chapter is designed to help you learn to analyze your child's unique needs and then develop ways to take care of them.

Providing a Supportive Home Environment

From birth onward, most children are masters at making their physical needs known. They wail when they need to be fed, squawk when their diaper needs changing, and shiver when they need an extra blanket. Like any parent, you undoubtedly learned to interpret these signs early on and to take care of your child's physical well-being. But besides having physical needs, all children have a variety of emotional needs that may not be so obvious. Perhaps most importantly, they need to feel loved and accepted in order to feel good about themselves and their abilities.

For children with Tourette syndrome, the need to develop feelings of self-worth is just as acute as it is for other children. But because their TS often makes them feel different or as if something is wrong with them, it can be harder for them to develop good self-esteem. By providing a supportive home environment, you can help your child with Tourette syndrome conquer negative feelings about herself and to feel like a valuable part of her family and community. The sections below describe some specific strategies that are often helpful.

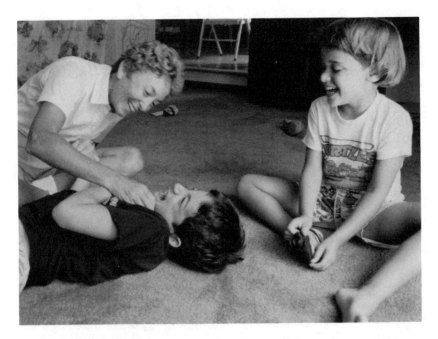

Coping with Tics

One of the best things you can do for your child's emotional well-being is to make sure she feels comfortable having tics at home. Children with TS may hold back their tics when they are in public because they do not want to seem different from other children. They need to know that there is at least one place where it is always acceptable for them to release their symptoms. Furthermore, helping your child feel comfortable with her tics lets her know that your family accepts her and her disability, which is crucial to the development of her self-esteem.

Constantly pointing out tics or blaming your child for having them only increases stress and usually makes tics get worse. Conversely, ignoring your child's tics usually helps relieve the stress she feels and therefore helps to reduce tics. Professionals usually advise parents to ignore their child's tics. There may, however, be times when you want to briefly acknowledge a tic to let your child know that you understand what she is going through and accept her disability. For example, if your child has a new shoulder tic, you could say, "I see that you are shrugging your shoulders. Let me know if you would like a massage tonight."

Ignoring tics is sometimes easier said than done. Phonic tics in particular can be very disruptive. Some parents wear ear plugs or listen to a portable radio or tape player to help them ignore tics. In addition, having your child listen to music can sometimes have a calming and quieting effect on tics. Experiment with all styles of music. Music with a constant beat may be more soothing than relaxation tapes for some kids. Because many children with Tourette syndrome need to hear favorite songs over and over again, make sure your child's tape recorder or headset has a rewind mechanism.

Listening to music may also help diminish your child's tics when riding in the car. Another strategy to use when traveling is to involve your child in activities that help her block out stressful stimuli and focus on something else. For example, you might give your child a tablet and crayons or play guessing games with the odometer, clock, or things you see outside.

If your child has a socially unacceptable tic or compulsion such as spitting or licking others, it may be possible to substitute a more socially acceptable tic or compulsion for the less desirable one. For example, a child with a spitting tic may be able to change the tic to a swallowing tic or other mouth or tongue tic. A child with a compulsion to lick others might learn to lick her teeth instead. And a child with coprolalia might be able to substitute a word such as "fork" or "fu" for the swear word she might otherwise say.

Just as the ability to control tics varies with each individual with TS, so does the ability to successfully substitute symptoms. It may help to talk to your child about possible substitutions. Children can often describe what tics feel like or what movements or sounds they need to make to "satisfy" a tic. Trust your child if she says she cannot substitute a particular tic. As children grow older, tic substitution sometimes occurs more easily, and many adults with TS learn to use it as a coping strategy.

If your child's tics cannot be reduced or controlled, then it is up to your family to accept that fact. Some people with uncontrolled disruptive tics have said that keeping a sense of humor and allowing others to do the same works best in these situations. You and your child should also understand that there may be times when a family member needs to go into another room and shut the door to get away from the tics. For example, if your child's tics disrupt a sibling's concentration so that he cannot focus on a book report he is writing, he should leave the room, just as he would if a television were disrupting his concentration. As discussed later in this chapter, if there are times when you feel you simply must have a break from coping with tics, you can also benefit from respite care services.

Rarely, children with TS may have self-injurious tics such as head banging, eye poking, picking their gums, or burning themselves. These tics cannot be ignored, and you should seek professional help immediately from your child's physician or a mental health professional. They can advise you whether a change in medication or an attempt at symptom substitution may help.

Providing Structure, Consistency, and Routine

Providing structure, consistency, and routine are important for all children. But they are even more important for children with TS, especially those who also have ADHD or OCD. Children with OCD often have a need to know what will be happening throughout the day. Surprises can be stressful for them, and may cause anxiety and increased symptoms. Children with ADHD, on the other hand, can become anxious and hyperactive if they are not involved in directed activities. Many things in the environment, but especially unexpected events, can overstimulate them. In order to stay calm and in control, children with these symptoms need daily events to be predictable.

The keys to providing your child with the predictability she craves are structure, routine, and consistency. Providing structure basically involves setting well-defined boundaries for behavior and activities. Your child needs to understand what she is expected to do, when, and how. When your child is at home, it is often up to you to tell your child what she can or should be doing by planning after-school and evening activities; outside the home, a structured school or day care setting can help. During summer vacation, you can help to keep your child's day structured by enrolling her in a YMCA or community recreation center program.

Developing routines, or a set way of doing things, helps to reduce surprises that may be stressful to your child. Generally, the more sameness in your child's life, the better. If your child can get up at the same time each morning, sit in the same spot at the breakfast table, even eat the same cereal every day if she so desires, she will feel more secure. Occasionally, of course, routines must be broken. For example, instead of coming straight home after school, your child may need to go to the dentist. When changes are necessary, keeping a family events calendar in a prominent location can help your child prepare ahead of time.

Being consistent in your parenting style is also important in providing predictability. Not only should you try to handle specific situations the same way each time, but you and your spouse should try to handle situations in the same way. If you have differing ideas about parenting, work together to develop a system that combines the strengths of both. For example, if you are more permissive than your spouse by nature, you should still follow through on decisions your spouse makes regarding discipline, even if you personally disagree. First, your child will be less likely to play one parent against the other if you can present a unified front. And second, your child will not be confused as to what is expected of her.

Keeping an Eye on Your Child

All babies and young children require close supervision to ensure their personal safety. As children grow up, they usually become more cautious and responsible for their own well-being. Children with TS, however, may continue to need a great deal of supervision as they get older. This is because they are often impulsive and have a tendency to wander beyond their boundaries. For parents, constantly supervising an active child can be very tiring. It may help to limit the amount of time your child spends on stressful activities that may worsen her symptoms. If she starts losing control, try to redirect her energies into another activity. For example, if she becomes overexcited while playing computer games with friends, send her outside to swing or ride her bike. Setting and enforcing physical boundaries inside and outside your home may also help. An enclosed backyard, a bedroom, or a special nook or cubby can give your child privacy, time to unwind, and relaxation. The idea is to provide specific areas where you child will not be overstimulated and where she will gain a clear understanding of where she fits into her environment.

If you take the time to let your child's siblings, friends, and neighbors know about your child's impulsivity, they can keep an eye out for her outside the house. Sitters can also help to relieve you of some of your supervising duties, especially if they know that you are not far away.

Occasionally, you may wish to make some alterations to your home to avoid persistent problems. For example, if your child always helps herself to snacks when you are not looking, you may want to lock up all the junk food in a separate cabinet and leave the healthy food readily accessible. If your child has a compulsion to climb out of windows, you might install bars on the upstairs windows that snap out in case of fire. If your child frequently gets into dangerous situations, talk to your physician or a mental health professional about ways of dealing with your child's behavior.

Providing a Physical Outlet

By providing your child with opportunities to take part in exercise and sports, you can help her reap both physical and emotional benefits. Many children with TS have fewer tics when they

are actively involved in a physical activity. Some experts believe this is because exercise produces or increases certain brain chemicals (endorphins) that have a calming effect. If your child also has ADHD or sensory integration problems, she may find exercises such as climbing, jumping, spinning, or swinging very

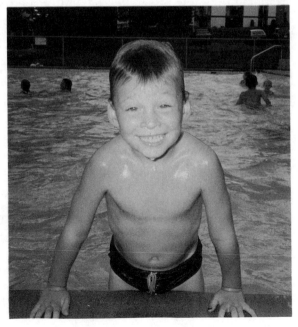

calming. This is because children with these problems often have a need for the increased stimulation of their movement (vestibular) sense that these activities provide.

At home, there are many ways you can encourage your child to work off energy. A mini trampoline or an old mattress in a play area may work indoors. Outside, you may want to install a basketball hoop, swing set, climbing tower, or a soccer goal.

In the sports arena, there are numerous individual and group activities that can benefit your child. Swimming is one of many individual sports that works well for children with Tourette syndrome. It teaches a life skill, involves the whole body, and provides a physical outlet for excess energy. It can be enjoyed either competitively or recreationally. Your child may feel comfortable swimming in a public pool, but if she prefers warm water, check for area hospitals that have therapeutic pools or facilities for people with handicaps or chronic illnesses. Other good choices of individual sports include skiing, ice skating, roller skating, dancing, biking, and jogging.

If going to group lessons makes your child too anxious, consider arranging for a few private lessons. After she feels more secure in her ability and surroundings, she can be worked into small group lessons. Be sure to discuss your child's symptoms with all teachers before classes begin.

Some kids with Tourette syndrome do well in team sports, but don't push your child if she doesn't. There are many stress factors inherent in team sports, and stress is what many children with Tourette syndrome need to avoid. Of course, some children will insist on pursuing an activity even if it makes their symptoms worse. If this happens, you will have to weigh the pros and cons of her continuing, and perhaps discuss it with the professional who is treating your child's TS.

As with any activity, there is a chance that your child may become compulsive with her chosen sport. If so, encourage her interest and try to use it to enrich other facets of her life. For instance, if your child likes to play baseball, encourage her to explore books on baseball. Or if she loves ballet, try introducing her to classical music. If your child is so compulsive about a sport that she becomes overtired, you will need to limit the time she is actively participating and promote quieter, related activities such as score keeping, charting, or reading about the sport.

Discipline and Behavior Management

Teaching appropriate behavior is a perennial concern for parents. Indeed, it is one of the most important responsibilities of parenthood. All children need to learn how to get along with others and how to follow rules of safety. They need to learn, for instance, not to dart out into traffic and to ask to borrow another child's toy.

When your child has TS, teaching appropriate behavior can be especially difficult. Your child is inherently unable to control certain socially unacceptable behaviors because of the nature of her disability. Although she may understand that some of her motor and verbal tics or obsessive-compulsive behaviors are unacceptable to many people, she cannot control them. She might also be impulsive, hyperactive, aggressive, disorganized, or socially and emotionally immature, making her even more prone to do things that others see as "misbehaving."

As a parent, you must decide which behaviors society will need to learn to accept and which behaviors your child will need to learn to control if she is going to live in the community. The behaviors that are referred to in this section as "inappropriate" are those that can cause physical or emotional harm to your child or to others and destruction of property. Examples include hitting other children, slamming doors, hanging out windows, stealing, punching holes in walls, doing karate kicks on windows, and the like.

Once you have identified which behaviors you want to discourage and which you want to encourage, you must then find the combination of behavior management strategies and discipline that works for your child. "Behavior management" is a general term for techniques used to help children learn appropriate behavior. Some examples of behavior management include praising desired behavior, ignoring unacceptable behavior, and punishing inappropriate behavior. "Discipline" refers to the rules and standards for acceptable behavior that parents establish for their children. Discipline forms boundaries within which children learn to act and behave appropriately.

Often, traditional behavior management strategies do not succeed with children with Tourette syndrome. Many parents of children with TS consistently follow the guidelines for good behavior management, yet their children still have persistent behavior problems. As the parent of a child with multiple motor and phonic tics, ADHD, and OCD, I was perplexed for many years until I finally figured out why the usual methods didn't work. Most of the behavior management strategies suggested to parents do not address the problems that arise when a child does not have normal control of impulses and may have very compulsive behavior as well. This realization started me on the road to finding some answers to how to handle children with neuro-behavioral problems.

The reason many traditional behavior management systems do not work well with many children with Tourette syndrome is that they are only "reactive." Parents respond or react to their child's actions by giving some kind of consequence that may or may not relate to the behavior they want to change. For example, two siblings might be playing a board game on the floor, when a third sibling runs into the room and slides into the game, scattering the game pieces all over the room. A reactive strategy might be to send the culprit to his room for a five-minute "time-out." Professionals assure us that if these kinds of consequences are given repeatedly and consistently, behavior will change. But if the culprit in this instance has a compulsion to run in the house, a compulsion to slide into games, or often acts impulsively, a reactive strategy may never change his behavior.

If the typical *reactive* types of discipline are not right for your child, you may be more successful with a *proactive* approach. Rather than waiting for your child to do something wrong and then reacting, you try to set up the environment to prevent undesirable behavior from occurring. In the example above, the siblings could be told to play their game on a table instead of on the floor. Meanwhile, their impulsive sibling could be redirected to an activity such as playing basketball outdoors that would not give him cause to run into the game board.

Over the years, my husband and I have found that such proactive strategies really work. For example, our son went through a period when he kept slamming the clothes chute door. At first, we tried reactive methods, punishing our son every time he slammed the door by giving him "time outs." When that didn't stop the behavior, we tried taking away privileges, but that didn't work either. We finally decided that the behavior was very compulsive and resistant to change. Taking a proactive approach, we removed the chute door for several months. By the time we replaced the chute door, our son's compulsion to slam it was gone.

Obviously, you cannot always change the environment to accommodate your child, but you may still be able to use a proactive approach. For example, for several weeks my son had a compulsion to throw chairs in his classroom. Two possible proactive approaches would have been to remove all the chairs from the room or to nail them to the floor, but that would have caused too much disruption for the other children. Instead, we used a less intrusive proactive approach and removed our son from the room until he was able to control his compulsion. We placed him in a smaller, less stimulating room where he was able to calm down and regain self-control more easily.

Aside from benefitting your child, a proactive approach can also help you. In deciding how and when to deal with your child's inappropriate behaviors, you will no longer need to ask yourself which behaviors are due to Tourette syndrome and which are not. Nor will you need to sort out which behaviors are caused by medications. As long as you use proactive strategies, you do not have to differentiate between causes of misbehavior. You simply try to prevent it before it occurs, regardless of cause. Instead of punishment, the emphasis is on setting up the environment for success, praising acceptable behavior, and redirecting unacceptable behavior.

Crucial to the proactive approach is cultivating the type of supportive environment described earlier in this chapter. If you can avoid stressful situations while providing structure, routine, and consistency, your child will have an easier time controlling her actions. It is especially important that discipline be clearly defined and consistent. If rules keep changing, your child will be confused. But if your child knows what to expect, there will be fewer variables and unknowns, and she will feel less stress.

The sections that follow offer a number of proactive strategies for helping parents of children with TS manage challenging behavior.

Cues and Redirection

Redirection means changing your child's focus of attention when she has lost control, or is about to lose control, of her behavior. It can be accomplished by physically moving your child from one place or activity to another or by suggesting another activity for her to do.

For children with TS, redirection works best when used *before* they have begun to behave inappropriately. This makes it important for you to learn to recognize the *cues* or signs that your child is on the verge of losing control. Cues might include more frequent vocal or motor tics, an increase in hyperactivity, an angry facial expression, or uncontrolled giggling. Redirecting your child quickly and calmly will help her regain control before she loses it completely.

My husband and I often use redirection to cool down my son's anger. For example, when my son is playing informal team sports, he frequently gets angry if he doesn't perform up to his expectations of perfection. His anger usually starts with yelling and accusing someone else of cheating. Depending on the situation, we try to redirect him either by having him sit quietly for a while in a safe area, or by having him move over to the swings for a few minutes. If he remains angry, we insist that he not play the sport for the remainder of the afternoon and help him select another activity, such as score keeping or playing a completely different game. If we didn't redirect him at this point, his anger would probably increase and he would start throwing equipment or rocks, or kicking something across the yard, without concern for anyone else's safety.

If your child is older, you might see signs of frustration while she is trying to do her homework or work on a project. Encourage your child to take a break, and suggest what she could do for a few minutes to calm down. For example, you could ask her to move the lawn sprinkler or taste the chili you are making. Be sure to praise your child for helping you afterwards. To help your child feel as if she is an active part of the plan, discuss with her, in advance, why she might need to be redirected and how you might redirect her.

Redirecting OC Behaviors. Learning to use redirection is especially important if your child has obsessive and compulsive symptoms. Children with OC symptoms often become frustrated because they are "obsessing" on something that it is too difficult for them to do. In these cases, it can be helpful to try to channel the obsession into something they can do more easily, but still feel satisfied. For example, if putting together model airplanes is too difficult for your child, suggest that she draw airplanes or do some library research on airplanes.

Redirection may also be used to channel your child's OC symptoms into something more productive, whether or not she is feeling frustrated. For example, if your child is obsessed with horses, try to turn her obsession into a learning opportunity. Give her opportunities to play with toy horses, read about horses, draw horses, go to a farm and watch horses, and arrange for a horse ride. Use obsessive behaviors to develop talents such as music, dance, or art. A child who is compulsive about practicing the piano, for example, might be encouraged to become an accomplished musician. There are several famous sports figures who have Tourette syndrome and acknowledge that their OC symptoms helped them achieve their success.

Redirecting can make a significant difference between your child feeling out of control and her feeling good about herself. Take the time to get to know your child's cues, and experiment with different types of redirection. Remember, however: redirection should only be used with relatively harmless OC behaviors. If your child's symptoms are socially unacceptable, self-injurious, or harmful to others, they should be dealt with by a neuro-psychiatrist who specializes in working with OCD. As Chapter 3 explains, there are several medications that can often improve OC symptoms. Symptom substitution may help as well.

Time Outs

Aside from redirection, another method of helping your child regain control is the "time out." To use "time out," you and your child agree upon a "safe place" where she can go when she is about to lose control or is already behaving inappropriately. Ideally, you can help your child learn to recognize her own cues that signify she is in danger of losing control of her behavior. She can then take responsibility for her own behavior and retreat to her "safe place" long enough to regain control. When your child has already lost control, you may need to take her to her "safe place" and stay with her, perhaps helping her to calm down by stroking her back or using soothing words. "Time out" should be explained to your child as a positive way to calm down, rather than as a punishment for bad behavior. You may wish to re-label it "calm time" or "relax time" if your child already associates "time out" with punishment.

Handling Transitions

Children with TS and OC symptoms or ADHD may have trouble making transitions when they are physically or mentally involved in something else. That is, they may find it difficult to end one activity and move to another or start a new task. It is often frustrating for parents to have to constantly nag at their children to get them to do something or go someplace.

If your child has trouble with transitions, it may help if you provide visual reminders of what she needs to do and when it needs to be done. For younger children, charts with pictures work well. For example, you might design a chart with pictures of each morning task: get dressed, eat breakfast, take pills, brush teeth, put on jacket. Then hang the chart in a visible location. As your child completes each task, she can check it off on the chart. Once your child knows her numbers, it is easy to use a digital clock for visual cues. Tell your child what time she should do specific tasks and, if necessary, write the time and task on a chart. Be sure to praise your child for each task completed. Charts are particularly helpful when there is a change in routine. For example, when your child returns to school in the fall, it may be difficult for her to change from her leisurely summer schedule to a more organized, fast-paced, get-ready-for school routine. Using a chart on which she can check off tasks as she completes them and/or visual cues such as pictures of a toothbrush and toothpaste may help her organize her morning more efficiently and get off to school with minimal fuss.

Older children can design their own lists of what they need to do, together with a time schedule that will help them get the tasks done within an appropriate amount of time. Using charts in this way can not only provide needed structure for your child, but also teach her to be responsible for herself.

At times, you may need to give verbal reminders about transitions. Allow enough time for your child to complete what she is doing or to put it aside in a way that is less stressful for her. For example, if you want your child to go shopping with you, you might tell her she must be ready to leave in thirty minutes. Ask her if she needs help getting ready or ending her activity. If your child resists, let her know the consequence of not being ready in thirty minutes. For example, you might tell her that for every additional minute you must wait for her, she will lose that amount of play time later. When fifteen minutes are up, remind your child again and tell her you will give her a reminder five minutes before you will leave. When the time is up, it's time to go. Insist that your child accompany you, even if—as my son does—she tells you that she can't leave to go shopping because she is "obsessing" on something. The fact is, I know my son would be ready in two minutes if I said we were going to play video games. Understanding your child's special needs *is* important, but following through with consistent discipline will help your child learn her boundaries.

Modeling Appropriate Behavior

Children learn behavior from their parents, so in essence, we are all teachers. If we want our children to behave in a certain way, then it is important for us to behave the same way. For example, you cannot expect your children to be kind and cooperative with each other if you and your spouse are constantly fighting and criticizing each other. If you use physical punishment such as spanking, then the chances are good that your child may hit others to try to get her way.

Because children with TS often have trouble controlling their impulses, it is especially important for parents to model non-violent behavior. You and your spouse should learn to discuss your differences using calm, non-threatening language, so that your child can hear and see how it is done every day. In addition, regularly praising family members and friends will encourage your child to be respectful of others.

Praising Your Child

Children with TS often hear so many negative comments about their symptoms and behavior that they start to believe that they are bad people. To counteract this misperception, catch your child being good and praise her whenever possible. Try to be specific when praising your child; tell her exactly what it is that you like. If your child has cleaned up her room, you might say, "Mary, your room looks really nice. Cleaning your room shows that you care about your belongings. Also, it gives me more time to play with you." Be careful not to dilute your praise with subtle criticism. For example, if the way your child has made her bed isn't up to your adult standards, don't say, "That's a pretty good job even though the bedspread is crooked." Instead say, "I'm proud of you for making your bed without having to be reminded."

To encourage the least stressful sibling relationships, remember to praise all your children. Each needs to feel special and worthy. Praise your children for their kindness and cooperation, tasks completed or attempted, bravery in new situations, and other accomplishments. Sometimes I give my children or their friends paper medallions with special inscriptions for doing something well. For example, I've made awards for "1st place room cleaner," "Best cooperative play for one hour," "1st place diver," or "Gold award for bravery for staying overnight at John's house."

Children like to hear that they are good. It makes them feel proud and accepted, and also makes it more likely they will repeat the behavior they have been praised for. You may want to keep a "Special Person" notebook in which you list the things your kids do well each day. This list can be reviewed with each child at night before bed. Likewise, your children can make "I'm Proud of Me" books and share their positive experiences and feelings with the family.

Reward Systems

Volumes have been written on using reward systems to shape children's behavior. But the basic principle behind reward systems can be stated quite simply: You can either reward your child for not doing something you don't want her to do, or you can reward her for doing something you want her to do.

Before you try using a reward system, you must first decide what behavior you wish to reward, then decide how the system will ensure your child's success, and finally, pick a reward. Here is an example of how you might do this:

Let's say you want your child to stop hitting her sister. That means the behavior you want to reward is any behavior that does not involve hitting her sister. To ensure your child's success, you must devise some way to reward her even if she frequently hits her sister. You might have to start, for example, by giving your child a star for every thirty minutes that she does not hit. If she receives six stars in a day, then she may receive a sticker, balloon, or whatever reward you decide will inspire your child. (Ideas for rewards are endless, but some professionals advise against using money or food for rewards.) If your child easily earns six stars, you may want to gradually increase the number needed for a reward. If your child cannot earn six stars, you will need to back up as far as necessary for her to achieve success. As your child's behavior improves, you can increase the stakes for getting the reward, remembering to praise your child even if she has a more difficult day.

If your child is older, you might award her points that can be used to "purchase" something from your family store. The list of items available and number of points needed to buy them can be posted on the refrigerator. These rewards can be services that others will perform, such as Dad cleaning the child's room for one hour or Mom taking the child to a park to fly a kite. They may also be special privileges, such as being allowed to stay up one hour past bedtime or choosing a video to watch. My children often picked going to the car wash with me as a reward. Reward systems are only limited by your creativity and your child's desires.

While you are using a reward system, remember that it is only a temporary measure. Ultimately your child must perform the desired behavior without receiving any more reward than praise and self-satisfaction. Although some unacceptable behaviors may return when you discontinue your reward system, others will not. It is worth a try to experiment with reward systems to break the pattern of unacceptable behavior.

Handling Aggressiveness and Anger

If your child has trouble controlling aggressive behavior or she experiences prolonged anger and severe temper tantrums, safety can become a pressing problem. Seek professional help for your child immediately. Try to find a neuro-psychiatrist who is knowledgeable about TS-associated behaviors and medications, and who does not blame your child for her behavior.

Your child's doctor will teach you specific ways to deal with her anger and frustration, but there are some general strategies that can help many children. Once again, it is easier to prevent an inappropriate behavior from occurring rather than react to it once it has begun. For example, if your child is aggressive with other children, limit the time she spends with friends. End the play period while your child is still in control. Let your child know that her play time with friends will increase as she shows you that she is able to play appropriately. Some professionals recommend that everyone in the family refrain from watching all television programs and movies that are violent and use abusive language, including most cartoon shows. They also recommend removing both real and toy guns and weapons from the home.

Because you cannot prevent all frustrating situations from occurring, teach your child a variety of ways to express herself and handle frustration. For example, you might set up a safe place for her to go to calm down. The area might have pillows, a mattress, stuffed animals, or other unbreakable objects. The area should be as free of visual and auditory distractions as possible. Let your child remain in her area for as long as necessary for her to feel that she is back in control.

Being held helps some children with Tourette syndrome regain control, but other children become more angry or aggressive. Some children want to be left alone, which is fine if you've provided a safe place to go. Other activities that may calm your child include having a back massage, swinging, rolling into blankets, crawling into a box, taking a shower, or soaking in a bathtub.

If you can, try to redirect your child's anger before she loses control. Have her draw a picture of her anger, write a couple sentences about appropriate behavior ("I will say kind things to my sister"), or say three nice things about the enemy ("Amy is good at drawing). The first tries may end up crumpled and tossed, but eventually your child will settle down as her focus shifts from internal stress to external expression.

Whatever strategy you use, keep reassuring your child that she will calm down, and praise her when she does. Remember that using physical punishment to teach a child to use non-violent behavior does not work. Reversing aggressive behavior takes time, supervision, appropriate role models, and sometimes, professional help.

Once your child has regained control, allow her to make amends for her behavior. She may apologize, share a toy, color a picture, or do whatever makes her feel okay about herself again. Don't expect or demand immediate remorse. Although many children will do something to make amends quite naturally, others need to be taught how to do this. Your child may need to repeat the same mistake many times before she understands why it is wrong. But if you allow your child to learn from her behavior, ultimately she will learn to be responsible for her actions and their effect on other people.

Your other children also need to learn how to deal with their sibling's anger. Teach them to quietly move away from their brother or sister if they see she is losing control, and to notify you that this is happening. Going to another room or to a friend's house may provide them with safety and security until your child with Tourette syndrome has calmed down. If your child with TS is a threat to the safety of other family members, professional intervention is needed. Your child may need to be removed from your family until she is on medication that improves her symptoms or has learned to control her aggressive behavior. There are hospital and residential treatment programs that can help your child learn to cope with her symptoms in non-violent ways.

Other Strategies for Daily Care

Building Self-Esteem

One of the most important goals of parenting is building self-esteem—feelings of self-worth and self-acceptance—in all of our children. High self-esteem is a vital component of good mental health. To a large extent, it determines how willing people are to set high goals for themselves, as well as how hard they try to meet those goals. In fact, research shows that high self-esteem is more important to professional and personal success than high grades in school or a high I.Q.

Children with Tourette syndrome are often very intelligent, and are quite aware of their inappropriate behaviors, tics, and noises. They are also very much aware of other people's reactions to them. As a result, they may feel different, unaccepted, and left out, and their self-esteem may suffer. Because you don't want to add to these feelings of differentness, you should make sure that your daily care routine is aimed at building self-esteem and understanding.

Behavior Management and Self Esteem. How you manage your child's behavior on a daily basis can have a major impact on your child's self-esteem. You must, at all costs, avoid making your child feel as if there is something wrong with her for not being able to control tics and other symptoms associated with her TS. By using the proactive, positive behavior management techniques described earlier, you can avoid punishing your child for behaviors that are out of her control. And as long as you use techniques that help her succeed in following through on family rules, her opinion of her own abilities will rise. It also helps if you can let your child know that the purpose of discipline is not to punish her for unacceptable behavior but to help her learn to act appropriately and build self-control. In other words, be sure to convey the message that you want her to learn to make wise decisions about her behavior and you believe she is fully capable of doing so. This will help her understand that she is a loved and accepted part of the family, and will, in turn, boost her self-esteem.

Protection vs. Overprotection. It is natural for parents to want to protect their children with TS from negative reactions from people in the community and to rush to their defense when they are blamed for actions they cannot control. But sometimes it is better to let your child take care of herself rather than to intercede. Knowing where to draw the line between protection and over-protection is essential to building your child's self-esteem.

When your child is young, you will certainly want to protect her from harassment and inappropriate punishment for her symptoms. As she grows older, however, you must encourage your child to learn about TS, her own particular symptoms, and how to deal with other people. (See the section on "Handling Others' Reactions," below.) As she becomes able to communicate about her disorder to others, you must allow her to make her own way in the community. Otherwise, if you try to shield your child from all undesirable situations she might encounter, you risk sending her the message that she can't make it on her own in the real world.

Recognize When Your Child Needs Help. Educators and parents often remark that some children with TS use their TS as an excuse not to do something that they are capable of doing. But if TS really does interfere with a child's abilities, it can be damaging to her self-esteem to be accused of not trying. If your child is having trouble doing something, it may be worthwhile to look for alternate ways to allow her to succeed. For example, a boy in third grade claimed he couldn't take spelling tests because he had TS. The teacher got angry at the boy, and blamed the parents for being overprotective of their son. In reality, the boy had great difficulty writing due to tics and sensory-motor problems. When the boy was allowed to dictate the answers to someone else, he was able to take spelling tests. The point is that the boy was correct in his initial statement, but he was not able to elaborate all the intricate details of his problem. Obviously, it is far better to make minor adaptations that allow your child to succeed than to let her wallow in feelings of failure.

Let Your Child Make Choices. Children with TS are always being reminded of what they cannot control—their tics and behaviors. Allowing your child to make choices for herself is a good way to focus instead on the control she has over many aspects of her life. Daily choices such as what to wear, what movie to attend, and what to buy for a birthday party should be encouraged. Asking your child's opinion on many topics from how to fix a broken appliance to what she thinks about current events can also help strengthen her sense of competency and control.

Focus on Your Child's Talents and Abilities. All children with TS have unique talents and abilities. One may excel in art, while another may be a computer whiz. It is vital to your child's self-esteem that you give her frequent and positive feedback about her areas of special talent and ability. This helps offset the feelings of failure your child may have because of her symptoms and her inability to be like everybody else.

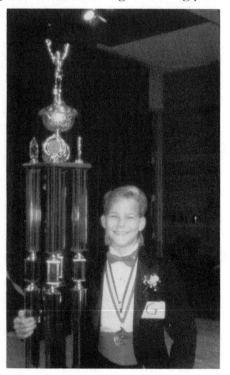

Mealtimes

Many children who have TS with ADHD or OCD have trouble behaving at mealtimes as their parents would like them to. One reason is that children are often left to their own devices while Mom or Dad is busy in the kitchen. This may be fine for most kids. But children with TS start losing control while they are waiting for dinner if their time is too unstructured. Furthermore, if a child has ADHD, she will have trouble sitting still at meals. And if she has obsessions about certain foods, planning meals can be challenging.There may be no way to eliminate mealtime madness altogether, but a few tricks can make mealtimes more pleasant.

One technique that can help make mealtimes more manageable is to give all your children specific mealtime chores such as setting out napkins, plates, and glasses. You can remind your children who is responsible for doing each chore by listing the chores on a chart. You might also let your children prepare easy meals and serve them. If your child with Tourette syndrome is focused on her responsibilities, she is more likely to be in control of her behavior.

To avoid arguments and confusion about who will sit where during meals, have your children draw names for seat assignments or assign them on a rotating basis. Let your children know how long the assignments will last. Have them make place cards. If your child has an obsession about where she must sit, accept that this is not harming anyone, and, if possible, work around her need.

Wherever your child with Tourette syndrome is seated, don't expect her to sit for very long if she has ADHD. Instead, establish basic rules of conduct during meals. For example, tell your children they may eat only when sitting down in their assigned place at the table, they must pass food instead of throwing it, and they must use utensils to eat. If your child feels she must move around during a meal, tell her specific things she can do, such as walking around the living room twice or standing by her chair, but don't allow her to eat unless she is sitting in her assigned spot.

Remember that the more structured and calmer the mealtime, the easier it will be for your child to stay in control. Some families find that if they defy the experts and watch TV during meals, their child has better control. This brings a little peace and sanity to their mealtimes. It does not, however, help the child learn to behave appropriately at meals served away from home. (For tips on eating out, refer to the section on "Restaurants" below.)

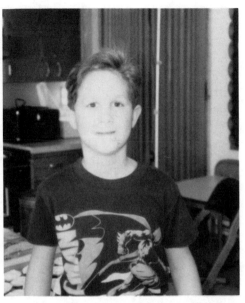

If your child with Tourette syndrome will only eat certain foods, you should work together to develop nutritious menus. Often, if you provide the foods that she feels she *must* eat at each meal, she may eat other foods as well. And she may eat foods that are closely related to foods that she refuses to eat. For example, your child may not eat yellow vegetables, but she may eat green vegetables. In addition, your child may eat a greater variety of foods if they are served on a specific plate that she likes. Limiting between meal snacks to fruits and vegetables may give your child the nutritional supplements that she isn't getting at mealtime. If you are unsure whether your child's nutritional needs are being met, enlist the help of a nutritionist.

In addition to having idiosyncratic food preferences, some children with Tourette syndrome may also have allergies or sensitivities to certain foods, additives, or dyes. Experts disagree as to whether and to what extent allergies actually affect symptoms of Tourette syndrome. But some experts think allergies sometimes make symptoms worse. For example, some children may have an increase in tics, increased hyperactivity, persistent runny nose, skin irritations, or a general feeling of restlessness. Many people with TS say that their tics get worse if they consume caffeine. Others claim their symptoms increase after eating foods with certain yellow or red dyes. Because of the waxing and waning of the disorder, it is often difficult to make determinations by observation alone. Professional allergy testing by a pediatric allergist may be helpful if you suspect that your child is reacting adversely to certain foods or airborne substances. If your child is hyperactive, don't assume that sugar is the culprit and automatically switch to diet products. Artificial sweeteners may cause more problems for some children with Tourette syndrome than sugar. In any case, if you are considering eliminating something from your child's diet, be sure to consult a nutritionist or your child's physician to see if a nutritional supplement is needed.

Finally, a word about special meals. Don't invite guests unless they are familiar with Tourette syndrome and associated behaviors. Adding another person to the table changes routine and adds stimulation. If guests are expected, let your child know ahead of time, review the family rules, discuss any changes in the normal meal routine, and remind her that she can go to another room if she feels she is losing control. Have holiday meals at noon, if possible. The longer everyone has to wait, the greater the anticipation and excitement. For a child with Tourette syndrome, that usually means more tics and other symptoms. If your child must wait, it may help to involve her in structured activities, such as making the table centerpiece, place cards, or window decorations. If your child is older, let her cut vegetables or prepare dessert.

Dressing and Clothes

Dressing can pose special problems for you and your child if she has ADHD or OC symptoms in addition to Tourette syndrome. Children who have TS with ADHD often have trouble organizing themselves enough to select their own clothes and get dressed in a limited amount of time. Those who have TS with OC may become obsessed with wearing a specific item of clothing or a specific color of clothes. One way to ease these problems is to help your child set out her clothes before bedtime. It is usually easier to resolve the issue of what to wear at night rather than during the morning rush. This gives you time to wash your child's favorite shirt or mend the only pair of shorts that she will wear.

Your child may also have trouble accepting new clothes if she has OC symptoms. If so, try laying the clothes out in her room for several days before you ask your child to put them on. Pre-wash the clothes so they feel softer and smell more familiar. Some kids are very sensitive to touch and need very soft fabrics. They are excellent recipients of "hand me down" clothes. Remember to cut out all tags, and don't be surprised if your child can't stand the feel of synthetic fabrics, synthetic thread, wool, or lace.

Some children with OCD have difficulty making seasonal transitions in clothing. For example, as the weather grows cooler, some kids persist in wearing summer clothes. One idea is to have them start the transition by wearing their summer clothes under warmer clothes. As they become accustomed to wearing the new seasonal clothes, they will usually discontinue wearing the summer clothes underneath. When my son started first grade, he wore his bathing suit and a shirt to school for two weeks before he was able to change to shorts and jeans. His teacher says she never even noticed. We often have so many issues to deal with every day, it is important to play down those that are less significant.

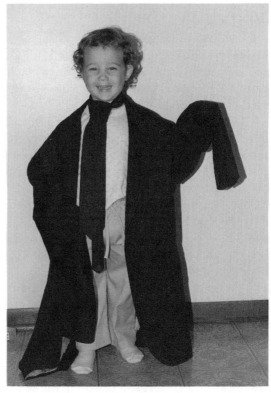

Sleep

Most parents wish their children would sleep from 8 p.m. to 8 a.m. each day and wake up refreshed, clear-headed, and happy. When your child has Tourette syndrome, the reality is that this is very unlikely. To begin with, medications used to control tics or other symptoms may cause sleep problems. Some drugs make kids sleepy and others keep them aroused. Sleepiness may occur during the day, and arousal at night. In addition, some children get more hyperactive as they become fatigued. And children with OCD may have trouble getting to sleep until everything feels just right and all rituals have been performed. For example, a child might need to prepare for bed by doing certain things in a specific order. Pillows may have to fluffed and re-fluffed and sheets and blankets may have to be loosened or tightened.

You can't make your child fall asleep, but you can determine what time she must be in bed, ready for sleep. Most kids with TS are very active and need a good night's rest, and so do you, the parents! Besides, keeping to a consistent bedtime helps satisfies your child's need for routine.

Often a bath or a back massage before bed will help your child to relax. Be sure to tell her what she can do in bed and what she can't. Playing a tape softly or looking at books are usually calming activities. You may want to purchase a vibrating pad, carried by most discount stores, and let your child rest on it. (The vibration provides tactile stimulation which is relaxing for many children.) Jumping on the bed and shooting Nerf balls are examples of activities that should not be allowed. If you can ensure that your child's bedroom is quiet and remove distractions that are too stimulating, it will be easier for her to settle down.

To help your child get used to a calming bedtime routine and to get ready for bed independently, use a chart or reward board until the routine is well established. List each thing that your child should do to prepare for bed, such as: take a bath, brush teeth, put on pajamas, select clothes for next day, read a story with Mom or Dad, listen to tapes, lights out. Give your child points that can be redeemed for rewards later when she completes each task on her chart. After your last hug and kiss, wish your child a good night and let her know that you'll be nearby, but it's now your private time.

If your child keeps leaving her room, redirect her back to her room and praise her when she settles down. Remember that many kids with Tourette syndrome and ADHD don't want to miss out on anything, and may challenge you for quite a while. If you let your child know the rules, routine, and possible consequences—such as an earlier bedtime the next night—it will be easier for her to follow through.

Sometimes sleep problems may be caused by emotional stress. If you suspect this is the case, encourage your child to share her concerns and frustrations. A caring hug may ease her tension.

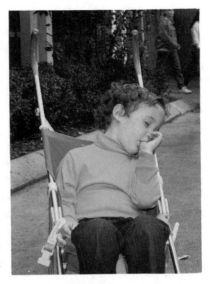

Finally, as mentioned above, sleep problems may be linked to your child's medication. An adjustment in dosage or time of ingestion may bring relief. Be sure to report significant sleep changes and difficulties to your child's physician, and don't make any adjustments in medication without his or her advice.

Organization

Many children with Tourette syndrome and ADHD have trouble organizing their belongings and their time. Besides making it difficult for them to make transitions or get dressed in the morning, this lack of organizational skills can affect everything from how tidy your child keeps her room to how well prepared she arrives at school.

To help your child get organized and keep organized at home, try using masking tape or pictures to label where things are supposed to go. For example, label dresser drawers "underwear," "T-shirts," and "socks," and label shelves in her room or play area "books," "crayons," and "paper." If your child is supposed to help with kitchen chores such as putting away dishes or groceries, you could also label those shelves and cabinets. If there are certain activities you'd like to restrict to certain places in your house, it may help to mark off play areas on the floor. For example, use tape to mark off an area where building blocks are permissible. These visible boundaries and visual cues will usually help your child understand where things belong.

How you communicate with your child can also affect her ability to get organized. When you are giving directions to your child, especially if she has ADHD, make them simple and specific. For example, instead of saying, "Put your clothes away," you could say, "Put your socks in your sock drawer." When that task is completed, praise your child, and then say, "Put your underwear in the underwear drawer," and so on. Many children like to take care of their belongings and help with family chores but are overwhelmed if the directions are too vague.

To help your child get organized for school, designate a specific place for her to assemble the things she needs to bring to school. You might make a checklist of items needed every day. Then make a note each day for additional things that your child must take. Whenever possible, have your child get her school things ready for the next day at night before she goes to bed. If she takes a lunch from home, make a menu for the week so the lunch can be ready to go without a fuss.

Aversion to Odors

Because TS is a sensory disorder, it sometimes affects the sense of smell. As a result, some children with Tourette syndrome are very sensitive to certain odors. Smells that may be agreeable or only mildly offensive to you may be intolerable to your child. Listen to your child's complaints and eliminate the odors if possible. There are now many fragrance-free products that can make your life easier. When it is necessary to use something with an odor offensive to your child, try to use it when she is out of the house. For example, clean your oven when your child is at school and open windows and use a fan to remove the smell more quickly. If you plan to paint, it may be a good time for your child to visit Grandma. If you wear perfume or aftershave lotion, and the smell bothers your child, wait to put it on until you have left the house. Some of these strategies may be a little inconvenient, but irritating your child's senses can increase stress and may cause an increase in symptoms. For example, one older child with TS told me that he gets a feeling of restlessness and general irritation when he is near someone wearing perfume.

Your Child in the Community

When you and your child are out in the community, you often confront problems that you don't need to deal with at home. Unlike at home, you cannot always set up the environment to make it easier for your child to control her symptoms. And particularly if your child has ADHD, the stimulation from unfamiliar people and places may send her into a frenzy. At times you and your child may feel as if everyone is staring at you—and you could be right.

Difficult as it can sometimes be to brave an outing into the community, it is important not to let Tourette syndrome take over the lives and activities of everyone in the family. Your child with TS needs to feel like an important, accepted part of the outside world, and so do your other children. All of your children need to learn how to get along as independently as possible in the community.

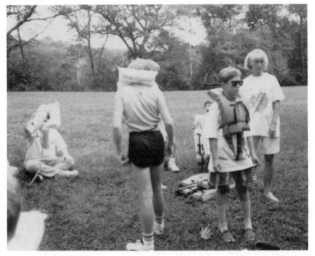

How your child adapts to life outside the home depends largely on you, the parent. If you appear to be at ease with your child in public, she is more likely to feel comfortable as well. By following your lead, she will learn to handle stares, comments, and potentially awkward situations. Friends and strangers will also take their cue from the respectful way you treat your child. Some strategies that may be useful in integrating your child into the community follow.

Educating Others

Many problems children with TS encounter in the community arise from others' ignorance about Tourette syndrome. Other children may tease or make fun of your child, while adults may scold her for misbehaving, because they don't realize she can't control her tics and other symptoms. Consequently, as your child's community gets larger, it becomes important to educate people about TS so they will understand your child's symptoms and behaviors.

Although the media has done much to increase public awareness about TS, it is up to you to educate the people who come in contact with your child. In the process of trying to answer other people's questions about TS, you will find yourself learning more about the disorder, your child's particular symptoms, and how best to deal with them.

Although you can wait for people to ask you questions, it is often preferable to educate others before your child gets into new situations. Again, this really depends on the severity of your child's symptoms and how they affect others in the community. Because my son's symptoms are so obvious, we usually hold inservice sessions for all of his school classmates, teachers, friends, neighbors, relatives, and teammates. Our son wants others to know about his disorder, so that he doesn't have to constantly answer questions about his tics and behaviors. On the other hand, some children don't want anyone to know about their TS. It is up to you to determine if it is in your child's best interests to tell people.

If you decide to "inservice" and educate, the national Tourette Syndrome Association has many prepared pamphlets and videos about TS that you can purchase. (See the Resource Guide for the address of the national TSA.) The Minnesota chapter of TSA has an educational video available that addresses the symptoms of TS as well as the associated behavioral aspects (ADHD, OCD, and developmental delays). If you ask, your local newspaper may run an article on TS. Your local radio and cable TV stations may help you produce a talk show on TS. Educating the public about such a complex disorder is not easy, but it is necessary to ensure more understanding and acceptance of Tourette syndrome.

Handling Others' Reactions

Many parents feel anxious about doing things in public with their child because they worry about how others will react to their child's TS symptoms. Although you cannot predict how strangers will respond, you can rehearse a variety of strategies that can help you and your child through awkward or potentially embarrassing situations.

In general, there are three ways to deal with strangers' questions and comments. 1.) You and your child can ignore the comment. 2) You can acknowledge the tic without explaining the cause ("I have a tic which makes me jerk my head; I don't do it on purpose"). 3) You can educate the person about Tourette syndrome ("I have Tourette syndrome and licking my lips is a tic I can't control").

Some people carry informational brochures about TS (available from the Tourette Syndrome Association) or hand out cards that they have had printed with a brief explanation of TS and a phone number to call to get more information. It may help to "role play" different scenarios with your child. Act out many possible remarks people could make about your child's tics, and let your child practice different positive responses rather than reacting in a negative or aggressive way. For example, if your child gets a very red, chapped face from a rubbing tic, you might mimic, "Hey kid, did you fall into a vat of tomato sauce?" First, your child could try ignoring your comment. She could then try offering a general, neutral explanation such as "My face is chapped." Finally, she could attempt to explain a little bit about Tourette syndrome: "I have Tourette syndrome. Rubbing my face is a tic. It makes my face chapped."

Sometimes children with TS unintentionally insult or upset a stranger with inappropriate touching, name calling, or other behaviors. In these instances, it is often best to tell that person that your child has Tourette syndrome and give a very brief explanation of the disorder. Although your child should not have to apologize for having an impairment, most people will expect an apology. You and your child should discuss this possibility and do what is comfortable for you.

Planning Ahead

There are some places you can go where your child's symptoms will be more noticeable and disruptive than others. For example, your child's tics may go unnoticed at a baseball game, but attract quite a bit of attention at a library. This does not mean that you should avoid all potentially troublesome settings, but that you should minimize stressful situations by a little advance planning. Some strategies for handling specific situations are outlined below.

Movies and Concerts. In any kind of quiet social gathering, it is usually best to prearrange a place that your child can go if her symptoms become disruptive. For example, at movies or concerts, your child can go to the lobby or into the restroom if she feels she is losing control. Taking seats on the aisle, toward the back, is usually a good idea.

Use your best judgement when deciding on concerts and movies. If your child has ADHD, she will be more likely to sit still if the movie holds her interest. Disruptive symptoms will probably not be noticed at a rock concert, but may cause problems at a symphony. Outdoor concerts are less stressful and less likely to exacerbate symptoms.

Rather than chance an embarrassing situation, some people with disruptive tics prefer to watch video tapes or listen to music at home with a few friends. Although you and your family understand coprolalia, most people do not, and a movie theater or concert hall is not always a good place to start educating them.

Restaurants. Eating out can be especially stressful if your child gets overstimulated or is hyperactive. You may be able to prevent some potential problems if you reduce waiting time by ordering ahead, picking a buffet or fast food restaurant, or selecting a restaurant with a video arcade or other form of kids' entertainment. It may also help if you bring crayons and paper or a puzzle book to use during the wait for service. Seat your child next to and across from people who will help her stay in control, rather than near a child who may overstimulate her. Be sure to review the rules of eating out before you go and when you arrive at the restaurant. Again, many children with TS need to know very clearly what they can and cannot do in a given situation.

If your child starts to lose control, take her outside or into a quiet area for a few minutes, so she can settle down. If all else fails, be prepared to leave. On the rare occasions when our family goes to a restaurant that may be difficult for our son, my husband and I usually drive in separate cars. If our son has to leave, he goes with one parent while the other remains at the restaurant with our daughter. Although it is hard not to blame your child for this inconvenience, you have to remember that overstimulation makes the symptoms worse, your child is not deliberately trying to drive you crazy, and she usually feels worse than anyone else. Your child needs encouragement, not reproach.

Shopping. Tics and vocalizations often get worse at a shopping mall. Children with ADHD quickly become overstimulated, and children with OCD always find some obsession to cause them to run ahead, bounce around the floor tiles, or hide in the clothes carousels. To minimize these problems, take your child shopping only when necessary and only when the stores are the least crowded. Be sure to call ahead to see if the desired items are in stock. If you haven't already, you might also want to look into catalog shopping.

If your child "needs" everything in sight, this can pose problems in grocery stores, drug stores, self-service shoe stores, and other types of establishments with a vast array of products to choose from. These types of stores are also overstimulating for many kids with Tourette syndrome and ADHD. For many of them, the aisles alone hold great attraction as race tracks. To reduce problems, tell your child ahead of time where you will shop and exactly what you intend to purchase. If your child will be picking out something to buy, try to decide on the exact item or reduce the possibilities to only a few before you leave home. Save your browsing for a shopping trip by yourself. When shoe shopping, try to find a store where shoes are kept in the back room and your child must sit in a chair to be waited on. Be sure to praise your child for what she does well, such as staying with you or calmly selecting her shoes, and tell her how much you enjoyed the shopping trip with her.

Libraries. You may feel especially reluctant to enter a library with your child. But all the public librarians with whom I've spoken insist that everyone is welcome in a library. They encourage anyone with any disability to use the facilities. Furthermore, they point out that public libraries are not really as quiet as many people think because kids are often using computers and doing group projects. Still, if you or your child feel you are too conspicuous, librarians are usually willing to make accommodations. For example, they might allow your child to use a conference room if she feels she is bothering other people. You might also plan to visit the library during the hours when it is less crowded.

Changes in the Teen Years

The teen years for any child bring many changes to the family. When you have a child with Tourette syndrome, these changes can be especially dramatic. Depending upon the course of your child's symptoms, daily life for your family may become either more or less difficult.

In some children with Tourette syndrome, ADHD symptoms begin to decrease during adolescence. Children may become less hyperactive, and their ability to focus and stay on task improves. Many teenagers develop a much better capacity to understand Tourette syndrome and can become advocates for their own needs. These kids can also become positive role models for younger children with Tourette syndrome.

Other children, unfortunately, have increased symptoms in the teen years. It is important to understand that these changes can make your child feel different and lonely. Listen to your child and

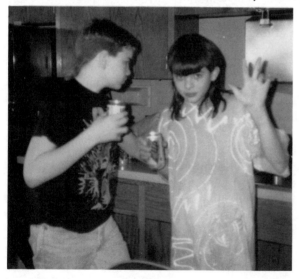

encourage her to talk about her feelings. If you can find a support group for teens with Tourette syndrome, your child may find it very helpful. You might contact your local chapter of the TSA to see if such a group exists in your area, or they may help you set one up.

Because of changes in body hormones, your child's medications may need to be adjusted or changed. Medication checks should be scheduled at regular intervals with your child's physician. Be sure to tell your physician about changes in your child's emotions, sleep patterns, attitude toward school, family, and peers, in addition to reporting tics and other symptoms. Any of these can indicate that a change in medication is needed. School refusal and depression are not uncommon in teens with TS and should be treated by a professional. Sometimes a medication change or psychological or psychiatric counseling is needed. Chapter 3 provides more information on medications used to treat TS.

During the teen years, you should also alert your child to the hazards of recreational drugs. Because Tourette syndrome is a disorder involving brain chemicals, some street drugs can be more dangerous for people with Tourette syndrome. Since there are still so many unknowns about how drugs affect the brain, tell your child to say "no" to all street drugs. Remember, too, that substances such as caffeine and alcohol can also have undesirable effects on your child's symptoms, and their use should be discussed with your child's physician.

If your child has coprolalia or symptoms that could be misconstrued as intoxication, make sure she carries cards that give a brief explanation of Tourette syndrome and the phone number of your child's physician, the local Tourette syndrome organization, or the national Tourette Syndrome Association. You can also purchase a medic alert bracelet and have information about your child's disorder engraved on the tag. These cards and tags can come in handy if your child is ever stopped by a law enforcement official and has symptoms such as uncontrolled swearing, walking in unusual step patterns, punching, kicking, spinning around in circles, or falling to the ground.

You can ease some of the changes in the early teen years if you prepare your child for her progression from elementary to secondary school. Have her help you educate her new teachers about Tourette syndrome and her particular symptoms. If your child has organizational difficulties, this would be a good time to ask the school to provide an extra set of textbooks to be left at home. Work with your child to set up a good time for homework. Some kids with Tourette syndrome need free time before homework to relax, let out tics, or run off energy. Others, particularly those with OCD, may feel a need to do homework right away. If you see that your child is overwhelmed with homework, work with her and the school to plan reasonable expectations. Chapter 7 provides more detail about how to make adjustments in your child's school program to accommodate her special needs.

One final issue that is extremely important to teenagers is friendships and dating. As your child's interest in the opposite sex increases, she may find that the interest isn't always returned. Many teenagers simply do not want to associate with anyone who seems different. Educating peers about Tourette syndrome may help, but for many, the need to conform outweighs compassion and sensibility. Reassure your child that as she gets older, she will meet many people of both sexes who are more understanding and accepting of people with disabilities. Acknowledge what Adam Seligman, a young man with Tourette syndrome, observed in an article written shortly after his graduation: "High school is not a place noted for the maturity of its inhabitants." In the meantime, encourage your child to pursue activities that interest her in school and in the community. People who share similar interests and talents may be more able to see beyond the symptoms of Tourette syndrome. Lastly, be prepared to accept friends that may seem "weird" to you at first. Kids who don't quite "fit in" often find each other, and very special friendships can develop.

Taking a Break from Child Care

When you have a child with Tourette syndrome, spending quality time alone with your spouse or friends is very important. Parents have a tendency to get so involved in the welfare of their children, they forget about nurturing themselves. B.C. (before children), most parents had many interests and hobbies. Take time to pursue those activities and share your talents with others. Eat properly, get enough sleep and exercise, keep yourself healthy, and try to find something to laugh about every day. Keep your own stress level down. Treat yourself to a massage, a concert, or a movie. Don't feel guilty about taking time for yourself. You deserve it!

Finding competent sitters who are comfortable with your child can be a challenge, but don't give up. Although you may have difficulty finding a teenaged babysitter in the neighborhood who is skilled enough to deal with your child's special needs, there are many other avenues. Students in special education, occupational therapy, or nursing programs at nearby colleges, as well as vocational school students, often make excellent sitters. Your local branch of ARC may also be able to recommend competent sitters with experience caring for children with disabilities. And don't overlook other parents of children with Tourette syndrome as a source of names.

Some families of children with Tourette syndrome need more than an occasional evening away from their child. These families can often benefit from *respite care.* Respite care gives parents a respite, or break, from caring for their child. In the most common form of respite care, your child goes to the home of a qualified caregiver on a regular basis, usually for a weekend, but sometimes for longer or shorter times. You may also be able to request respite care on an emergency basis, with little or no advance notice. Don't be surprised if your child behaves differently at the respite home. A change in environment can reduce behavioral difficulties on a short-term basis or increase them.

"In home" respite care is another option. If you qualify, a trained person comes into your home on a pre-set schedule to relieve you or to help you with child care.

To find out about respite care in your area, contact your county social service agency or local TSA chapter. Eligibility criteria vary, but in many counties you must qualify by showing a need for the service. Fees are usually on a sliding scale and based on family income. Some private social service agencies, such as those run by churches, may also have respite care programs.

Don't be afraid to ask for help. The daily stress of living with a child with Tourette syndrome can sometimes be overwhelming, even for the best of parents. In addition to "out of home respite care" arranged through our county, I get help from a wonderful woman who answered an ad that I ran in our local newspaper. She comes to our home four mornings per week before school and has restored order and sanity to my life. You, too, may find that an experienced helper can make your daily life more enjoyable.

Conclusion

A newspaper reporter recently came to our house to write a story about our son. She had heard about his TS, ADHD, OCD, developmental delays, and sensory motor problems. I don't know what she expected to see, but she said she was pleasantly surprised to meet a boy who is bright, creative, full of zest for life, and blessed with a great sense of humor. It was a wonderful reminder that our children with Tourette syndrome are kids like all other kids, with special gifts and talents, who must be nurtured and loved and given all the opportunities that life has to offer.

It is true that you must make special accommodations for your child with TS, and daily life may seem more complex. But by trying the strategies presented in this chapter as well as others that you discover, daily life certainly can be manageable, not to mention enjoyable. Take pride in yourself and your parenting skills. You're doing great if you can even find the time to read this book.

Parent Statements

There doesn't seem to be much information out there which definitely spells out what doesn't work, why it doesn't work, and what does work.

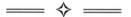

It takes so much involvement to stay on top of planning things for my son that I'm often "drained" in my free time.

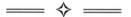

Most recreational activities that people like are unstructured and loud. For my son, these things are extremely challenging. Ball games, family birthdays, state fairs are all a challenge. He is at such a high emotional state and seems to be at odds with his body. People talk to him and he answers with an unrelated comment or says nothing.

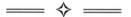

At a ball game, I take him for a walk or to get refreshments a lot. He counts all the bathroom stalls and blow dryers in the men's and women's restrooms and compares the number of each.

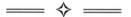

Punishment and time-out don't work for Robby. He doesn't understand them, because he didn't get out of control on purpose. It's as if his computer is overloaded with stimuli. If *we* allow the computer to become overloaded, we know what will happen. Pro-active behavior management techniques are so much more successful.

═══ ✧ ═══

Once when he was thrashing around on the kitchen floor, I held him—so he thrashed me around with him! But I told him I was there and wouldn't leave him, and that I loved him and he was a good little boy. That was what he needed then, and I had to stay with him for nearly an hour. It made me more determined than ever not to ever let him down, but to support and reassure him and "be there."

═══ ✧ ═══

The hyperactivity and compulsive behaviors are draining. But it helps when you understand why your kid is acting that way.

═══ ✧ ═══

Michelle's self-esteem greatly improved at TS Camp. She was impressed with the cool teenagers with TS. The acceptance she received there gave her quite a boost.

═══ ✧ ═══

The baby books can really throw you off. So can books on such things as the strong-willed child or on how to discipline. Usually these books do not acknowledge that other things such as neurological problems may be influencing behavior.

═══ ✧ ═══

There's no getting around the extra amount of energy needed to parent a child with TS, especially if he has complications such as LD or OCD.

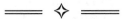

He's got the impulsiveness, the obsessive thinking, the anger from having been treated unkindly. I worry about how he will end up. I

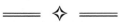

hope my best efforts will be enough to make things come out all right in the end.

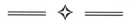

Every once in a while I feel like I should give him a damn good spanking and everything will be OK. But it doesn't work that way. We have to accept that we have a child with a handicap, and we have to work with that.

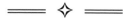

A lot of people don't understand. When we're in a restaurant or store and he gets hyper or throws temper tantrums, they really give us the looks.

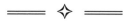

Because she doesn't have the inhibiting factors that most people have, other kids can and will manipulate her, and she'll be the one to get in trouble.

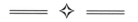

The single most important thing you can do for your child with TS is to build up his self-esteem

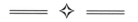

Remember the ABCs of Tourette syndrome. A: *Accept* the fact that your child has TS. *Accept* the tics and noises, the impulsivity, the immaturity. Your child may have little control over his symptoms, but you can have control over your reactions to them. B: *Build* your child's self-esteem. C: *Choose* your fights. Ignore the ignorable. Figure out ways to cope or get around the really disruptive tics and behaviors. Concentrate on those which are a danger to your child or others and ignore the rest.

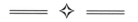

Tourette syndrome is an explanation for unacceptable behavior, not an excuse. Kids with TS have to have consequences for their

behavior, but the consequences must be appropriate to the amount of control the child is able to exert over his symptoms and behavior.

═══ ✧ ═══

My son doesn't like to talk about TS. He doesn't think he'd have any friends if they knew.

═══ ✧ ═══

Remember the 5 R's of Tourette syndrome. 1) Reduce stress—provide structure, no surprises, no timed tests. 2) Realistic expectations—when tics are at their worst, don't expect behavior or school performance to be on the same level as when tics are mild. 3) Reinforce good behavior—there's no such thing as too much praise or affirmation. 4) Redirect unacceptable behavior. 5) Remove your child from the scene—as a last resort, but without anger or blame.

═══ ✧ ═══

Punishment makes the person who punishes feel better. Discipline helps the person who committed a mistake realize what he did wrong and learn from his mistakes. Discipline involves teaching. Punishment is easier, but it usually doesn't do any good.

═══ ✧ ═══

In order to think proactively, you have to put away conformity and use common sense and creativity. Parenting then becomes more exciting and rewarding.

═══ ✧ ═══

Show your child by your own "self-praise" that it's OK to say to others that you did a good job. It's even OK to say that you're totally awesome!

═══ ✧ ═══

FIVE

✧

Children with Tourette Syndrome and Their Families

CARL R. HANSEN, JR., M.D.*

Parents often have no idea what they're getting themselves into when they decide to start a family. They may be caught off guard by the many responsibilities that parenting brings, as well as by changes in their routines and priorities. But although raising a family may be challenging at times, most parents feel that the rewards far outweigh the demands. In fact, most parents find that providing a safe and harmonious family life for their children is one of the most rewarding experiences of life.

Family life for parents of children with Tourette syndrome is not always more challenging than it is for other parents. Especially if your child has very mild symptoms of TS, you and your family may not run into any special problems. But for many parents, having a child with TS complicates the already complex job of raising a healthy, happy family. Stresses and strains within the family are different, if not greater, than they are for other families. Relationships can become strained, for example, if tics such as spitting or obscene gestures are directed at other family members, or if family members continually have to explain TS symptoms to people outside the family. And both parents and children may need to develop

---

* Dr. Carl R. Hansen is a child, adolescent, and adult psychiatrist at the Hansen McLeod Neuropsychiatric Clinic in Golden Valley, Minnesota.

special coping strategies in order to live peaceably and productively with one another.

How well your family adjusts to having a child with Tourette syndrome depends primarily on you, the parent. Children, other family members, and friends will all follow your example. Indeed, how you treat all of your children will send them important messages about their own place in the family and in society.

Because the parent's role in family life is so crucial, this chapter begins with a discussion of some common problems that can make it harder for you to give your family the guidance it needs. It then reviews problems that other members of the family may encounter, and suggests ways you can help family life run more smoothly.

Feeling Good about Yourself As a Parent

Having a child with TS does not change your ability to be a good parent, but it may change how you look at your ability. Because of the many ways TS and associated difficulties such as ADHD and OCD affect your child and your relationship with him, your self-confidence may plummet—even if you have successfully raised other children. You may, for example, feel as if it is your fault that your child's social skills lag behind other children's. You may blame yourself if your child cannot follow rules when playing a game with other children his age, or if other children in the neighborhood do not want to play with him. Then, too, repeated frustration at not being able to get your child to "behave" can make you feel like a failure. Even though *you* understand that your child's tics and other behaviors are out of his control, you may blame yourself in front of friends, family members, or teachers.

If feelings of failure persist too long, parents sometimes take it out on their child through inappropriate discipline. Or they may turn away from their child, immersing themselves in their work, outside activities, or even alcohol or drugs to escape the pain. At a minimum, they are likely to feel depressed and wonder why they should keep trying so hard.

Obviously, learning to cope effectively with the special challenges that confront your family is crucial. For this reason, the next section offers suggestions to help you recognize and begin to work around some problem areas you may encounter.

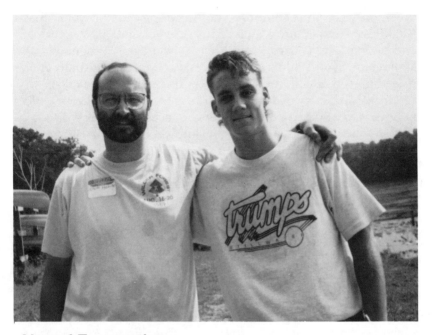

Altered Expectations

Parents tend to judge their success as parents by the success of their children. But when your child has Tourette syndrome, his accomplishments may seem to lag behind other children's. In the neighborhood, tics and associated conditions may lead to problems making friends and to delayed social development. In the classroom, tics, learning disabilities, or attention problems may make it harder for your child to make progress in some academic subjects. Your child stands out—but not for the reasons you would have hoped.

All parents must learn to reconcile reality with fantasy—to see that in place of the idealized, perfect child they dreamed of, they have a flesh-and-blood child with his own unique set of strengths and weaknesses. For parents of children with TS, it is especially important to acknowledge your disappointment and frustration. You cannot accept your child's weaknesses and vulnerabilities unless you work through your feelings about them and acknowledge that the problems are part of your child's underlying condition. Denial of your feelings makes it harder to move ahead and cope with these problems. At the same time, you do not want to dwell too much on what your child *can't* do. Focusing only on your child's weaknesses and failures can lead to overwhelming disappointment and hopelessness. It can also prevent you from recognizing and appreciating your child's many successes—and there usually are far more things that children with TS *can* do than they *can't* do.

Indeed, the key to dealing with your feelings about your child's failures is to work with him to achieve success. Chapter 4 discusses why success is so important to your child's self-esteem. But helping your child achieve and celebrate successes can also give your self-esteem a boost. Consequently, when you help to reduce the stress that increases your child's symptoms, or steer him toward activities in which he is more likely to succeed, you are helping yourself while you help your child. For example, your child may find the beginning of school especially stressful. But if you anticipate the problems your child typically has on the first day of school, you can take steps to minimize them—perhaps by taking your child to visit his classroom and teacher to aquaint him with the new surroundings before school starts. Likewise, if your child wants to be in athletics but has a hard time taking turns, you might guide him toward individual sports such as swimming or running. The less frustration and failure your child experiences, the more successful everyone in the family will feel.

Most parents do not have to make a conscious choice about many decisions that will enourage their children to succeed. These values are passed from one generation to the next. But when you have a child with special needs, you have to make many conscious choices about many details of daily life. Having to plan out so many details in advance can complicate your life in the short run, but in the long run, choosing to work with your child to help him succeed is one that you are not likely to regret. Consult Chapter 4 for specific strategies for building success into the daily life of your child.

Concerns about Appearances

To outsiders, children with TS often look as if they are "misbehaving." For example, children with TS may have tics that cause them to spit or to make faces at others. Or if they have OCD or impulsiveness associated with ADHD, they may be unable to control the urge to touch things in a store. Although you may understand that your child cannot control his behavior, you may still

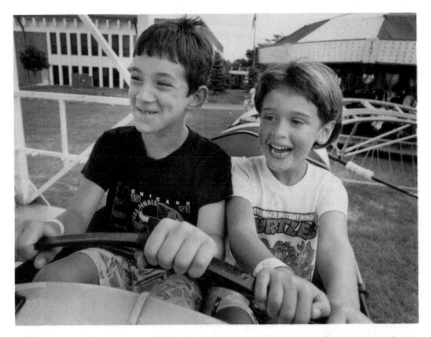

feel inept as a parent when you see other children doing exactly as their parents say. Unsolicited comments and advice from others about what you are doing "wrong" can further undermine your confidence in your abilities as a parent.

As Chapter 4 discusses, there are many strategies you can try to help your child behave appropriately. But there also may be many behaviors your child simply cannot control. Once you are confident that you are managing your child's behavior properly, it may be necessary to stand against criticism in the confident knowledge that you are doing what is best for your family. Your family just may have to look different than the average family on the block. For example, you know that asking your child to suppress tics is asking for trouble. Even if he is able to hold his tics in for a time, the effort of doing so can dangerously increase stress and make it harder for him to concentrate on what is going on around him. OCD behaviors, too, often cannot be controlled. Consequently, your family may need to ignore swearing that other families would punish, or ignore compulsive behaviors such as poking others, stomping, or opening and closing doors. Or you may need to do things in a way that looks a little odd to others. For example, if your child constantly pokes his sister when riding in the car, it may work better for a parent to sit in back with him.

This is an area where your child's well-being must take precedence over your own concerns about appearances. In the end, what matters is not what onlookers think about your abilities as a parent, but the knowledge that you are doing what is right for your child.

Looking after Your Own Needs

Because of your child's TS, you may need to devote more time and energy to caring for him than you would have otherwise. For example, if your child has trouble making friends, you may spend a great deal of time arranging play opportunities or playing with him yourself. Or if there is a danger that your child may harm himself or others because of symptoms of impulsiveness or aggressiveness, you may need to supervise him very closely. If tics or other symptoms interfere with his ability to learn, you may also have to make numerous trips to his school to help plan his educational program. And if your child has separation anxiety or cannot tolerate any change in routine, you may be a virtual hostage to his needs; even leaving him with a babysitter for just a few hours may seem out of the question.

Demands like these have a way of sidetracking parents' goals for themselves. You may, for example, find yourself weighing career advancement and opportunities against your child's needs. You may even change or lose jobs because you feel you must be free to respond to crises at home or at school whenever they occur. You might also have to put plans for further education on hold, or say good-bye to any kind of a social life.

Although there are many reasons why you might find your role limited to being the parent of a child with TS, this is not a healthy situation. If you feel as if your child is consuming all your time and energy, you may turn your anger, resentment, and frustration on your child—or on your spouse, if you feel he or she is not doing his or her share of the childcare. Frustration at your child can get in the way of acceptance; frustration at other family members can lead to disharmony in the family and make it harder for everyone to support one another and work together as a team.

A social worker may be able to help you work out a compromise between your child's needs for care and supervision and your own needs for fulfillment. You should be able to locate a social worker through your county Human Services department, or through the special education program at school. Finding a respite care provider can also give you some breathing room. As Chapter 4 explains, respite care is skilled childcare provided by a worker trained in looking after children with special needs, and may be available for a day, weekend, or longer, if needed. Most importantly, you and your spouse need to work together to make sure that each of you has some time to devote to your own needs for growth and independence. Often one partner in a marriage winds up shouldering the majority of childcare responsibilities—either because he or she does not work outside the house, or because his or her job has more flexibility, making it easier to look after the children's needs. In general, there is nothing wrong with this arrangement, unless the spouse with primary childcare responsibilities always gets stuck looking after the children, even when the other spouse is around to help. For example, if a wife quits her job to take care of her child with TS, but her husband keeps his job and continues moving up the career ladder, it is essential that the couple work out some way for the wife, too, to have a life outside the family. The husband might offer to stay home with the children in the evenings while his wife takes classes or joins a bowling league, or he might take over childcare responsibilities on the weekend so she can work on a novel. These are issues that you and your spouse must discuss openly and often, whenever one or both of you feels overwhelmed by the demands of raising a child with Tourette syndrome.

Being the parent of a child with Tourette syndrome takes more adaptation than usual. And the changes you will need to make likely won't come without anxiety and frustration. Accepting that your family life will be different than the Cleavers' is the first step in successful family management. If you don't change how you look at and work with your child, you will only meet greater frustration and failure. You may find it helps to remind yourself that you are doing things differently to increase your child's—and your own—success. And you will definitely discover that love for your child can help you weather seemingly unbearable difficulties and crises.

Parents with Tourette Syndrome

Parents who have TS themselves may encounter special problems in coping with the challenges of child care. When their child first begins showing symptoms of TS, they may feel as if they are reliving their own childhood. Especially if they were misunderstood as a child, painful memories they have long suppressed may be awakened. They may remember instances of emotional or physical abuse at the hands of teachers, parents, or other children, or times when they were laughed at or shunned. Some parents may have nightmares or flashbacks or become less able to cope with their own symptoms. They may also feel guilty or sad about passing TS on to their child. These feelings may make it harder for parents to see their child's situation objectively or as distinct from their own life.

Your children's attitudes toward your Tourette syndrome can also affect your relationship with them. Just as parents wish for perfect children, children wish for perfect parents. They often idealize their parents, even in the face of extreme problems or illness. If you have TS, your children may deny the presence of the disorder or prevent their friends from meeting you to keep alive the fantasy-perfect parent they have described to others.

Often, frank and complete discussion of concerns with a mental health professional or members of TSA support groups can help allay anxiety and other painful emotions. Medications may also be helpful. Parents who have symptoms of severe depression—suicidal thinking, changes in appetite or sleep, loss of energy—should consult a psychiatrist. Coping may not be easy, but most parents with TS are eventually able to come to terms with their feelings and get on with their lives.

It is worth remembering that adults with TS often have a special talent as parents of children with TS. They have a special empathy and understanding of what it is like to have TS, and can offer their child tried and true methods of coping with TS symptoms. They often feel driven to see that their child does not have to go through the same negative experiences they faced as a child, and can become dedicated advocates for their child at school and elsewhere. Most importantly, they can serve as a positive role model for their child, demonstrating through their actions and attitudes that children with TS can grow up to be successful members of their community.

Family Life

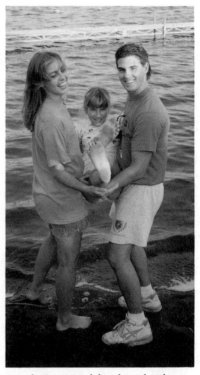

Although TS may sometimes dominate your time and attention, it should never be allowed to become the focus of your family life. If everyone is to feel like equal and contributing members of the family, they must be treated that way. Everyone deserves to have their needs and problems taken seriously *and* to have their talents and strengths nurtured. And everyone should share equally in family obligations and chores. Otherwise, their self-esteem will suffer and they may have trouble developing to their full potential.

For the sake of all members of the family, it is important to strive for as normal a family life as possible. Of course, you do not want to push your child with TS into situations that he finds particularly stressful. But you also do not want to keep your family cooped up in the house, thereby sending the message that there is something "wrong" with them. As a family, you need to go out to eat, to shop, to see a movie, to attend a concert, to visit an amusement park, to fly a kite in the park—to do all the normal activities that other families do. These normal activities help all family members develop social skills and expand their world. They also provide the good times that help everyone weather conflicts and crises when they arise.

How much your child's TS contributes to conflicts and crises within your family will depend to some extent on the severity of the tics and other problems. When tics are very mild, they may have little or no impact on family relationships. But symptoms such as loud vocal tics, compulsions to touch others, or impulsive behavior can definitely affect the way family members interact. The empathy and compassion that members of your family have for one another can also make a tremendous difference in how everyone gets along. Because you, the parent, can have a profound effect on family relationships, the next section discusses how you can help keep friction to a minimum and foster the atmosphere of understanding and acceptance that everyone needs to grow.

Siblings

Brothers and sisters can grow up to be the best of friends or mortal enemies—or anything in between. Exactly what kind of relationship develops depends on many factors: common interests, differences in age, personalities, parental guidance. In other words, your child's TS alone is probably not going to make or break his relationships with his brothers or sisters. It may, however, present special challenges for your children to deal with in getting along with one another. Some of the most common problems are discussed below.

Embarrassment. Children often want others to believe that their family is perfect or at least just like any other family. But when a sibling has tics or other unusual behaviors it is impossible for a child to hide the fact that his family is different. Siblings may discourage their friends from coming over to the house for fear that their brother or sister with TS will embarrass them. They may also refuse to join in family activities if their brother or sister's behavior often attracts unwanted attention. Embarrassment frequently becomes a major issue during early adolescence when children feel an acute need to conform and fit in. During these years, they are very self-conscious about *any* difference, including braces or eye glasses, so having a sibling with TS can make them feel as if they really stand out.

There is probably no way to keep siblings from feeling embarrassed, but you can help them to cope with their feelings of embarrassment. First of all, you need to teach your children that all people are different, and if someone makes fun of them or their sibling, it is not their problem, but the problem of the person who is doing the ridiculing or harassing. Second, help your children understand that it is their sibling's TS symptoms that are embarrassing them, not their sibling himself. He is not deliberately behaving this way to draw attention to your family, and in fact, would give anything to be able to stop. It is also important to help your children realize that embarassment is perfectly natural, but also survivable. You can do this by being honest about your feelings and creating an atmosphere of open communication. For example, after an awkward incident, you might say, "Boy, was that embarrassing. Did you see that man's face when Bob poked him?" Encourage everyone, including your child with TS, to share their feelings, and to see the humor, if any, in the situation. Finally, encourage your children to educate their friends about TS. If friends accept your child with TS and understand that he does not do these things on purpose, siblings are less likely to be embarrassed when your child discharges tics in front of their friends.

Fighting and Aggression. Because of your child's tics and other behaviors, sibling relationships may sometimes be strained to the breaking point. Away from home, your other children may witness "inappropriate" behavior from your child with TS and may feel real or imagined pressure to make their sibling straighten up. Of course, since the tics are involuntary, your child *can't* shape up. But especially if your child persists in coprolalia or violent or aggressive talk, increasing frustration may lead his siblings to try to beat him out of his tics. Likewise, if your child has a tic that causes him to poke, kick, pinch, or slap his siblings, tension is guaranteed to mount and may lead to fighting. The daily tension can lead to longstanding resentments and scapegoating. Whenever something goes wrong, siblings may blame your child with TS, even if it has nothing to do with his TS. For instance, a sibling may blame the child with TS for not being invited to a birthday party, when he may just have been overlooked. In addition, some children have long memories and bear grudges over their sibling's inappropriate behavior. Eventually, they may take steps to "pay back the wrong" they think was done to them by fighting with or picking on their sibling with TS.

To help your other children handle the urge to fight with their sibling with TS, it helps once again to let them know that you understand their feelings. Let them know that you, too, think it is unfair that they have to deal with strange behaviors on a daily basis, and that it is understandable that they would sometimes lose their temper. Talking about problems as they occur can help to diffuse rising anger. For example, if your child's tics are disrupting family TV time, talk openly about the problem and try to work out a solution. And giving your other children plenty of individual time and attention when they are *not* fighting makes it less likely that they will become angry because their sibling seems to get all the attention. A sibling might also benefit from talking to a counselor about how he feels about living with a brother or sister with TS.

Children with TS can be on the giving as well as on the receiving end of fighting. If a child with TS has difficulty controlling anger, he may be more apt to take out aggressive impulses on siblings. He may push siblings around or lose his temper easily. Although your child may not be able to control these impulses, his Tourette syndrome should not be considered an excuse to victimize family members. If family members must continually fend off impulsive or aggressive behavior of a child with TS, their psychological well-being can suffer.

Whenever necessary, you must take swift and protective action to prevent siblings from being injured. When your child with TS is younger, you should step in and divert him to some other activity, such as running or bike riding. As your child grows older, help him learn to recognize signs that he is losing control and take action to extricate himself from the situation. As Chapter 4 discusses in more detail, you can plan safe activities that give him the opportunity to release his emotions. If aggression is a significant problem, you may need to work with a psychologist who is knowledgeable about the neurological nature of TS and associated behavioral difficulties.

Disruptive Symptoms. As earlier chapters discuss, it is important to ignore your child's tics and other symptoms as much as possible in order to keep stress to a minimum. But sometimes this can be easier said than done. Your child's tics will change over time and some may be difficult to ignore. He may make loud noises while siblings are trying to watch TV, he may kick furniture, or he may have to have all the cupboard doors open all the time. In addition, some symptoms may seem to be directed at a particular member of the family. For example, he may spit at his sister or poke her shoulder. Teaching your other children to simply leave the room if they cannot ignore a symptom may work in some, but not all cases.

Many children with Tourette syndrome have delays in social skills or sensory integration problems that make it difficult for them to observe boundaries. Consequently, they may follow their siblings around the house or into their rooms.

Your child has a right to have his tics, but your other children also have a right to concentrate on their homework, a game of chess, or a favorite book without being constantly distracted. When tics and other TS behaviors are too overwhelming to ignore, siblings must have a place where they can get away from it all (and lock the door, if necessary). Everyone needs privacy occasionally. You must also teach your child with TS to respect his siblings' needs to occasionally be alone. Keep explaining why he must leave them alone and keep enforcing boundaries as often as it takes. During periods when tics are especially severe, you may want to arrange for respite care for your child with TS or time away for his siblings to give everyone a break.

Handling Siblings' Needs

Your other children need to be treated as children in their own right—not just as siblings of your child with Tourette syndrome. Unless they are appreciated for who they are, their confidence in themselves and their abilities will suffer and they may have difficulty reaching their potential. True, their needs may not seem quite so dramatic as those of their sibling with TS, but they still deserve your serious attention.

Because having a child with TS can reduce the amount of time you have to devote to your other children, being able to recognize siblings' needs as they arise is especially important. Many of these needs will be no different than other children's, but others will be directly related to having a brother or sister with Tourette syndrome. For the sake of your children's emotional well-being, none of them should be neglected.

Information. In order to cope effectively with the challenges of living with a sibling with Tourette syndrome, your children will need regular doses of information about TS. Information can be the best antidote to fears and frustrations. It also gives siblings the background they need to deal with questions from classmates and friends. Furthermore, understanding how and why their sibling with TS behaves as he does can help brothers and sisters respond more appropriately. For example, if they understand that their sibling cannot control his coprolalia or aggression, they may be able to ignore this behavior instead of starting a fight.

Your children's information needs and abilities to absorb information will change as they grow older. Depending on the severity of their sibling's symptoms, preschool children may not even notice that their sibling is different. If they do notice symptoms, they may

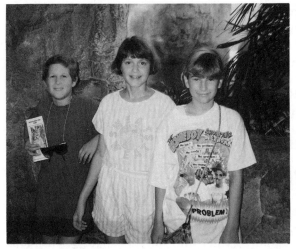

wonder if TS is a disease that their sibling will die from, or if they can "catch" TS by drinking out of the same cup. At this stage, what they need most is calm reassurances and the chance to see that their sibling is more like them than different.

As children reach school age, they become ready and able to understand a great deal about TS. They can be told that Tourette syndrome is caused by a problem in the nervous system, that their sibling does not do these tics on purpose, and that they should ignore symptoms as much as possible. They can also benefit from watching children's videos from the national TSA. "Stop It, I Can't" is a good one for this age group.

In the teenage years, siblings may become preoccupied with the genetics of Tourette syndrome. They may wonder if they carry the TS gene, and what the chances are that they will have a child with TS. They may benefit from reading literature from the TSA on genetics, teen issues, or any other aspect of TS. The TSA also has a variety of videos targeted at teenagers and adults.

Communication. Even when children understand in theory what TS is and how it affects their sibling, they may still have trouble handling TS on an emotional level. They may feel resentful because their sibling is allowed to get away with behavior that they are not, sad because he is different than other children, and jealous because he seems to get more attention. Often, children keep these emotions bottled up because they think their feelings are "bad" or that their parents already have their hands full dealing with their sibling with TS.

Obviously, you can't do something about a problem if you don't know about it. This means that if your children don't come to you with their problems, you will have to be alert to clues that something may be troubling them—for example, fighting at school, worsening grades, or depression. In the beginning, you may have to do a little probing to find out what is at the root of these outward signs of emotional difficulties. The key is to help your children understand that you care about their feelings and will consider and respect them. As they begin to open up, you can let them know that the emotions they have are normal and understandable. You can help them understand that it is vital for all family members to talk about their feelings, as well as about any conflicts that are developing.

If your family was not in the habit of communicating openly before your child was diagnosed with Tourette syndrome, the lines of communication are not going to automatically open afterwards. Many families have great difficulty dealing directly with one another. If you and your family simply cannot seem to discuss your feelings, it may help to get family counseling from a mental health professional with expertise in Tourette syndrome.

Balance. Sometimes parents think it's OK to focus exclusively on their child with TS for a while, just until things "settle down" and they have more time to spend with their other children. This kind of thinking, although understandable, is wrong. Tourette syndrome is a chronic condition that cannot be cured. True, because of the waxing and waning, symptoms will sometimes be milder than they are at other times. But your other children's needs most likely do *not* wax and wane, and can't be conveniently scheduled for the times when tics are least disruptive.

In order to feel as if they are worthwhile and important, each of your children needs individual parental attention. When parents spend much more time with their child with TS, other children may feel jealous or unloved. These feelings fuel sibling rivalry. Your other children may misbehave to get your attention, on the grounds that negative attention from you is better than no attention at all.

To keep your other children from feeling neglected, try scheduling time each week to do something special with each child. It doesn't have to be anything elaborate—you might take turns taking your children out to lunch, or to the library, or out shopping. Be sure also to ask *all* of your children how their day went.

As part of your balancing act, you should make sure that each of your children is given his fair share of responsibility around the house. Each child needs to experience the satisfaction of a job well done and feel like a contributing member of the family. Perhaps your child with TS has difficulty focusing his attention on a chore long enough to complete it. But if you avoid giving him chores because of this problem, your child will not learn responsibility and siblings will resent the special treatment you give him. Each child in your family should be given jobs corresponding to their age and ability levels, and they should be expected to do their best at their jobs.

Finally, keep in mind that while children want to be given equal treatment, they also want to be treated as individuals. Sometimes special needs and talents *will* need to be taken into account when meting out privileges and responsibilities. Ideally, all your children would be given the same privileges and responsibilities once they reached a given age. For example, at age eight, they would be allowed to stay up until nine o'clock, ride their bike to school, and use the microwave oven to make popcorn. But because children's talents and weaknesses vary widely, it is not always possible to treat each child exactly the same. Your child with TS, for instance, may not be able to be left at home without adult supervision at the same age as his siblings, or may not be able to handle full responsibility for a pet. In deciding what your children can and cannot do, be sure to consider their talents, disabilities, judgment, and maturity.

Organization. Chapter 4 discusses how important organization is for children with Tourette syndrome. Having a predictable, settled routine can help reduce tics and problems such as over-stimulation arising from attentional problems. But organization is also important for your other children. *All* children (and adults) become frustrated, angry, and confused if their home routine is chaotic. Consequently, your family should try to follow a daily routine that is fairly constant on both weekdays and weekends. Meals, bedtime, play time, and homework time should basically come at the same time every day. When changes in routine are necessary, you should anticipate them and plan for them in advance. If you can anticipate a particular problem before it arises, you can take steps to deal with that problem. For example, if your child has an exciting birthday party to attend, and you know there is a possibility he will become overstimulated, make sure that the rest of the day will be relaxed and on schedule.

Individuality. One of the constant refrains in this book is that your child with TS is a child first, and only secondarily a child with Tourette syndrome. Your other children, too, are children first—not just the brothers or sisters of your child with Tourette syndrome. Each child in your family needs the opportunity to develop as an individual—to discover his own interests outside of the family and to pursue them with friends who share those interests. In other words, your other children need to be allowed to make their own friends. They should not always be forced to act as a playmate for their sibling with TS, whether or not he has friends outside the family. Experiencing social acceptance and success within the community is vital to your children's self-esteem.

In developing a sense of individuality, your children will also develop a sense of their own specialness—or what sets them apart from others. Your children may learn they have distinctive talents and abilities that make them special, but also distinctive problems and disabilities. For example, your child with TS may be gifted in academic subjects such as math, science, and reading, but have substantial delays in social and emotional development. His brother may be unusually articulate and persuasive when speaking to a group, but have great difficulty putting his thoughts on paper. It is important that you help each of your children understand and accept that everyone has both strengths and weaknesses and to encourage them to pursue their special interests and talents. But it is also important not to let special talents in one area blind you to serious problems in another that need to be worked on. This goes for all your children—not just your child with Tourette syndrome.

Although the main purpose of this chapter is to focus on potential family problems and their solutions, it would be unfair to imply that sibling relationships are always more challenging when

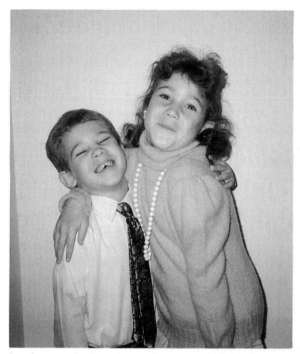

one or more children has TS. In fact, having a brother or sister with TS can have many positive effects on siblings. For instance, having a sibling with Tourette syndrome helps many children grow up to be more tolerant of all people who are different. They learn that aggressive behavior need not always be answered with aggressive behavior, and that they can walk away from potentially dangerous situations. By working out compromises with their brother or sister with TS, many siblings also hone their problem-solving skills. Most importantly, however, when siblings learn to see their brother or sister as a person first, rather than someone whose major characteristic is TS, they learn invaluable lessons about the essence of humanity.

Your Marriage

When you have a child with TS, it is important not to let your marriage take a back seat to your responsibilities as a parent. Your child's well-being, after all, depends on the survival of your family, and the survival of your family depends on the survival of your marriage. Fortunately, many couples find that having a child with TS strengthens their relationship in the long-run. Jointly facing the challenges that TS brings and working together to meet their child's needs can bring them closer together than ever before. Other couples, however, find that their relationship suffers when a child with TS joins the family.

Having a child with TS *does* put some unusual stresses on a marriage. Dealing with tics and associated problems for months and years on end can wear patience thin and fuel intolerance. And constantly putting forth herculean efforts to gain acceptance for your child in the community can leave you feeling too burned out to give your marriage the attention it needs to flourish. But too often TS is blamed for marital problems that have their roots elsewhere. The fact is, the presence of any chronic disorder in a family tends to bring out and intensify *existing* problems—not to create new ones.

Marital discord and breakup can usually be traced to core problems with communication, roles, or intimacy.

Communication

Chapter 2 discusses common emotions parents have when a child is diagnosed with Tourette syndrome. Because these feelings are often painful or are perceived as being shameful, many parents have trouble sharing them with their spouse. Other parents may think that if they ignore their feelings, they will go away. Unfortunately, denying or hiding these feelings can drive you and your spouse apart.

Honest communication is at least as important for you and your spouse as it is for siblings. It is crucial that both partners feel free to express all of their feelings, including feelings about their needs, their family life, or raising a child with TS. It is just as vital that these feelings be validated or supported by a caring spouse.

Active listening is the key to good communication. This involves setting aside time to listen to each other without making value judgements or blaming or criticizing your spouse. You don't have to agree with your spouse; just let him or her know that you respect his or her feelings. It may help to remember that feelings are only feelings, and neither good nor bad. There are many popular self-help books on communication in marriage you may wish to refer to.

Roles

Having a child with TS may bring added family pressures. Parents often have to spend time and energy taking their child to doctors or couselors, attending meetings at school, or supervising their child at home and in the community. Consequently, as mentioned earlier in the chapter, parents need to put some thought into decisions about family roles. One spouse or the other should not have to bear *all* the pressures related to having a child with TS. You and your spouse need to recognize that you may not be able to rely on traditional roles or do things the way your parents did. The husband, for example, needs to be more than breadwinner and disciplinarian, while the wife often must be more than homemaker and nurturer. Sometimes spouses naturally gravitate to the parenting tasks they do best. More often, however, they need to formally figure out an equitable division of the responsibilities involved in keeping their family running smoothly. This is another area where being able to communicate openly is a godsend.

Intimacy

An intimate relationship is one that is based on trust, sharing, and closeness. Intimacy in marriage strengthens parents for the emotionally draining task of nurturing and supporting a family. It helps them feel that they are not alone in the struggle to raise a healthy family. Intimacy is especially important in families with children with TS, as more energy is often needed to keep up with their children's day-to-day needs.

When you have a child with TS, time is often the biggest roadblock to increased intimacy. Because you may need to spend a disproportionate amount of time taking care of your child's medical, educational, and social needs, you may have less time available to spend with your spouse. It can be a vicious circle. The less time you have for intimacy with your spouse, the more isolated and exhausted you feel; the less energy you have, the harder it is to cope with the demands of parenthood. You must therefore make it a top priority to schedule some regular, unpressured time to work on your relationship with your spouse. Although this will reduce the *quantity* of time you are able to spend with your child, it will increase the *quality* of time you devote to him as you and your spouse recharge your emotional and physical batteries through intimacy.

Some couples are able to work out their problems on their own. Others may find it helpful to consult a mental health professional, especially someone who is knowledgeable about the effects of TS or other chronic disorders on emotions and relationships. All couples benefit from developing an outside support network. It can help take away some of the feeling that "we're doing it all alone." This support can come both through formal arrangements—from babysitters, respite workers, or support groups—or more informally, from neighbors, friends, and extended family. Chapters 2 and 4 provide more information on developing support networks.

Single Parents

Divorce is never something to be entered into lightly. When a child with TS is involved, it can make day-to-day life considerably more difficult for both parent and child. A single parent has limited relief without a spouse to step in and help out with child care. Financial concerns, too, can be overwhelming. Parents may find their jobs in jeopardy because of the amount of time they need to spend on doctor visits, school conferences, and therapy sessions, and the cost of medications can be considerable. Then, too, the changes in routine that divorce brings can cause a child's tics and other symptoms to worsen.

Still, divorce sometimes is in the best interests of the family. For example, if one parent has significant problems with alcoholism or drug addiction or is abusive to the children, then the other parent alone could likely provide a more supportive home environment.

In working out a divorce settlement, it is essential to keep both the financial and emotional costs in mind. For example, if the child with TS currently receives medical benefits under the terms of one parent's insurance, provisions should be made for that coverage to continue. Otherwise, the child with TS will likely lose substantial health benefits, and new coverage would probably be unobtainable because Tourette syndrome would be considered a pre-existing condition. Likewise, if one spouse has been abusive, legal action may be necessary to protect the children from harm after the divorce.

During the divorce process, counseling for spouses and children is often helpful. Most children become depressed and angry when their parents divorce. This can be even more of a problem for children with TS who have problems controlling aggression and anger. Children with TS may also worry that it was their tics and other behaviors that drove their parents to divorce, and they may therefore be consumed with guilt and remorse. A divorce can be especially hard on children with TS if it results in changes in routine. For example, if they are shuttled from one parent's house to another, they may find their daily life too confusing to handle. Often, professional counseling is essential to help children with TS through this period. Chapter 3 offers tips on finding a mental health professional with expertise in counseling children with TS. Your child's school might also have a children's divorce group.

Parents, too, often need help coping with emotions after a divorce. Some may need to seek counseling from a mental health professional in order to cope with the day-to-day demands of their family life and jobs. Respite care and a support system of family and friends can also help parents cope with the extra demands of single parenthood. In addition, some parents find it worthwhile to attend a single family support group.

Often, remarriage may appear to be the logical solution to the woes that accompany being a single parent. But dating and marriage are like a double-edged sword for most single parents of children with Tourette syndrome. On the one hand, there is the hope that a new spouse will be able to provide the emotional and financial support everyone in the family so desperately needs. On the other hand, there are the internal conflicts and self-doubts that can arise. For example, parents may feel that they are undesirable because they have a child with TS, or because they themselves have a tic disorder. Some worry that after marriage, the romance may fade and that antagonism toward their child or themselves may arise as in their previous marriage.

The effects of dating and remarriage on the child with TS must also be considered. Dating and marriage produce major changes in the life of the family. These changes can lead to considerable anxiety in the child with TS, and as a result, tics may become worse. Problems may also result if a parent's new spouse or boyfriend or girlfriend does not understand Tourette syndrome. He or she may try to discipline the child with TS for tics or other behaviors that seem disrespectful or abusive, but are really out of the child's control. Obviously, no one should be allowed to discipline a child with TS until he or she understands the condition and has learned what management strategies are effective. Remember, no child or adult deserves to be mistreated, and it is up to the parent to take steps to ensure the safety of the family.

If you decide to remarry, professional counseling is often helpful. Family counseling with a psychologist or social worker can speed the adjustment period by helping everyone in the family develop better channels of communication. A counselor can also help spouses develop more systematic parenting—helping them decide in advance what behavior management strategies they will both use. It is also helpful to keep the medical and educational professionals involved with your child with TS informed about any changes the family is going through. They can provide support and help develop a treatment plan if it becomes necessary. For example, if your child has difficulty adapting to a new step-sister after your remarriage, they can devise strategies to help him adjust.

Conclusion

Having a child with Tourette syndrome adds a new dimension to family life. All family members need to learn coping strategies and confront challenges that they would not otherwise encounter. But family life need not—in fact, *should* not—revolve around the child with TS. True, your family may need to make many adaptations, both individually and together, to accommodate your child's special needs. Remember, however, that other family members also have needs that are equally important. And just as your family pulls together to solve the problems that Tourette syndrome brings, they should also pull together to solve all the problems that face your family. As a parent, you call the plays. It is up to you to see that everyone feels like a welcome, valued member of the team.

Parent Statements

My husband and I want to support our son by understanding his behavior in public, because nobody else really understands why he acts the way he does. We try to avoid problem situations when possible, or else we constantly keep close tabs on his needs.

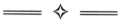

One of the hardest things for siblings to learn is that they may have to ignore behaviors from their brother or sister with TS that would be considered inappropriate behavior if they did it.

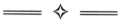

Our family finds it best to just expect the unusual from Robby—so long as he doesn't hurt himself or others—and to try to ignore these things.

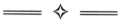

I enjoy life with our own family—watching TV, shopping, having pizza nights—and try to forget about the wishes of people outside the family.

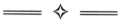

We have to avoid large gatherings. Crowds tend to escalate Sally's behaviors. We opt for activities such as going to the park. We also belong to a health club. Swimming is one of Sally's favorite activities.

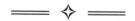

I come from a dysfunctional/abusive family. I know the pain of abuse and neglect, and I promised my beautiful, perfect newborn son a fun and happy childhood. It's almost horrifying to watch him go through so much misunderstanding and pain. My dedication to him has not been able to spare him. The final irony is to have so many professionals and nonprofessionals assume I must be causing these problems with some sort of faulty parenting style.

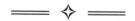

The therapist said, "Oh, 'impulsiveness.' That's a convenient excuse people use to continue lazy parenting."

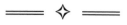

We try to control the high energy of our children, and yet, as adults, we'd do anything to have more energy.

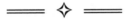

One neighbor suggested I get a life and quit paying so much attention to Laura. Some suspect you are under-involved and neglectful; others suspect you are over-involved and smothering.

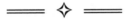

The incident which caused our family the most anger and frustration was when our sixth-grade son was benched for three days in Little League because he missed a practice to go to a support group for kids with TS! The coach knew all about our son's TS. We had spoken to him many times about his tics and how his medication made him sleepy. But all this coach cared about was WINNING and he only played his "best" kids, in spite of Little League recommendations. He went on to become a state champ with one of his WINNING teams. In our opinion, this "coach" was the biggest LOSER we've ever known. My son, at seventeen, is doing just fine. The coach is still playing with a handicap—his own short-sighted view of life. He's to be pitied. My son's the real WINNER now.

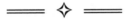

Most of the time, my kids get along great together. They're able to settle their differences pretty much on their own, and my husband and I rarely have to intercede.

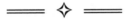

Although I am usually able to ignore Dave's constant vocalizations, his sister cannot. She is very annoyed by it, and it causes a lot of fights between them. I can't make her not be annoyed, and I can't make him stop the vocalizations. It's difficult for all of us.

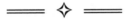

Our family has tried to maintain a happy, healthy, and normal lifestyle—which is not easy with the behavior problems. We agree that the tics are a piece of cake to deal with. Most important, we want Allen to know we love him and will stand by him always.

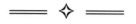

SIX

$\diamondsuit$

Your Child's Development

ROSANNE BREZDEN PAPADOPOULOS, B.M.R. O.T.M.,
GARY A. SHADY, PH.D., C. PSYCH., ROX WAND, MD FRCPC,
PATRICIA FURER, M.A.*

Doctor, professional athlete, teacher, parent . . . these are some of the professions held by adults who have Tourette syndrome. Their stories serve as a reminder that Tourette syndrome does not necessarily limit an individual's potential. Nonetheless, when a child is diagnosed as having Tourette syndrome, parents generally worry about the effect that this disorder might have on their child's life. They often wonder if their child will develop "normally" or master skills as well or as quickly as other children.

Unfortunately, it is impossible to predict exactly how Tourette syndrome will affect any one child's development. Like all children,

* Rosanne J. Brezden Papadopoulos received a Bachelor of Medical Rehabilitation (Occupational Therapy) from the University of Manitoba. Presently she performs clinical duties within the Tourette Syndrome Clinic and research duties within the Occupational Therapy Department of St. Boniface General Hospital in Winnipeg, Canada. Dr. Gary A. Shady is Senior Psychologist for Child and Adolescent Psychiatry, St. Boniface General Hospital. He is also Director of the TS Clinic at this hospital and an Associate Professor in the Department of Psychiatry, University of Manitoba. Dr. R. Rox Wand is the Medical Director, Child and Adolescent Neuropsychiatric Disorders Clinic, St. Boniface General Hospital. He is an Assistant Professor in the Department of Psychiatry, University of Manitoba, and a Consultant Psychiatrist at the Child Guidance Clinic of Greater Winnipeg. Patricia Furer was a psychology associate within the Department of Child and Adolescent Psychiatry at the St. Boniface General Hospital and the research coordinator of the TS Clinic. She is presently completing her Ph.D. at the University of Manitoba.

each child with TS is unique. Some acquire skills at the same rate or even faster than other children do, while others may lag somewhat behind. Usually, however, Tourette syndrome is associated with some common strengths and weaknesses in development. Exactly how Tourette syndrome will affect your child's development may depend on many factors, including the severity and type of tics, the presence of associated conditions such as attention deficit hyperactivity disorder (ADHD) or obsessive-compulsive disorder (OCD), and the support your child receives both at home and at school.

This chapter will provide a framework to help you understand your child's development. It explains what development is, and describes what is generally considered "normal" development, as well as some of the developmental areas with which your child may have difficulty. It also provides suggestions as to how you can help your child overcome developmental difficulties and reach her full potential. Many of these suggestions have actually come from parents of children with Tourette syndrome, and you will undoubtedly be able to add to the list.

What Is Development?

Your child was most likely given a diagnosis of Tourette syndrome because you and your physician realized that she was not showing the usual signs of expected growth or change. Perhaps she took much longer to become toilet trained than an older sibling did, could not seem to control her temper as well as other children her age could, or had trouble learning to hold a crayon and scribble. In other words, in some way she did not seem to be "developing normally."

Most children grow and acquire skills, or *develop*, according to pretty much the same timetable. That is, there are certain skills that most children acquire by a certain age. For example, most babies can wave bye-bye by about ten months of age, can walk with their hand held at around twelve months, and can say ten words at eighteen months.

When a child successfully accomplishes a basic developmental task such as waving or walking, this is usually referred to as reaching a developmental *milestone*. In so-called "normal" development, there is a wide range of ages at which children can achieve milestones. Children can attain some milestones slightly ahead of or behind other children who are the same age and still be considered to be developing normally. For example, although walking typically begins at twelve months of age, many healthy children begin walking much later, and some develop this skill considerably earlier. In fact, it is unlikely that any child reaches every milestone at precisely the "normal" time. Thus, do not be concerned if your child does not develop each new skill at exactly the "correct" age suggested by this or any other book. Because it is helpful to have some idea of normal expectations, however, Tables 1–6 provide samples of some typical milestones.

Not only do children usually reach particular milestones at particular times, but normally they also reach these milestones according to a predictable sequence. For example, in learning to climb stairs, a child may first retreat from the stairs, then look at them with curiosity. Next, she may attempt to climb with support and eventually without support. The reason milestones emerge in sequence is because each milestone attained lays the groundwork for the next, more complex milestone.

Once again, children may sometimes learn skills outside of the normal developmental sequence. But there are a few basic developmental principles that hold true for all children. For example, they develop "from head to toe." As a result, they are able to focus their eyes on a toy before they are able to use their hands to play with it. Likewise, their movements develop "near to far"; they can control movements closer to the center of their body before they can control their limbs. That is, body control develops before hand control. For example, an infant may be able to show excitement only by wiggling or jostling around, while an older child may drum her fingers.

General rules aside, it is important to keep in mind that there is a tremendous variety in rates and styles of development. This is because all development depends a great deal on biological programming. In other words, a child's genetic makeup sets the foundation for growth and acquisition of skills. For example, inheriting a musical aptitude may have an effect on choice of interest, hobby, or career. Other factors such as environment, culture, and psychological makeup are also important. The effect that the availability of toys or books can have in motivating a child to read and learn is just one example. Because so many combinations of factors can occur, no child's development is exactly the same as another child's development. One child, for instance, may move carefully through each step of learning to talk, while another child may seem to pick up language skills in a short "outburst" later on. Remember, how quickly your child learns to do something is not as important as how well she can eventually do it.

Areas of Development

Just as the skills a child learns in school fall into different subject areas, so too do the skills she learns during the course of development. Human development is most often divided into six categories: 1) gross motor; 2) fine motor; 3) cognition; 4) language; 5) social; and 6) self-help. Within each of these categories are expectations for the achievement of tasks. To help you identify possible developmental problems in your child, a brief description of normal development within each area is provided below.

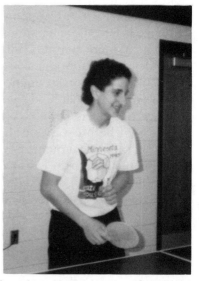

Gross Motor

In gross motor development, children learn to control their bodies through the use of large muscles such as those in the legs, arms, and abdomen. Rolling, sitting, crawling, and walking are examples of basic gross motor skills which later develop into more advanced gross motor skills such as running and climbing. Because these types of skills enable the child to "master the environment" and explore the world around her, they play a crucial role in development in other areas. Table 1 shows the ages at which children typically master some important gross motor skills.

Table 1

Gross Motor

Months (approx.)	Activity
1–3.5	Lifts head
2–4.5	Sits up with support
3–7.6	Stands, holding on
9.5–13	Stands alone well
11.8–14.5	Walks well
14.5–23.8	Throws ball overhand
20.6–33	Jumps in place
22–35	Pedals tricycle
37–66	Balances on 1 foot, 10 seconds
43–65	Catches bounced ball

Fine Motor

In fine motor development, children learn to use smaller muscles such as those in their hands and face to make precise, detailed movements. Focusing the eyes, drawing, and buttoning clothing are all types of fine motor tasks. Fine motor skills lay the foundation for later development of academic skills such as handwriting, as well as self-help skills such as those described below. See Table 2 for examples of the ages when fine motor skills are usually attained.

Table 2

Fine Motor

Months (approx.)	Activity
1.5–3.8	Brings hands together
3.2–5.5	Reaches for object
5–8.5	Passes small object hand to hand
7.2–11	Grasps objects with thumb & finger
11.8–25	Scribbles spontaneously
18.4–35	Copies vertical lines
40–62	Draws human, 3 parts
49–73	Draws human, 6 parts

Cognition

Cognition is the ability to reason and solve problems either with words or numbers. In the early stages of cognitive development, a child learns about the concept of object permanence—that an object continues to exist when it is out of sight. Prior to this, the child may have believed that "out of sight" meant "out of mind." Also in the early stages, the child learns the principle of cause and effect—that, for example, if she shakes her rattle, it will make a noise.

As the child's improving motor skills increase her ability to explore, she learns all sorts of information about her environment. In the first year, for instance, an infant usually learns that objects have weight, size, taste, and feel. By about the age of two, the toddler shows the first stirrings of imagination. She may pretend that her stuffed animals are alive, or convince herself that a monster is lurking under the bed. Over the next four or five years, the child gradually becomes able to think in more abstract terms so that at age seven, she no longer needs to touch or look at something to think about it. For example, she can picture in her mind what her parents will do if she makes a mess in the kitchen. In later childhood, the child masters more complex abstractions, such as those required to solve mathematical equations or think of metaphors. Table 3 summarizes the ages when important cognitive skills are usually mastered.

Table 3

Cognition

Months (approx.)	Activity
.5–4.6	Shows preference for visual patterns
.6–2.5	Responds to bell
3.4–8.6	Turns to voice
6.2–14.5	Discriminates between shapes (circles, crosses, triangles)
13.6–21.5	Points to 1 named body part
14.6–26	Follows directions
26–38	Gives first and last name
30–50	Understands cold, tired, hungry
34–58	Recognizes colors

Language

Through language development, children gradually learn one of the most vital skills in modern society, communication. Usually, comprehension of language, including words or gestures, comes first. Later, the child develops the ability to communicate her own messages through appropriate gestures, words, or written symbols.

For example, a child generally understands the word "milk" long before she is able to request a drink herself. This ability to understand words and gestures is known as *receptive language;* the ability to use language to communicate is known as *expressive language.*

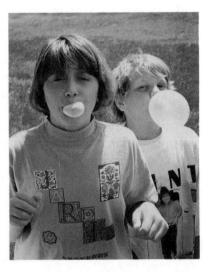

The first signs that a child is experimenting with language are commonly vowel sounds such as "ah" or "uh," at around twenty-eight weeks of age. Usually within a month after that, consonant sounds such as "ma" and "da" appear. At around eight months, a child typically astounds her parents with "mama" and "dada," and at around eighteen months, she has a ten-word vocabulary. Generally, by the age of three a child is talking in three-word sentences and has a vocabulary of five hundred words. By six, the child may have a vocabulary of up to two thousand words and can grasp very complex sentence constructions. Table 4 provides additional examples of language skills.

Table 4

Language

Months (approx.)	Activity
1.5–5.5	Squeals
5.5–10	Says "Dada" or "Mama"
6–11.5	Imitates speech sounds
11.8–20.5	3 words other than mama or dada
14.5–25	Combines 2 different words
20–35	Uses plurals
35–72	Defines words

Social

As a child develops socially, she learns to get along with others, as well as to respond with appropriate emotions. Usually even very young infants take an intense interest in others around them. As early as two months of age, they may smile and watch others' movements. By about eight months, they can recognize family members and are often frightened by strangers, especially when left alone with them ("separation anxiety"). During the preschool years, children learn the difference between genders, begin to recognize feelings in others, and react to others with varied emotions such as shyness or anger. Also during these years, children progress from playing by themselves, to playing beside other children, and eventually to playing together with other children in the same activity. By five or six, children are able to form special friendships and show increased independence. All of these social skills help children to fit in and become functioning members of society. See Table 5 for more examples of social skills.

Table 5

Social

Months (approx.)	Activity
1.5–5	Smiles spontaneously
5.5–9.5	Initially shy with strangers
6.5–10.5	Plays peek-a-boo
10.5–14.5	Indicates "wants"
12.5–18.5	Imitates housework
14.5–23.5	Helps with simple household tasks
17.5–20.5	Hugs a doll
22.5–58	Separates easily from mother

Self-Help

At birth, babies are totally dependent on others for their survival and well-being. Through the development of self-help skills such as feeding, grooming, and dressing, they gradually learn to do things for themselves and become more and more independent. Self-help skills can develop early in life, particularly when children are given opportunities to act independently. For example, when physically able, a child can learn to use a spoon instead of being "spoon-fed," so long as others at the table don't mind the mess. Not only does tolerating this type of independence help a child reach developmental milestones, but it also helps parents boost their child's self-confidence and self-esteem—both of which can make learning new skills in all areas easier. Table 6 shows the ages at which children usually achieve some major self-help skills.

Table 6

Self-Help

Months (approx.)	Activity
4.5–8.5	Feeds self crackers
9.5–16.5	Drinks from cup
13.5–21.5	Removes own garments
13.5–22.5	Uses spoon, spilling little
20.5–34	Puts on own clothing
30–50	Buttons up
34–62	Dresses without supervision

Sensory Integration

Besides the six recognized areas of development described above, another area known as *sensory integration* also affects growth and learning. Sensory integration refers to a child's ability to take in, organize, and make use of information received from all body sensations—sight, hearing, touch, taste, smell, movement. A sensory-integrated brain is essential for almost every human activity. For example, eating a banana re-

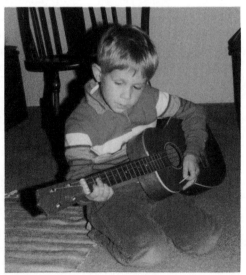

quires that sensations from our eyes, nose, mouth, skin on our hands, and muscles and joints in our arm, hand, fingers, and mouth all be sorted and organized by our brain.

Because sensory integration is what enables us to perceive the world around us, it is vital to learning in all areas. A well-integrated system helps children take in information through their senses and learn from it in an organized way. This helps them act or relate to the world in a manner that is likely to create successful and healthy interactions. Sensory integration occurs automatically and differently in all children. As with other areas of development, some children progress more quickly than others.

The Development of Children with Tourette Syndrome

Most children with TS are born following a normal pregnancy and delivery. But in the preschool years before tics appear, parents sometimes notice mild, subtle differences in their child's behavior compared to that of other children in their family or other children they know. Then, as the child becomes a toddler, overactivity, aggressive behavior toward peers, temper tantrums, seemingly excessive separation anxiety from parents, or excessive rituals bordering on compulsive behavior, may start to develop. When concerned parents report these behaviors to pediatricians or family doctors, they are often inaccurately told that these are passing phases of development that the child will quickly outgrow. There is a great deal of variety in how children with Tourette syndrome develop during these years, however. Many children who develop tics at the average age of seven have no unusual pre-tic phase of development or behavior.

Now that your child has received the diagnosis of Tourette syndrome, medical specialists may still be reluctant to predict exactly how the disorder will affect your child's development and functioning. This is first of all because the range of symptoms in children with TS can vary so widely. In some children with TS, the only symptoms are motor and vocal tics. Other children may have obsessions, compulsions, hyperactivity, learning problems, frequent mood swings, or aggressive or self-mutilative behaviors. The symptoms present in any one child will wax and wane, as will the motor and vocal tics. All symptoms will have varying degrees of severity at their peak of activity. The effects on the child's development will vary depending on frequency and severity of symptoms. For example, a child with only mild tics and no associated conditions may have only a few problems in development and adaptation, while a child with severe tics, obsessive-compulsive disorder, and attention deficit hyperactivity disorder may have more obstacles to overcome in many areas of development. Although every child with Tourette syndrome *is* unique, generally the disorder has at least some effects on social, emotional, and academic development. It may also impede development of sensory integration, cognition, fine and gross motor coordination, and language skills.

The sections below review some of the ways Tourette syndrome *may* affect a child's development. But remember; all children do not have the same developmental concerns. Your child may have many of these problems, but then again, she may have few, if any, of them.

Motor Development in Children with Tourette Syndrome

Some children with Tourette syndrome have no motor problems except in controlling their tics. Most often, however, children or adolescents with Tourette syndrome have a history of poor fine and gross motor coordination. For example, they may be sloppy eaters or have poor bicycling skills. They may not have any obvious developmental delay in reaching motor milestones, but often they have what professionals refer to as "soft signs," which suggest subtle neurological problems. These signs include:

1. awkward body postures during physical activities;
2. poor balance;
3. "floppiness" in body and limbs during movement;
4. difficulty identifying right and left or with activities such as bowling or basketball in which both sides of the body must be used in a coordinated way;
5. clumsiness due to perceptual-motor problems (difficulty perceiving the world around them with their senses and then responding with a motor movement).

Researchers have also found that children with Tourette syndrome often have a disrupted sense of touch. They may be *hyper-reactive* (over sensitive) or *hypo-reactive* (under sensitive) to sensations on their skin. Characteristics of hyper-reactivity include such things as: seeming to feel pain more than others, reacting with anger to an unexpected touch from behind, avoiding play with messy things, and distinctly preferring certain textures of clothing. Hypo-reactivity affects touch sensations much as wearing a pair of gloves does. Children who are hypo-reactive may feel pain less than others and seem "fumbly" when trying to pick up small objects.

On a day-to-day basis, motor development problems may lead to difficulty in physical education class or reluctance to join in-

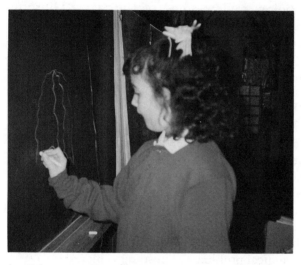

tramural or team sports. The child may feel left out of playground or neighborhood games, and feel more comfortable with individual activities or indoor, sit-down pastimes such as computer games. As a result, she may lose out in developing good overall physical health, as well as social and peer relationships that often happen during sports. Additionally, children who are hyper-reactive might avoid working with papier-mache, finger painting, or taking part in other activities that require them to touch gooey or slimy materials. And children who are hypo-reactive might have more difficulty drawing or playing a musical instrument.

In addition to the potential problems described above, children and adolescents with Tourette syndrome often have poor fine motor control. This can result in difficulty in handwriting, dressing, grooming, eating, and arts and crafts. There are several reasons for hand control problems, including hyper/hypo-reactivity to touch and poor motor control. The most common cause of hand control problems is poor visual-motor processing, or difficulty using input from the sense of sight in making movements. For example, poor visual-motor processing can impair handwriting by making it difficult to organize input about the shape and size of letters or lines on the paper in order to make accurate movements with the arm, wrist, and fingers. Tics, or the child's attempt to physically hold back an arm or hand tic, can also contribute to handwriting problems. Symptoms of ADHD and OCD can add to motor problems. Hyperactivity may exaggerate problems of clumsiness and contribute to accidents, while poor attention makes it more difficult to complete tasks calling for sustained handwriting. Likewise, rituals such as continually erasing work or counting certain letters may get in the way of completing a writing assignment.

Depending upon the nature of your child's motor problems, your child may benefit from occupational or physical therapy.

Occupational therapy (OT) is aimed at helping a child develop her motor and other skills so she can better cope with her day-to-day activities. For instance, an occupational therapist might help a child with TS improve handwriting skills by using a built-up handle on her pencil, teaching her to hold the pencil differently, or by playing visual-motor games such as maze drawing. Physical therapy (PT) focuses more specifically on identifying and treating problems with movement and posture. A physical therapist might help a child with TS with poor balance by having her sit on a tilt board, bounce on a large therapy ball, and work up to jumping, hopping, and running. Both OT and PT often combine treatment with play and therefore work on several areas at any one time. A therapy session concentrating on gross motor skills might include a trip through an obstacle course including a balance beam, scooter board (postural control), bowling pins and balls (visual aiming and motor accuracy), as well as floor mats for working on rolling or crawling. A therapy session focusing on fine or visual-motor skills might include maze-drawing, matching, and lacing or stictching, as well as finding buttons in a bowl of flour or playing with "monster goop" to work on touch response.

As a parent, you can help your child's skill development by encouraging her to attempt a variety of fine motor and gross motor activities. Choose activities to fit her strengths and limitations and be sure she is involved in the decision making. After all, she is more likely to succeed if she is motivated to try an activity. For example, if she enjoys playing in the water at the beach, then consider enrolling her in swimming lessons at the local pool; if she loves making "things," then have her join a craft club at a nearby community club; if she adores rock music, she might want to learn to play the guitar, piano, or drums. Where sports are concerned, remember that a thoughtful, non-competitive instructor or team coach who can balance fun and skill can make a tremendous difference to a child with TS. Above all, be patient and accept the fact that accuracy and perfection may never be accomplished, but your child *can* learn to compensate for and cope with motor problems.

Cognitive Development in Children with Tourette Syndrome

When a child is diagnosed as having Tourette syndrome, the parents often worry that intelligence will be impaired. Although Tourette syndrome can be very challenging for children and families to cope with, it does at least have the saving grace of *not* affecting overall cognitive or intellectual development.

Your child's cognitive abilities can be measured informally by evaluating how she copes with daily life or through a formal IQ test which compares her abilities with those of other children her age. Most children and adolescents with Tourette syndrome have average IQs. As in the general population, some children with Tourette syndrome are above average in intelligence, and some are slightly below. A small minority of children with Tourette syndrome also have mental retardation; that is, their cognitive capabilities are much less than average and affect skill acquisition and performance in all areas of development. The percentage of children with Tourette syndrome who have mental retardation, however, is the same as for the population as a whole. Tourette syndrome does not cause mental retardation.

Although Tourette syndrome does not diminish overall intelligence, it is frequently associated with problems with specific cognitive skills. It is important to remember, however, that for most people, cognitive abilities are not evenly developed across all areas. We each have areas of relative strength and weakness. For example, you may excel at working with numbers, but may be less comfortable writing business reports. Your spouse, on the other hand, may write reports and creative essays with ease but be unable to balance a check book. Thus, we each have more difficulty with certain cognitive skills than with others. The same holds true for children with TS.

Many children with TS share the same types of difficulties in cognitive skills, as can be seen both in their daily living and on IQ tests. We have yet to figure out exactly *why* children with TS tend to have these problems. Nonetheless, you may find it helpful to at least be familiar with the kinds of challenges your child may encounter.

Many studies have found that children with TS tend to have better verbal skills than they do visual-motor skills. That is, your child may have difficulty with skills that require good hand-eye coordination, such as handwriting. At the same time, however, she may have excellent verbal comprehension skills, enabling her to grasp the central message of a short story, for example.

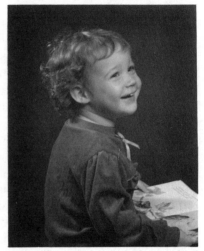

Children with Tourette syndrome may also find written arithmetic very challenging and often do better on oral arithmetic word problems. As a result, your child may have difficulty with mathematics at school, where these skills are typically taught and tested in a written format. She may, however, be quite capable of applying mathematical concepts to everyday life. In other words, she may have no problem figuring out how much change is owed when purchasing a candy bar, even though she cannot solve even simple written numerical problems, such as 12 + 28, on her math worksheets.

Another area that often is difficult for children with Tourette syndrome is taking timed tests. They often do relatively poorly when they are given time limits. This may be painfully obvious in the classroom where students are often given in-class tests or assignments to complete in, for example, twenty minutes. Your child may also run into this problem at home when given a time limit in which to dress or to complete a chore such as cleaning her room.

Children with TS, especially those who also have attention deficit difficulties or hyperactivity, may have problems with memory and concentration. These problems can affect cognitive development and performance both at home and at school. Your child may, for example, have great difficulty following even a simple set of instructions such as "wash your face, brush your teeth, and comb your hair." Children with these problems frequently forget one or two steps or seem to get distracted before the task is completed. Similarly, your child may have trouble remembering to do homework assignments or to bring home the textbooks required to do so. These types of problems can cause endless frustration for parents.

Besides interfering with the development of specific cognitive skills, the problems described above may also cause the intellectual potential of children with TS to be underestimated. This can occur for several reasons. First of all, some motor and vocal tics directly interfere with *performance* in various activities at home and at school. For example, if your child has a vocal tic involving the frequent repetition of her own words, an otherwise excellent speech can become virtually unintelligible. Thus your child's public speaking skills may be hidden by a tic. Secondly, tics may hamper your child's performance on an IQ test. For example, a severe arm-jerking tic might make it difficult for your child to accurately position a set of small blocks. So, even if your child has the visual and spatial skills required for this task, she would be unable to demonstrate these skills because of her tics. This would artificially lower the score on this part of the test, and your child's overall intellectual development would be underestimated. Finally, your child's intelligence and abilities may also be underestimated if the cognitive "dulling" effects of TS medications are not recognized.

These potential problems underline the importance of having your child's intellectual potential assessed by a psychologist who is familiar with Tourette syndrome and the medications used to treat it. It is also essential that professionals, teachers, and parents understand that a child's poor performance on a given task may be due to interference from tics or medication, rather than to a lack of ability or intelligence.

If your child has any of the cognitive difficulties described above, it is important that she learn to compensate for these problems. For example, children who have difficulty with handwriting (due to poor eye-hand coordination or because of an interfering tic) may be more successful if they learn to do their written work on a computer or typewriter. Teachers can assist children with difficulties in mathematics by permitting them to do at least part of the required work orally instead of in written format. Similarly, relaxing or eliminating the time restrictions on tests can be helpful for some children with TS. Finally, children who seem to constantly forget or to avoid responsibilities may benefit from strategies designed to help them get organized for everything from getting ready to school to completing household chores. You or your child might make "things to do lists" in homework books, diaries, or on write and wipe boards. As a parent, it may be necessary to impose organizational strategies upon your child's disorganized world in an effort to teach her to do the same for herself. Use your own creativity and enlist the assistance of your child's teacher and school in order to develop successful strategies to compensate for your child's difficulties.

Language/Communication Development in Children with Tourette Syndrome

Parents sometimes wonder whether their child's vocal tics can be traced to abnormal language development in the early years. In general, however, how speech and language develop when a child is young does not seem to have any impact on the types of tics which develop later in childhood or adolescence. In fact, children with Tourette syndrome usually have normal speech patterns. Their verbal tics "fit in" to normal speech rhythm and often occur at the same point where speakers normally hesitate or pause, such as at the beginning or ending of sentences. Typically, speakers stop during speech and often make unnecessary, non-verbal movements of their lips, tongue, and vocal cords, producing sounds such as "um" and "uh." Therefore, the verbal tics found in TS originate in "normal" behavior.

Once verbal tics develop, they are more likely to interfere with language expression, rather than comprehension. Research has shown that children and adolescents with Tourette syndrome often have good ability to repeat sounds they hear, good ability to remember what someone has said (except when long sentences are involved), and good understanding through their sense of hearing. At the same time, they often stutter, have trouble elaborating on a story or finding the right word, or use loud or pressured speech. So when telling a story to friends, your child may stutter at key phrases, talk very quickly, or pause while struggling to think of a word. Many of these difficulties arise because your child is placing a great deal of concentrated effort on holding back a vocal tic.

Interpersonal communication can also be disrupted if tics are expressed, rather than suppressed. This happens if tics involve word perseveration (repetition) or echolalia, and if the vocal tics are explosive (loud and distracting). Listeners become distracted and lose track of the conversation, as may the speaker if she has an attention disorder. This can be frustrating for both the listener and the speaker. The child with TS may lose her desire to communicate at all, which can lead to further language or social problems. It is easy to recognize the social and emotional anxiety that may result from communication problems for some children and adolescents with Tourette syndrome.

To minimize the effects your child's verbal tics have on language development, be prepared to be very supportive. To help her get used to communicating with others, encourage your child to play with peers—first on a one-to-one basis, and then in small groups. Allow her to speak for herself in conversations; do not answer for her. your child might also benefit from the help of a speech therapist.

Social and Emotional Development in Children with Tourette Syndrome

Years before your child developed tics, you may have noticed problems with social development. This is not uncommon. Although tics may begin as early as age one or two, they usually do not appear until after age five. Other problems, however, often start in the preschool years. These include temper tantrums, hyperactivity, aggressive behavior, and difficulty sharing. Often these types of difficulties run in families, and siblings may also have similar problems, although only one child actually develops TS. During the pre-tic years, the child who later develops Tourette syndrome also frequently has severe separation anxiety.

When a preschooler has any or all of these problems with emotional or social skills, her behavior may disrupt family life. Parents may believe that their child intentionally misbehaves at home and in the community. Parents' frustration may turn to anger, and they are likely to repeatedly, but unsuccessfully, correct and discipline their child. The child, in turn, is likely to resent the criticism and to feel isolated from other family members. Children who have little control over their behavior may feel intense frustration, which can interfere with various aspects of social and emotional development. Family relationships can become quite strained even before the onset of a child's first tics.

After the motor and vocal tics develop, additional challenges face your child and family. For example, you may initially think that your child's tics are a way of expressing anger toward you, other family members, or playmates. As a result of this misunderstanding, you may discipline or correct your child, and siblings or playmates may ridicule her for behaviors that are completely out of her control. This creates or adds to your child's frustration toward you, self-doubt as to whether she is really doing this deliberately, and isolation from normal activities with siblings or friends.

Once you know that your child has Tourette syndrome, some of these misunderstandings may be cleared up. But most families find that the motor and vocal tics, together with any attention deficit problems and obsessions and compulsions, disrupt the family and the child's social and emotional development in many ways. For example, your child will often try to hold back tics to appease parents, teachers, siblings, and peers. If she succeeds in controlling the tics and associated conditions while in school or other public places, she will have to release many tics once she is home, in the presence of family members. This often creates disharmony in the family, particularly when brothers and sisters demand equal leniency for their own disruptive behaviors. In addition, parents are often unsure whether the symptoms are willful behaviors for which their child should be held accountable, or are involuntary behaviors for which their child should be excused. This uncertainty puts additional pressure on family relationships. All these factors may add up to reduced opportunities for socializing and for developing social skills. For example, if family members are embarrassed by TS symptoms or their inability to make the child with TS "behave," they may limit their outings to public places such as restaurants or movie theaters or withdraw from other social and recreational activities.

As children enter adolescence, their "different" behaviors often increase: tics become more frequent or severe, obsessive-compulsive symptoms either worsen or are added to the repertoire of symptoms, and attention deficit hyperactivity disorders frequently continue unabated. Poorly developed social skills become much more obvious, and adolescents with Tourette syndrome seem to have more difficulty understanding and changing their behaviors. Families and peers often see them as immature or lacking in social skills. Just at the stage in life when the need for peer acceptance is greatest, your child may feel captive to a condition which appears bizarre to her friends. She may hesitate to join in normal adolescent activities such as dances, parties, dating, or part-time employment. As a result, she may feel isolated and lonely. Continuing academic difficulties may also worry her. The lower her self-esteem gets, the harder it becomes for her to seek out new opportunities in social relationships. As the parent of an adolescent with Tourette syndrome, you may frequently find yourself forced to act as your child's best friend, encouraging her to develop social skills, social relationships, and self-acceptance.

Whatever her age, you have a teaching role in helping your child learn appropriate social skills on a day-to-day basis. You can best help your child by concentrating on *gradually* improving her social skills. First reinforce "bits and pieces" or skills that are close to being right, then work up to more complete skills. For example, your child might often have trouble "reading" others' reactions to her behavior. She might not realize how frustrated she makes a playmate by refusing to share a toy. If she does consent to share— with or without a reminder from you—praise her enthusiastically. Because social development can frequently be interrupted or delayed if your child is ridiculed or unfairly disciplined, you also have an advocacy role. It is up to you to ensure that information about Tourette syndrome is available to your child's teachers and classmates. Providing this information may help demystify the bizarre behaviors which baffle children or adults unfamiliar with the syndrome.

In addition to increasing understanding of Tourette syndrome among teachers and friends, you can also enhance your child's social development by enrolling her in group therapy or recreation programs at facilities that treat children or adolescents with Tourette syndrome. Recreational or educational summer camp programs for children or adolescents with Tourette syndrome can also boost your child's sense of well-being and social skills. By sharing information and feedback with other children with Tourette syndrome, your child can learn new coping styles which may ultimately lead to better relationships at home and in school. The National Tourette Syndrome Association or a local chapter can help you find programs that can give your child a boost in social development.

Self-Help Development in Children with Tourette Syndrome

Many of the problems in other areas described above can, understandably, add up to poor self-help or daily living skills. For example, if your child cannot remember a simple series of instructions, she may have difficulty learning how to make her own breakfast, use the washing machine to do her laundry, or any number of self-help skills. If tics delay her social development, her ability to get along independently may be hampered. For example, she may be unable to deal well enough with strangers to make a purchase in a store, ask for directions when lost, or place an order in a restaurant. And, as mentioned earlier, poor fine motor control can lead to problems with eating, dressing, and grooming.

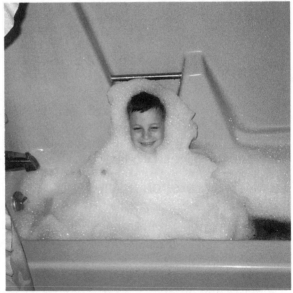

If your child has delays in self-help skills, occupational therapists can offer helpful ideas and suggestions. They are specifically trained in the area of self-help skills. To help your child with problems related to fine motor control, a therapist might, for example, recommend using built-up or thicker-handled eating or writing utensils. The therapist might also recommend bigger buttons or velcro on clothing, and a typewriter or computer.

In addition to other self-help delays, children with Tourette syndrome often have trouble becoming toilet trained due to developmental difficulties gaining bowel and bladder control. Children with Tourette syndrome and/or ADHD often seem to have daytime "accidents" up to the age of four. About one-third of children with Tourette syndrome continue to have problems with nighttime bed-wetting after five years of age. If your child has this problem, consult your family doctor to investigate options such as medication or nighttime "buzzer" systems.

One final area in which children with TS often have difficulties is sleeping. Although sleep habits are not themselves considered a self-help skill, poor sleep habits definitely interfere with children's abilities to help themselves. Children with TS may have one or several problems in sleeping: inability to take naps, day/night reversal, or night terrors. Sleep problems often interfere with a child's ability to learn in general. They may make it more difficult to:

- pay attention at school;
- "hang in there" when problems with peers or school-work become frustrating;
- slow down and not solve problems impulsively.

This list could go on and on. You need only think of *your* behavior on days when you have not had enough sleep! Chapter 4 discusses strategies for dealing with sleep problems.

Sensory Integration in Children with Tourette Syndrome

There may be sensory integration problems underlying some of your child's developmental difficulties. You may even have recognized some of these problems prior to the onset of your child's TS tics or diagnosis of ADHD or OCD. For example, your child may have had some problems in processing sounds—for example, language delay or difficulty listening. Or she may have had trouble with touch sensations, and consequently became anxious when people touched her or stood too close. Difficulty with movement sensations may have shown up as unskillful play, clumsiness, or poor coloring or cutting skills. Because of these problems, you may have suspected delays in various developmental milestones.

Sensory integration problems usually become more apparent when your child enters school. If your child has trouble organizing the many sensations bombarding her brain, she will have difficulty concentrating, sitting still, standing in lines, or taking part in gym class without hitting or pushing other children who may accidentally bump into her. Besides contributing to delays in other developmental areas, these sensory problems—added to the tics of Tourette syndrome—can very easily lead to poor self-esteem and poor relationships with family and friends.

You can help your child by encouraging her to take part in a wide variety of physical activities. The more exposure your child has to the sensations of the environment, the greater the chance that she will overcome sensory problems, or at least, develop coping skills to help her compensate for areas of weakness. It is important to begin with non-competitive, successful experiences, and a flexible instructor who can take your child's special needs into account. Professional help is also available from occupational or physical therapists with special training in working with sensory integration problems. These professionals can assess and treat your child's sensory problems and serve as liaisons with school staff concerning these problems, but you may still have to educate them about Tourette syndrome! Chapter 1 provides more information about the nature and treatment of sensory integration problems.

Helping Your Child Overcome Developmental Problems

At this point you may feel overwhelmed by the multitude of developmental challenges your child may face, and also by the importance of your role in helping your child with specific difficulties. You may not know where or how to begin to meet these challenges. The following guidelines may help you gain an overall picture of your child's development, and also to focus on the areas that will most help your child. You can use these guidelines in dealing with most problems your child may encounter.

Understand Your Child's Tourette Syndrome. Both you and your child should understand all aspects of your child's disorder so that you can make informed decisions when solving problems.

Treat Your Child as a "Normal Child." As much as possible, treat your child as you would any other child. Consider her strengths and weaknesses where appropriate, but give her all the responsibilities and limits she needs to help her develop into a responsible adult.

Have Realistic Expectations and Set Realistic Goals. This is an inherent part of good parenting. Expectations and goals need to be reasonable according to your child's age, strengths, and limitations to allow for challenge and success. Success in reaching early goals creates the energy and motivation needed for future goals.

Let Your Child Make Choices. Allowing a child to solve problems and choose for herself is essential to her self-esteem. Making choices helps her gain confidence in her ability to control her life and take responsibility for herself, despite her developmental needs.

Make Learning a Part of Daily Life. Try to teach social skills and life skills on a day-to-day basis as situations occur. "On the spot" learning teaches children to face problems, not avoid them, and figure out more successful ways of dealing with a situation so that next time it happens, the child has another choice. You might want to try role-playing the situation over again with your child to "try on" the new behavior.

Boost Your Child's Organization and Independence. Make use of any strategies and devices that will help your child become more organized or independent on a day-to-day basis. For example, use reminder books or charts or built-up handles on utensils.

Seek Help. Perhaps you are beginning to feel frustrated after reading some of the guidelines above. You may already have tried some of these strategies, but found that they never or rarely work. This may signal that you need some help in establishing a parenting style that works for your child with TS and your family as a whole. Do not be afraid to seek help, not only for your child, but also for your family. Your family doctor can assist you in finding a counselor, preferably one already knowledgeable about TS, to help your child and your family deal with the stress of coping with TS.

Obtain Needed Therapy Services. Occupational, physical, and speech therapists can help your child overcome a variety of motor, self-help, and sensory problems. As explained in Chapter 7, these services are available free of charge through your child's school if she qualifies for special education. You may also want to consult private therapists, especially if your medical or life insurance will cover the costs.

Your Child's Development in Adolescence and Adulthood

The end of childhood does not mean the end of development. Most people, including those with Tourette syndrome, continue to grow and learn all through their lives. True, early milestones lay the foundation for most major skills, but there are also important developmental goals to be met in adolescence and young adulthood.

In the teen years, children continue to tackle challenges in cognitive, physical, and social development. For example, they master increasingly complex academic subjects, become more skilled in athletic pursuits, and learn to maintain long-term friendships. Gains made in these areas are often directed at achieving independence. As a result, adolescents may feel more anxious when development does not go as expected. By the same token, however, their confidence seems to grow more rapidly than in childhood, because when they succeed, they truly feel that they have reached their goals "on their own."

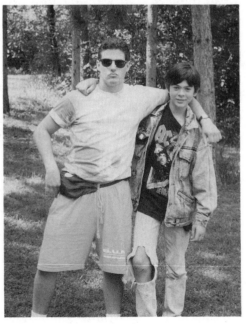

In reaching independence, adolescents with Tourette syndrome may need to overcome more than the usual number of obstacles. Some typical social problems at school were touched on earlier. But teenagers with Tourette syndrome may also have problems with dating or with fitting in or being accepted on the job. Often, following what appears to be the "mature" course of action does not help. For example, telling other employees or supervisors about Tourette syndrome seems a positive gesture, but has been known to cost some teenagers their jobs. Likewise, being open about Tourette syndrome symptoms with a girlfriend or boyfriend would seem to be the best avenue, but can be extremely difficult for adolescents who have been ridiculed or rejected during their childhood.

These barriers to full independence can, of course, be surmounted. Three factors are especially important in helping teenagers with Tourette syndrome make the final step to independence. First, your child must strike a reasonable balance between early successes and failures. For example, it is not necessarily a bad thing to start learning a musical instrument and then lose interest. Everyone can learn from mistakes. However, your child will likely feel better about giving up on music if she then takes up a sport or other leisure-time activity that she enjoys and sticks with for a reasonable length of time. Second, your child needs a real sense of support and encouragement from others—both inside and outside the home. Much of this support will come from you, the parent. But remember, teachers can also be strong advocates for your child and help out by teaching others about this disorder. Often, you need only give teachers the opportunity to learn about Tourette syndrome to enlist their support. And finally, your child herself must have access to a reasonable flow of accurate information about Tourette syndrome and its real or fictitious limitations. This kind of self-education about Tourette syndrome helps your child feel as if she has some control over a disorder that, by its nature, cause considerable difficulties in controlling movements and vocalizations.

Given this kind of head start, the chances are that your child will either conquer most developmental differences or learn to compensate for them satisfactorily. She will have every reason to hope for optimal employment, good relationships with friends and family, and good self-esteem. Most importantly, your child can grow up to be a healthy adult, capable of reaching her potential.

Conclusion

No two children develop in exactly the same way. Inborn strengths and weaknesses, as well as outside influences, all help to determine how quickly and easily children reach milestones on the way to adulthood. Your child, too, will follow her own path to maturity. Most likely, her path will not take her too far afield from other children's, although her Tourette Syndrome may make development more challenging.

As a parent, there are many steps you can take to minimize the effects of Tourette syndrome and associated disorders on your child's development. You can seek help from professionals with expertise in treating developmental delays. You can work with teachers to develop the educational program and classroom atmosphere best suited to your child's learning needs. And you can support your child's efforts with information and understanding. Remember, if you believe in your child as an individual whose Tourette syndrome is only one aspect of her total being, your child will also be more likely to see herself as someone with abilities, rather than disabilities.

Parent Statements

Children with TS seem to learn in big jumps, not in gradual, sustained progression. If your child is given the right kind of help, by the time he reaches high school, his behavior and ability to learn could be at an acceptable level.

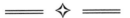

Kids with TS often seem to be two or three years behind their peers socially and emotionally. They prefer to play with younger children rather than children their own age. *Accept* this symptom of TS. By the time your child is an adult, he'll have developed his own way of fitting in. Love him and build up his self-esteem. He'll catch up in his own time.

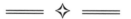

My son sometimes has problems with sensory integration. He doesn't seem to be aware of what's going on around him. He doesn't pick up clues about how to act, what to say, what's appropriate. He's like someone in a foreign country who doesn't know the language or the customs. He's not deliberately being obnoxious or outrageous. He really doesn't know any better and has to be carefully taught what's right and what's not. It's not his fault that he's out of step with the rest of the world. It's part of this neurological impairment called Tourette syndrome.

Concentrate on the abilities of your child with Tourette syndrome, not the disabilities.

The hardest thing is that we have a child who doesn't look like he has a handicap. But he acts extremely immature at times, trying to hide his tics by acting like a five-year-old. It's difficult, but we have to keep moving forward. We want to keep our son on the right track and work with his handicap.

TS can be compared to an electrical system that "shorts out" when it is overloaded, or to a computer that shuts down when it is overused. Kids with TS tend to shut down when they are bombarded by too many stimuli, too many directions, or too much activity. Anything that can be done to simplify your child's day, structure his activities, or help him to focus on only the most important skills or concepts to be learned will be helpful.

Kathy's handwriting is so messy that she has to take a lot of her tests orally.

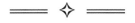

My son is so good at echolalia, I think it could lead to a career in international translation.

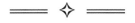

My son has incredible muscle tone from all his motor tics. That plus his high energy level makes him an asset on any sports team.

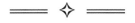

Give value to obsessions and channel your child's interests into positive endeavors.

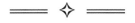

After six months of Sensory Integration therapy, my nine-year-old son is learning how to write, and his overall coordination has improved dramatically. He is learning how to stop and plan his actions rather than just acting impulsively.

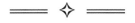

She used to lash out at anyone who touched her. After Sensory Integration therapy, she is much more tolerant of touch and has learned what kind of sensations and touch calm her down.

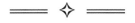

I never thought Dave would be able or willing to play a team sport. We were thrilled when he joined a soccer team in fourth grade. He's always enjoyed individual sports, but participating on a team was really an achievement for him.

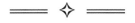

Although many children who have TS seem to have developmental delays, the same kids also have incredible talents in certain aspects of their development. It is up to parents and educators to nurture these special gifts and help each child reach his academic, social, and creative potential.

═══ ✧ ═══

SEVEN

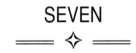

Educational Needs
of Children with
Tourette Syndrome

LARRY BURD, M.S.*

For some children, Tourette syndrome poses no special problems in the classroom. They keep up with the class in most, if not all subjects, discover special talents and interests, get along with most of their teachers and classmates, and eventually graduate with the academic, social, and vocational skills they need to fit into the adult world. But many children with TS cannot glide through school quite so easily. Because of their tics and other symptoms, they sometimes need extra help to achieve their potential in school.

The amount and type of help your child needs will depend on a variety of factors. First, your child may face special challenges in school, depending upon the severity of his tics and his attitude toward them. For example, if your child has loud, disruptive vocal tics or unusual motor tics such as touching or licking others, classmates may avoid or tease him. This can interfere with the development of social skills. And regardless of how disruptive your child's tics are, he may have trouble learning if he expends a great deal of energy suppressing them. He may concentrate so much

---

* Larry Burd is an assistant professor in the departments of Neuroscience and Pediatrics at the University of North Dakota School of Medicine. He is also an education specialist in the Child Evaluation and Treatment Program at the Medical Center Rehabilitation Hospital Clinic in Grand Forks, N.D. He has published over twenty-five professional papers on TS.

effort on not making sounds and movements that he has no energy left to accomplish his school work.

Conditions often associated with Tourette syndrome can also lead to problems in school. For instance, about 40 percent of children with Tourette syndrome have a learning disability in addition to their motor and vocal tics. Most often, these learning disabilities cause reading difficulties. Handwriting, spelling, and math problems are also very common. Attention deficit hyperactivity disorder (ADHD) is another condition that can make learning more difficult for children with Tourette syndrome. If your child has trouble concentrating his attention, shutting out distractions, or following instructions, he will obviously have problems learning.

Obsessive compulsive disorder (OCD) is yet another problem

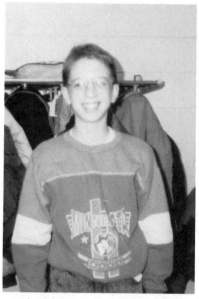 often associated with TS that can cause difficulties in the classroom. If your child must deal with obsessions, or unwanted, intrusive thoughts or images in school, he may have trouble concentrating. Compulsions, or actions your child feels a strong need to do, may also interrupt his work. For example, if your child has to silently count to 13 each time he thinks about the number 7, he will have difficulty completing his math assignments. If he is required to keep working when he feels he has germs on his hands and wants to wash them for the twentieth time that day, he may not be able to work as rapidly as he or the teacher would like. Many children with OCD have problems switching quickly from one task to another. They often feel they haven't finished the first task completely or that the work is not perfect or nearly so. As a result, they may become frustrated or irritable when they are asked to do something different or their schedule is changed.

Despite the long list of possible problems, few children with Tourette syndrome have all of them. In fact, about 50 percent of children with Tourette syndrome have educational problems that require only minor adaptations to allow them to make satisfactory progress in school. The other half can be helped through special educational programs tailored specifically to their needs. In time, the educational problems of many children in both groups become less severe. For about 60 percent of children with Tourette syndrome, educational difficulties peak between the ages of eleven and thirteen, then gradually begin to decrease.

To help you ensure that your child's school experience is as positive as possible, this chapter discusses how TS can cause problems for your child both inside and outside the regular classroom. It explains the concept of special education as well as why this may sometimes be the best route for children with Tourette syndrome. Finally, the chapter offers some specific solutions to common educational problems, and describes ways you can work with the school to help your child make the most of his school years.

The Right Educational Program for Your Child

Because Tourette syndrome can affect a child's abilities to learn in so many ways, there is no one right educational program. Discovering what is best for *your* child may take some trial and error. Most often, children with Tourette syndrome start out in a regular classroom with their classmates of the same age. Extra help is usually needed only if they fail to achieve at the level of their ability in social, emotional, or academic areas.

Even if your child's grades are good and his teachers do not report any special difficulties, it is wise to monitor your child for problem areas once a diagnosis of Tourette syndrome is made. If he is having academic, social, or emotional problems in school or at home, he should be evaluated to determine the extent of the problem and to develop an appropriate intervention plan. This evaluation should be conducted by a "TS team" made up of you and your spouse, your child's physician, school personnel, and a resource person with expertise in developing management strategies for Tourette syndrome and the associated behaviors. Request that your school form a TS team if one is not already available. Figure 1 illustrates the TS team concept.

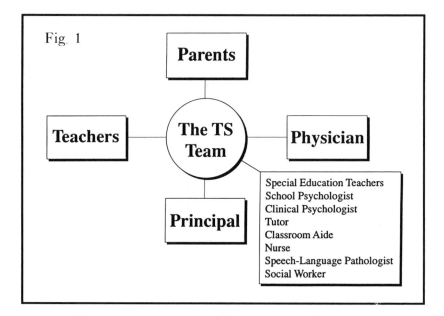

Fig. 1

Parents

Teachers

The TS Team

Physician

Principal

Special Education Teachers
School Psychologist
Clinical Psychologist
Tutor
Classroom Aide
Nurse
Speech-Language Pathologist
Social Worker

From an academic standpoint, the TS team needs to evaluate reading, spelling, math, and handwriting skills, as well as your child's ability to pay attention and concentrate. From an emotional standpoint, the team should look at how well your child accepts his disorder and how it affects his relationship with his teacher and the development of his self-image. Finally, the team needs to evaluate your child's social abilities: how well he gets along with others in his class, on the playground, at lunch, and with his siblings.

Once this evaluation is completed, the TS team should meet and recommend one of two courses of action. They will either recommend that your child continue in the regular classroom with adaptations made for his special needs, or they will recommend that your child be considered for special education outside of the classroom. As a member of the team, it is your responsibility to decide whether these recommendations or parts of them are appropriate for your child. Each of these options is discussed below.

The Regular Classroom

Within the regular classroom, your child may have academic or social problems that keep him from reaching his full potential. The TS team should work together to develop strategies to help him overcome these problems while remaining in his regular class. This should be the first option for children with problems in school.

Of course, before the teacher can understand how Tourette syndrome is affecting your child educationally, she needs a basic understanding of what TS is and is not. Too many adults misinterpret motor and vocal tics as nervous mannerisms or deliberate misbehavior. They often believe a child can control his tics—an impression that seems to be borne out when they ask the child to "quit it," and he is temporarily able to suppress his tics. Because attentional problems may vary in severity, the teacher might also incorrectly assume that since a child worked for twenty minutes on Tuesday, he should be able to do so every day. Most teachers see only four or five children with Tourette syndrome during their entire teaching career, and may therefore also have many other misconceptions.

To make sure all school staff involved with your child understand his specific symptoms and needs, the school should have a yearly inservice program on TS for all school personnel involved with your child. This session should be conducted by a knowledgeable professional such as a representative from the nearest TS clinic or a teacher experienced in working with children with TS. You should also be present so that you can answer specific questions about how TS affects your child. The inservice should explain not only the symptoms that your child has now, but also the full range of symptoms and behaviors that may appear in the future. This is important because symptoms sometimes change from year to year and many symptoms present at the beginning of the year will not be present at the end of the year. In addition to discussing your child's problems, you and school personnel should have an opportunity to discuss proposed interventions, or ways of handling TS behaviors in class and of helping your child adjust and learn. These inservice sessions should be repeated on a yearly basis, since teaching the second grade teacher about Tourette syndrome does not help the third grade teacher. A video on TS is not sufficient for an inservice program, although videos and pamphlets can be used to supplement the program and provide examples of TS symptoms. The cost of inservice training *should* be a school responsibility. If your school doesn't readily agree to pay the costs, contact the TSA or other parents for help convincing the school district of its obligation.

Handling Symptoms in the Classroom

Educating the teacher about Tourette syndrome not only makes her more sensitive to your child's educational needs, but also to his emotional needs. Most importantly, it can help her understand that by ignoring your child's tics, she can help reduce stress and, as a result, the number and intensity of your child's tics. And because of the teacher's unique position as a role model, it is important for her to set an appropriate example. If the teacher ignores your child's tics, your child's classmates are much more likely to be able to ignore them.

Even if everyone in the class successfully ignores your child's tics, your child may still be quite aware of his own sounds and movements. Although this self-consciousness may lead your child to try to suppress his tics, this is not a good idea as a general rule. Suppressing multiple motor and phonic tics requires considerable amounts of attention and effort. If your child expends much of his mental energy and attention on holding back tics, he may not be

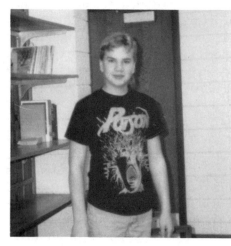

able to concentrate and work up to his ability in school. Consequently, you should work with the teacher to develop ways for your child to release his tics in relative privacy. For example, your child might be seated near the classroom door so that whenever he feels the need, he can get up, walk down the hall for a drink of water, and discharge his motor tics. Or the teacher might allow him to periodically walk to the front of the classroom and sharpen a pencil or go into the bathroom to discharge vocal tics. But remember, as important as these strategies are, it is just as important to have the teacher set an example by ignoring the tics and concentrating on getting the class's assignments completed. If your child's tics are quite disruptive, he may be prescribed medication. This may or may not enable him to control his tics. If it does not, the next step may be to try to substitute a positive behavior that is incompatible with the tic. That is, your child can be taught to do something that is similar, but more socially acceptable than a particular tic. For example, if your child has a spitting tic, he might be asked to try swallowing instead. If he licks other people, have him lick his teeth. If he touches or pokes others, have him poke a rabbit's foot or some other object he has in his pocket or on his belt. This strategy often decreases the problem tic markedly. About a third of the time, the symptom will disappear over a few weeks. This type of symptom substitution should only be tried after considerable planning and discussion among the TS team.

Social Problems

Sometimes a child's symptoms may interfere with the development of normal social relationships. A child who has ADHD in addition to TS may often be "in trouble" because of his behavior. If he is walking around when he is supposed to be sitting down doing his work or he is talking when he is supposed to be listening, the other children quickly figure out that doing things with him will often get them into trouble too. As a result, many children may avoid the child with TS to avoid getting into trouble. Other children may also avoid your child if he has tics that attract attention, such as sniffing, barking, or snorting, or tics that involve kicking, touching, or patting others.

If your child's symptoms result in significant social difficulties, you, the teacher, and the TS team will need to develop ways to combat this problem. The first goal should be to design a positive and reward-oriented program focusing on the behaviors you would like to see *increase* in frequency. All too often, schools begin with a list of problem behaviors and concentrate on eliminating them. They count how many times Billy gets up out of his seat, how many spelling problems he doesn't finish, how often he talks out of turn.

But they do not keep track of how often he's sitting in his seat, how many spelling problems he gets done, or how often he holds up his hand or waits his turn before he talks. Clearly, these are the behaviors to focus on. The more attention is paid to a particular behavior, the more likely a child is to repeat it.

An important key in improving behavior is to determine what your child finds rewarding and link that reward with a behavior you would like to see more often. For some children, praise may be rewarding; others need more tangible rewards such as smiley faces or gold stars on their papers or permission to do something fun. Generally, school personnel should link one particular reward with each different behavior they want to improve. For example, rather than using tokens that can be exchanged for treats to reinforce four or five different behaviors, it may be better to reward one behavior with time playing computer games, another behavior with a special visit to the library, and a third behavior with tokens.

Rewarding behaviors can be quite time-consuming for teachers. First, because rewards are only effective if they are given consistently, the teacher has to make sure she rewards your child every time he does as he is supposed to. Second, to determine whether rewards are actually working, the teacher must count the frequency of your child's behaviors both before and after beginning the reward program. As a result, it is best if a teacher begins by concentrating on one or two behaviors at the most. It is unlikely that a classroom teacher by herself could deal with more than three behaviors at a time. After all, if she has too much to do, she may not be able to accurately record the behaviors or give rewards consistently—let alone teach the other members of the class.

Academic Problems

If your child is having academic difficulties, it is a good idea to first find out why. For example, if he has trouble finishing work on time, is it because he is using all his energy to suppress tics? Does he have a compulsion to erase the words over and over until they are perfect? Is it because his medications make him feel dull and slow his thinking? The TS team needs this information in order to understand the problem and develop an appropriate intervention strategy.

Many children with Tourette syndrome have academic difficulties not because they cannot *do* the work, but because they cannot *complete* it. As noted above, this could be due to tics, attentional problems, or obsessions or compulsions. Often it is helpful to break the work up into shorter segments. For example, instead of giving a child twenty math problems to solve, give him seven, five, or three at a time, several times a day. Then, as his work habits improve, the teacher can increase the number of problems she gives him each time.

Stress is another factor that can affect academic performance. The stress of taking a test, for example, may increase your child's tics and make it harder for him to concentrate. If so, it may help if the teacher gives him more time to finish or allows him to take the test in a separate room.

A peer tutor—a classmate or older child who is doing well in school—may also be able to help your child. The peer tutor can work with your child side by side during school, or help him after school. For example, a tutor might help your child do his work by reminding him to finish his last two problems or by setting a good example and not talking with your child when he is doing his seat work. A sensitive, accepting older tutor can also be very helpful in improving your child's socialization skills and expanding opportunities for social activities.

This section has provided only a brief rundown of ways to handle common problems within the regular classroom. For additional strategies that can be helpful both in the regular classroom and in the special education classroom, see the section at the end of this chapter on "Common Problems and Solutions."

Special Education

If your child has significant academic or social problems despite in-class modifications, he may be considered for special education. Special education is instruction that is individually tailored to meet the unique learning needs of children with disabilities. The goal of special education services is to enable children to learn as well as possible so that they are eventually able to live the most independent lives possible. Consequently, special education does not just focus on helping children overcome difficulties in academic subjects such as reading, math, and history. It also includes special therapeutic or other services designed to help children overcome difficulties in all areas of development. By law, a child's special education program must include all special services, or "related services," necessary for him to benefit from his educational program. These services are provided by one or more professionals trained in working with children with special needs. For children with Tourette syndrome, related services may include speech therapy, physical therapy, nursing services, inservice training, and a wide range of adaptations in a child's regular school program.

Special education is not an all or nothing proposition. Receiving special education services doesn't necessarily mean that your child will be sent to a different room all day—he might take all or part of his subjects in the regular classroom. For instance, if your child has a learning disability that makes reading harder for him, he may receive special help from a tutor or work on his reading with a learning disabilities teacher in a separate room. Then again, the teacher in the regular class may simply modify your child's materials or her method of teaching reading to help your child learn. Remember, the key is an individualized program to meet your child's unique needs.

The Assessment Process

Before your child can receive special education services, he must first be declared "eligible." As Chapter 8 explains, federal laws govern who can qualify for special education. Only children with a "handicapping condition" which prevents them from making appropriate progress in a regular classroom can receive special educational services at public expense. Children with Tourette syndrome may qualify for services if they have a learning disability, or they may qualify as "other health impaired." The important thing to remember is that once qualified, your child will be eligible for programming for the full range of his educational needs.

To determine whether your child needs and qualifies for special education, you or a school staff member must first make a referral for a special education assessment, often to the principal. This assessment cannot be conducted unless you give your permission. Once you give the go-ahead, your child's learning needs will be assessed, or evaluated, by a *multidisciplinary assessment team*. As the name implies, this team will be made up of specialists with different areas of expertise. Usually, the same professionals that are on the TS team are a part of the multidisciplinary team.

To evaluate your child's abilities in each developmental area, members of the team will observe your child, collect data on his performance in the classroom, interview you and your child's teachers about his strengths and needs, and give him formal tests. The goal of this testing is two-fold: first to identify problem areas, and second to identify areas of strength that could potentially be used to compensate for the difficulties. For example, if homework is a major problem area for your child but he enjoys being at school, he could stay after school for twenty minutes to work on his math rather than doing it at home. In identifying problem areas, the team members will also try to determine whether a learning disability or some other underlying problem is interfering with your child's progress. For this reason, the multidisciplinary team will request input from your child's physician about the diagnosis, other associated difficulties such as attention deficit disorder or obsessive-compulsive disorder, and side effects of any medication your child might be taking. It is also important that the physician provide information on the benefits of medications your child is taking so that the school is not misled by the apparent lack of symptoms. After all, the purpose of the medication is to suppress symptoms. But if school personnel don't observe the symptoms, they may doubt the diagnosis. This information is essential in the early phases of planning a program for your child. With your consent, the physician can send his report to the school, or he can provide the TS team with the essential information through a phone conversation.

After each team member has gathered information in his or her area of expertise, the team will meet to share their findings with one another. Together they will develop a comprehensive summary report of your child's strengths and needs in all areas. At this meeting, the team members will discuss with you what they have discovered about your child's learning abilities and disabilities. The team, including the parents, will also decide whether your child is recommended for special education. If you disagree with their recommendation, you may request a second assessment. Chapter 8 explains how.

Developing an Educational Plan

If your child qualifies for special education, the next step is to develop a plan to meet his unique learning needs. This plan, known as an Individualized Education Program (IEP), will be designed jointly by you and school staff at one or more IEP meetings.

Your child's IEP will describe each of the areas in which your child has learning problems, as well as how the school plans to help your child overcome these problems. For each area, precise, measurable, long-term goals will be set. For example, if your son has trouble spelling, a goal might be for him to pass the semester test. This overall goal would be broken down into smaller, short-term goals. For example, he might be expected to learn seven spelling words a week, or perhaps, two spelling words a day. If your child has difficulty concentrating because of ADHD, a long-term goal might be to complete ten math problems in fifteen minutes. As a short-term goal, he might be expected to do five in fifteen minutes, then gradually work up to six, seven, or eight in fifteen minutes. Short- and long-term goals could likewise be set for a child with the OCD symptoms of writing, erasing, and rewriting until the work is perfect. If the ultimate goal is to have him write all his spelling sentences without erasing, a short-term goal might be to limit him to eight erasures, then seven, then six, and so on. Use of a computer or typewriter might also help him make his letters "perfect," and therefore limit erasures. In choosing these goals, it is also important to choose rewards that will help motivate your child to work towards those goals. Sometimes, for example, it is helpful to reward a child with less work if he does as he is supposed to. For example, if your child has fifteen math problems and does ten in twelve minutes, he might be rewarded by being told he doesn't have to do the other five.

Goals to help your child with problems in areas other than academic subjects will also be set if the TS team agrees there is a need for additional services. For example, if he is having difficulty making or keeping friends, his IEP might include goals designed to help him learn to socialize. His IEP might call for him to select one classmate each week to go out with for a soft drink. He would then practice this set of skills until it goes well, then move on to another situation. Developing social skills is extremely important for children with Tourette syndrome. It may also be more difficult for them because they have a wide range of behaviors that are not completely under control. These behaviors may drive potential friends away. After all, most children quickly learn that if you hang around with Don and Don gets in trouble, you will also probably get in trouble at the same time. This is why it is so important that teachers focus on positive behaviors and try to ignore negative behaviors as much as possible.

Your child's IEP will specify who is to work with him on each goal. This might be the regular classroom teacher, the classroom teacher and a peer tutor, or a school aide. Or your child might need to work with a special education teacher or tutor specially trained in teaching children with special learning needs. The IEP will also specify where your child is to receive this instruction—within the regular classroom or in a learning resources room. Generally, children receive services outside of the regular classroom only if they cannot work up to their level of ability with the modifications tried in the regular classroom. If your child does need to leave the regular classroom, it may just be to work on one particular subject or one skill. For example, your child might see the learning disabilities teacher once a day for special help in reading, but receive all his other lessons with the rest of the class. If his symptoms are so severe that they cannot be managed in the regular classroom with adaptations or do not respond to medication, he may require longer periods out of the classroom. In some cases, teachers (who are human and have all the limitations that trouble the rest of us) simply cannot deal appropriately with a child's behavior. If another teacher is not available, and support and training do not help the teacher deal with the child's behavior, then some out-of-class placement may be the only practical option.

The following basic principles may help you or school personnel in designing an effective IEP for your child:

1. Focus on positive behavior. Try to build on your child's strengths. If he has good attention but poor handwriting, for example, it may help to have him use a computer or calculator for more of his work.
2. Set goals based on what your child can *usually* do, not on what he can do on his best days. This is especially important because of the waxing and waning of TS symptoms. When your child's tics (head turning, eye squinting) are at low levels, he will naturally be able to concentrate on his work better than when he turns his head thirty times an hour or squints twenty times every eight minutes.
3. Provide support and motivation to increase skills. Pay attention to positive behaviors and use positive reinforcement whenever possible. Be flexible—adjust the work load on more difficult days.
4. Expect performance to be variable. As his tics and associated behaviors vary, so will his performance in school.

In developing an educational program, it is essential to carefully weigh the pros and cons of all decisions. All members of the TS team should give thought to their decisions and to their short- and long-term effects on the child. As a parent, you should weigh the risks and benefits of anything proposed by the team before consenting to a program for your child. For example, are the benefits of special education greater than the problems? Is the benefit of medication greater than the side effects? This balancing process is difficult because each child is unique and each situation is different. Often if comes down to deciding to try a given strategy or program briefly and then evaluate the results. Figure 2 shows a process that schools can use to develop appropriate placement recommendations and interventions for a child with Tourette syndrome.

Monitoring Progress

By federal law, your child is entitled to receive special education until the age of twenty-one, if he needs it. But once your child begins receiving special education, it does not necessarily mean he will be in special education all his school years. Depending on your child's needs, the duration of his special education services may vary. Each year, you and the school personnel will review his progress at a meeting called an annual review. You will discuss whether he is learning faster or slower than expected, and whether the goals set in his IEP were too high or too low. Your conclusions will be incorporated into a new IEP for the coming year.

Every three years, at a minimum, your child will receive a *triennial evaluation*—a complete assessment conducted by the multidisciplinary team described above. After evaluating your child, this team will determine whether your child still has needs that require special education. If he does not, they will recommend that he no longer receive special education. You and your child's teachers may also request that your child be given a triennial evaluation sooner than scheduled if you think a special education placement is no longer right for him.

To Label or Not to Label?

Often when parents are asked to consider special education for their child, they worry about the possibility of the twin "stigmas" of having their child labeled "disabled" and given an out-of-class placement. Clearly, in the best of all worlds, children would not have problems like TS or attention deficit disorder. This, however, is

Fig. 2

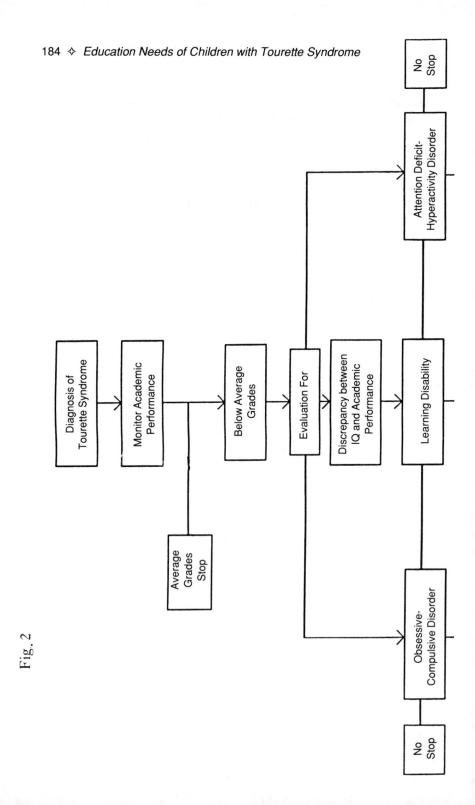

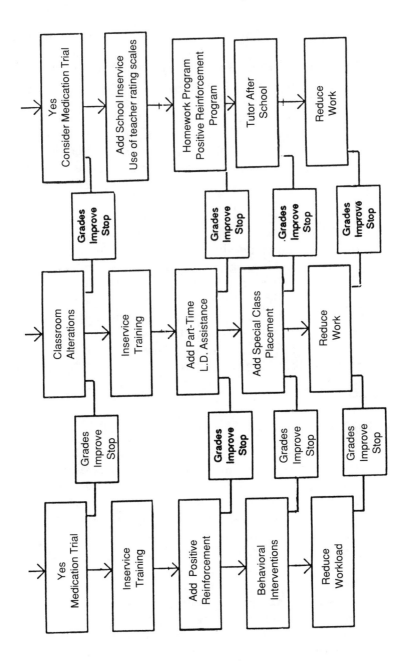

simply not the world we live in, and many children *do* require additional help in school.

Unfortunately, there is some stigma attached to anyone who is different and requires extra help. Even in the first grade, children can quickly recognize the top reading group—whether it's called the Bluebirds or the Beavers—and they can also recognize the "lower" reading groups. Differences are not something we should try to hide. Instead, we should try to equip children to see these differences *and* the inherent value in each person as an individual—whether they have difficulty with handwriting, reading, or sitting still.

It's true that requiring children to have a "handicapping condition" to be eligible for special education can be construed as labeling the child. But you could also view this as giving the child every opportunity to do his best and live up to his potential. Depriving your child of these services because you fear how he may react to a label may not be in his best interests. This is particularly true if your child will have significant academic and social problems if he tries to manage on his own, but could conquer these problems with additional help in school. Your child may even feel relieved to be doing something about a problem that he knows sets him apart from other children.

Common Problems and Solutions

There are no foolproof methods for dealing with the educational problems TS can cause. But there are many methods that are often effective, whether your child is taught in a regular education or special education setting. To help you and your child's teacher handle potential difficulties, some of these common problems and possible solutions are described below.

Tics

Tics and Stress. It is important that teachers know that stress often causes tics to become more frequent or pronounced. For example, taking tests, giving a speech, or being teased or punished may cause tics to increase. Increasing your child's involvement in enjoyable activities such as sports or music can help reduce stress. Often children with TS do not have as much time to do enjoyable things as other kids do. Parents should keep track of their child's free time and encourage their child to participate fully in available activities.

Waxing and Waning of Tics. There are several things teachers need to understand about the tendency of tics to wax and wane. First, they should know that even though symptoms will change over time and appear milder at some times than at others, this does not mean tics are under your child's control. Furthermore, if they ask your child to suppress his tics, he may feel increased stress and have less energy to devote to his school

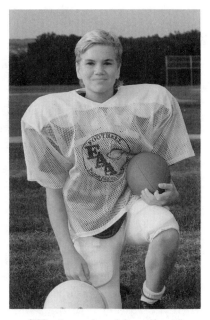

work. Second, if your child has severe TS, they should realize that it may be necessary to have two educational plans—a fall-back plan for those days when his symptoms are at their most disruptive, and another program for his average day. For example, on the most difficult days, your child may be given more breaks, more activities outside the class, and shorter assignments.

In setting overall educational goals for your child, it is important that you and the school staff consider how he does on an average day. If you go to a junior high basketball game, you might occasionally see a child make eight or nine shots in a row. This is not what you would expect or demand from this child at each subsequent basketball game. Rather, you would recognize that this is an unusual performance that was considerably different from the average performance. Likewise, on an exceptional day, a child with ADHD and TS might get his math done in class and stay seated during the entire class period. But on an average day he may complete ten out of fifteen math problems with four reminders and get out of his desk three times. Expectations should be based on his average performance, rather than on what he can do on an exceptional day.

Motor and Vocal Tics. The general rule for motor and vocal tics is to ignore them. Teachers should not encourage or reward your child for not having tics, as this may encourage him to suppress them. Instead, teachers should provide a place for your child to go to release his tics when necessary. Asking the teacher to explain Tourette syndrome and the difficulties your child faces may also help foster an accepting atmosphere in the classroom. Rarely, your child's motor tics may be a safety consideration—for example, in shop class or chemistry. In this case, the TS team may recommend an alternate activity for your child. Finally, if your child has tics that are particularly distracting to other children, there are several strategies to try. Consult with your physician about the use of medication, and with the other members of the TS team about behaviors that could possibly be substituted for tics such as kissing or pinching others.

Mental Tics. Some children with Tourette syndrome need to repeat words, numbers, or phrases to themselves. Children with these kinds of mental tics should be given extra time to come up with the response to questions, to complete assignments, and to refocus their attention from one activity to another. In addition, it often helps to break assignments into shorter segments. Making it easier for the child to predict what is going to be next may also increase his ability to complete his work. For this reason, the teacher and the TS team may need to work together to develop a schedule for the child that can be followed consistently.

Obsessive-Compulsive Behaviors

The most common obsessions and compulsions are listed in Table 1.

Table 1
Common Obsessions and Compulsions
Compulsions or Rituals

Placing objects just right
Touching things
Rechecking
Smelling

Licking
Erasing
Writing and rewriting letters until they are perfect
Washing hands repeatedly

Obsessive Thoughts

Mental echolalia—repeating words, phrases
  to oneself
Obscene thoughts
Counting or grouping
Sexual thoughts
Thinking about forbidden actions—standing on
  desk at school, kissing teacher, touching
  others sexually
Thinking about exposing oneself
Fear of hurting someone

The treatment of these problems is complex. Nearly always, a clinical psychologist and a physician will need to be involved, since medication can be very helpful. Chapter 3 discusses medical treatments that may be helpful in controlling OCD symptoms.

The first step in managing OCD behaviors at school is generally to develop an understanding of the symptom and its frequency. For example, writing and rewriting letters until they are perfect is a common symptom. To manage this symptom, the teacher needs to begin by counting how often the child erases his work, and then gradually limit the number of times he is allowed to erase.

In treating obsessions, it is often helpful to set time limits for certain tasks. For example, if it takes a child eight minutes to write two sentences, the time allowed should gradually be reduced by 10 or 15 second intervals. Although many children with OCD are very slow workers, they can often learn to work more quickly if their time is limited in this manner.

Behavior Problems

Anger or Aggression. If your child has difficulty controlling anger or aggression in the classroom, it may help if teachers allow him to channel his aggression into physical movement. For example, he might be permitted to walk down the hall for a drink of water or to lie down and pedal in the air. Relaxation techniques may also be helpful. If appropriate, a clinical psychologist can provide your child with a tape of relaxation exercises to keep in class and listen to with headphones when he needs to calm down. In addition, it is important to provide explanations for those likely to be the target of aggression. The TS team or teacher should lead the discussion with the other students, emphasizing that the child with TS cannot help his behavior, and that other children should not take his aggression personally. The TS team should be sure to let the other students know how to react and what to do if they witness aggressive behavior.

Restlessness. If your child is unable to sit still or fidgets constantly, he should be allowed to move about safely and freely as needed. Restlessness should be reported to your physician, as it is a frequent symptom of ADHD and is sometimes a side effect of medications used to control tics. As discussed earlier, a positive reward program can also be very helpful in encouraging your child to do his work and complete his assignments.

Difficulty Disciplining Your Child. If your child's behavior causes problems in the classroom, teachers should first try to control it with positive behavior management. That is, rather than punishing your child for inappropriate behavior, they should focus on the behavior they would like to increase in frequency. In particular, they need to understand that they should never punish your child for tics, because the stress of punishment may increase his tics.

It is essential to make sure behavior is managed the same way at home as it is at school. Otherwise, your child will get mixed messages about which behavior is acceptable and which is not. For example, if both parents and teachers ignore a child when he has a tantrum, the child is less likely to use tantrums as a way of getting attention. But if parents give in to their child's wishes when he has a tantrum at home, then he is more likely to resort to tantrums at school, too, even if teachers try to ignore his behavior.

Attentional Problems

Many children with Tourette syndrome also have attention deficit hyperactivity disorder. As a result, they may have poor concentration, be quite distractible, and have trouble finishing their work. In general, ADHD in children with TS can be handled the same ways it would be in children without TS. As with behavior problems, the best way to handle symptoms of ADHD is through positive behavior management. Teachers should focus on the behaviors that they would like to increase in frequency. For example, rather than counting how many times your child does not finish his work, they should count how many problems he completed and how many reminders were necessary to get it done.

Keeping frustration at manageable levels also helps. Your child should not be given more work than he can handle comfortably, and assignments should be shortened if he cannot complete them otherwise. Rather than guessing, the teacher should make sure the length of the assignment really is within your child's capability. Your child should be encouraged to complete tasks before being given any rewards. No child can be expected to develop appropriate work habits if he is overloaded with work and then punished when he cannot do the work.

As your child grows older, he will probably need extra help developing individual work and study skills. Using study guides or outlines provided by the teacher may help him stay focused while studying. Positive reinforcement will also continue to be important.

Some children with ADHD and TS may learn better outside of the regular classroom. It may be easier for them to concentrate and learn in a resource room where there are fewer distractions and where they can receive more individualized attention from teachers. This step may be recommended if your child fails to work up to the level of his ability and if modifications within the regular classroom do not improve his performance.

See the chart at the end of this chapter for more information on the symptoms of ADHD at different age levels and additional treatment suggestions.

Learning Disabilities

As mentioned earlier, about 40 percent of children with TS have learning disabilities. That is, there is a discrepancy between their ability to learn and their achievement which is not due to poor hearing or vision, poor school attendance, or limited proficiency in English. Learning disabilities affect three times as many boys as girls. The most common learning disabilities are in reading, spelling, handwriting, and math. Reading problems account for about half of all learning disabilities and may make it difficult for a child to say the words he reads (decoding difficulties), comprehend the words, or both. Spelling and handwriting problems are also very common and often occur together with reading problems or language disorders. Children with learning disabilities in math may have difficulty with calculation problems only, or have both calculation difficulties and difficulties with mathematical reasoning (understanding).

If learning disabilities are suspected, an evaluation by the multidisciplinary team described earlier is essential. This is because handwriting and math difficulties can also be the result of ADHD, and if so, will usually improve when treated with the medications discussed in Chapter 3. In the case of bona fide learning disabilities, the first step is usually to modify a child's regular curriculum. Your child may be able to make satisfactory progress with a tutor, reduced amounts of work, and positive reinforcement. With the emphasis on how much he is able to do, rather than on how much he can't do, your child's motivation may increase. Other in-class modifications might include oral tests and taped notes from the teacher for children with reading difficulties or the use of a calculator for children with calculation difficulties. Likewise, computers can help children with handwriting problems make considerable improvement in their ability to express themselves in writing. Most of these programs also have a spelling program which allows the child to use any word he wants without having to worry about how to spell it correctly.

As mentioned earlier, if in-class modifications are not enough to enable children with learning disabilities to progress in the regular classroom, they may attend classes in a special resource room for part of the day. There they can benefit from instructional methods and materials specifically designed to help children with learning disabilities. The Reading List at the back of the book lists several publications that describe these teaching methods in detail.

The education program for each child with learning disabilities must be individually tailored to his unique needs. It must also be reviewed at least once a year so that any changes necessary can be made. This is because most children's learning disabilities and tics become less severe as they reach adolescence. If their motivation and desire to do well are nurtured when they are young, their academic abilities will usually improve during adolescence and into adulthood.

Medications

As a parent, you need to ask your child's physician for detailed, current information about any medications prescribed for your child. If the teacher is to administer your child's drugs, make sure she understands how and when to do so. Be sure also to educate the teacher about the side effects and effectiveness of these drugs. Ask her to report side effects to you and to let you know if the drugs are having the desired result. The teacher should be especially watchful for signs of cognitive dulling, lethargy, seeming lack of interest, and decrease in coordination. If these side effects appear, have your child re-evaluated by his physician and find out whether medication can be adjusted or given in the evening. If necessary, ask the teacher to allow your child extra time for studying and test-taking, and request a tutor if appropriate.

School Phobia

A small number of children with TS develop a school phobia—a strong avoidance of school (not wanting to leave home and go to school). Children wake up in the morning complaining of headaches, stomach problems, or other vague symptoms that they hope will keep them home from school. Attempts by parents to get the child to school may result in clinging and loud, tearful complaints. The child may also voice a wide range of fears about going to school—for example, "I'm afraid of the teacher" or "The other kids tease me." In severe cases, children may miss months of school if this problem is not successfully treated. Even in milder cases, frequent absences can result in serious disagreements between parents and school personnel.

School phobias are sometimes caused in part by medications such as Haldol™ or Orap™ used to treat Tourette syndrome. If so, a change of medication may help. Often, however, school phobias require treatment by a team made up of the physician, a psychologist, school personnel, and family. See Chapter 3 for information on drug side effects, as well as on choosing and working with physicians and psychologists.

Social and Emotional Problems

Because of their differences, children with Tourette syndrome often feel isolated from their classmates. To help your child cope with loneliness or depression, the TS team should develop a plan to increase his self-esteem. For example, his teacher might praise him for even minor accomplishments and help him to recognize his special talents. All members of the team also need to encourage your child to participate in group and social activities.

Adults both at home and at school must make a concerted effort to prevent your child from being teased by other children. Teasing is tolerated far too often in the schools and is devastating to a child's self-esteem. When teasing occurs, it is not your child's fault. Rather, it results from the inability of teachers and other adults to control the behavior of other children. Teachers and principals must explain to other children that TS symptoms are not under your child's control, and that teasing will not be tolerated in school. Films from the TSA can be helpful in opening up discussions about Tourette syndrome in the classroom. All school staff must be aware of your child's TS so that when he is teased on the playground or in the lunchroom, they will know how to intervene. As a parent, be prepared to counter arguments from school personnel that it is not possible or reasonable for them to limit teasing. Ask the teacher how she would like it if her peers made fun of her in school and she was unable to use the bathrooms at school without the principal going with her. Ask the principal how she would feel if her peers pursued her home each night. School personnel must teach acceptance of differences, and school must be a safe place for each child.

If persistent teasing occurs outside the school, it is a more complex matter. You may be able to help by contacting the parent of the child who is teasing your child and politely explaining the situation to him or her. It often helps if you emphasize that you do not think the other child is deliberately being cruel, but that he just doesn't understand that the TS symptoms are really out of your child's control.

Because your child may have a variety of social and emotional problems related to school, it is important to encourage him to talk about his feelings on a 1-to-1 basis with you. You might also encourage him to join a peer group in which he can discuss his experiences with other children with Tourette syndrome (or other disabilities). The Tourette Syndrome Association can help you locate a group for your child.

Handwriting

Some children with Tourette syndrome have great difficulty with handwriting. These problems may be due to motor tics or related to the ADHD that many children with TS have. Solutions to these handwriting problems include allowing your child to use a tape recorder rather than requiring him to take written notes; permitting him to use a classmate's notes; assigning him oral, rather than written reports; providing him with a typewriter or word processor. Teachers should be especially flexible in designing alternate ways for your child to take tests. They might, for example, give essay tests orally. Or on computerized tests that require your child to fill in a small circle to indicate his answer, they might allow him to write his answers on a separate sheet of paper and then later transfer his responses to the answer sheet.

Homework

For children with Tourette syndrome, homework is often work not finished in school because of ADHD, mental tics, or handwriting problems. If your child routinely has trouble completing his schoolwork, work with your child's teacher to set a level where work can be finished in a timely fashion. For example, instead of expecting your child to do twenty math problems in a row, have him do three, then take a break, do three more, and then take another break.

Not surprisingly, the same problems that make it difficult for children with TS to complete their work at school also make it difficult for them to complete their homework. In addition, they often have trouble getting organized, getting started, and staying on task. As a parent, you can help your child with the organizational problem by setting aside a special place for him to do homework and making sure the area is kept stocked with pencils, paper, dictionaries, and other school supplies. It may also be helpful to set aside a specific time every day for homework. You might even want to establish a quiet hour for the whole family to spend reading or doing homework.

Although you may need to be more directly involved in your child's homework than you would if he did not have Tourette

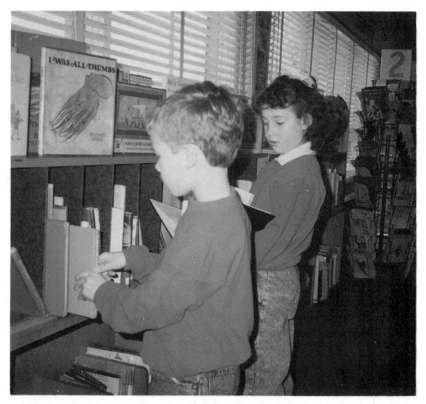

syndrome, it is important not to do too much for him. Don't let him take advantage of your extra help. Your aim should be to work with him to develop his skills so that eventually he can do the work independently.

Parent-School Relationships

Parents of children with Tourette syndrome often start out on the wrong foot with their child's school. Frequently, problems develop before a diagnosis of Tourette syndrome is reached. Even though parents insist that their child cannot control his behavior, schools may attempt to punish the child for his tics. Or schools may punish children who cannot complete their work due to ADHD or learning disabilities. Then, once Tourette syndrome is diagnosed, parents may feel the diagnosis gives a sense of legitimacy to problems the school has previously seen as willful misbehavior. They may have a strong desire to go up to school personnel and tell them what they *really* think about their past programs. As much as you may feel like saying "I told you so" to the school, this is a tactic that clearly should be avoided. Before you will be able to work together with school staff to develop the best educational plan for your child, you must develop a relationship based on mutual respect. This means you may have to forget many past wrongs so that you can look ahead to ways you can improve things for your child. Simply stated, what's past is past, and rarely does it do any good to continue to point out to the school that they were wrong and you were right.

A more constructive approach to dealing with the school is to try to foster an improved climate in which to meet and discuss changes. As discussed earlier, it is wise to arrange for an inservice training program to let school personnel learn about Tourette syndrome and how it affects your child. Showing one or two video tapes from the TSA and sharing this book may also help.

Once the school personnel have a better understanding of Tourette syndrome, try asking them what they think would be some appropriate programming suggestions in light of their new knowledge. Afterwards, sort through this information and select the goals and objectives and strategies which you feel are appropriate. In other words, don't criticize any inappropriate ideas the school has, but focus on those that are useful. This enables you to apply a little positive reinforcement to school personnel for their efforts. Next, contribute some of your own ideas of goals and techniques that would be helpful at school. By using this strategy, you can often uncover major areas of agreement where before it looked as though there was little common ground. This will also leave fewer points of disagreement to be resolved in developing your child's education program.

If your child is receiving special education services, both you and the school will, of course, have to follow the steps outlined in Public Law 94–142. (See Chapter 8 for a thorough explanation of this important federal education law.) In this situation, it is especially vital that school personnel recognize that you have valuable ideas to contribute to the IEP. To ensure that school staff take your suggestions seriously, you may wish to bring one or two people along to the meeting. A friend, experienced parent, or professional advocate can make sure you cover everything you want to cover and provide invaluable emotional support.

Even if you deal with all school personnel in exactly the same way, you will probably find that some are more accepting and supportive of your child than others. If you look back through your child's academic history, you will usually find that things went better with some teachers than with others. Try to enlist the support and help of the teachers who have had particular success in working with your child. Ask them to be involved in educational planning for your child as long as it's feasible and as long as they have ideas to contribute.

Above all, keep the lines of communication between you and your child's teachers open. Encourage them to let you know when your child is doing well *and* not so well in school. Many parents find it is helpful to keep in touch through regular meetings, through phone calls to the teacher, or by exchanging a notebook in which they and their child's teachers record progress and problems. Try to anticipate problems that might result from a change of medication—and let teachers know ahead of time. You need to make sure they understand that you are committed to helping them help your child, *and* to making the parent-professional partnership work.

Conclusion

Tourette syndrome can be a challenging disorder for schools, parents, and children to deal with. But with sensitive and knowledgeable planning, most children with Tourette syndrome can make good progress in school. As a parent, you can do a great deal to ensure your child's continued progress: first, by making sure that your child's motivation to attend school and learn remain high; and second, by advising school personnel of special learning needs and strengths that they may not be aware of. By enlisting the support of enlightened educational and medical personnel you *can* help your child learn the skills he needs to live up to his potential. No child deserves anything less.

References

Fisher, W., L. Burd, D.P. Kunce, and D. Berg. "Attention Deficit Disorders and the Hyperactivities in Multiply Disabled Children." *Rehabilitation Literature* 46 (1985): 250-54.

Burd, L., J. Kerbeshian, J. Cook, D.M. Bornhoeft, and W. Fisher. "Tourette Syndrome in North Dakota. *Neuroscience and Biobehavioral Reviews* 12 (1988): 223-28.

Burd, L. and J. Kerbeshian. "Symptom Substitution in Tourette Disorder." *Lancet* (1988).

Kerbeshian, J. and L. Burd. "A Clinical Pharmacological Approach to Treating Tourette Syndrome in Children and Adolescents." *Neuroscience and Biobehavioral Reviews* 12 (1988): 241-45.

Burd, L., J. Kerbeshian, M. Wilkenhaiser, and W. Fisher. "Prevalence of Gilles de la Tourette Disorder in North Dakota Adults." *American Journal of Psychiatry* 143 (1986): 787-88.

Parent Statements

This year our son is doing well at school, thanks to a combination of flexibility, routine, structure, and an understanding teacher.

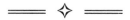

I think he gets on his classmates' nerves a lot. The teacher says his noise level (shrieks, shouts, and squeals) is loud, but she is easygoing about it.

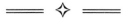

My son wasn't diagnosed with TS until the middle of fifth grade, but he had tics and behavior problems from the time he was three. His first grade teacher set the tone for his school career by promptly labeling him "Jumping John" at the beginning of the school year and staying on his case for the next eight months. I nominate her for the "Insensitivity Award" for that year!

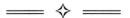

Because of her positive educational program and the care and concern of the staff, my daughter has gone from having very low self-esteem to being a success in school.

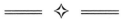

He's very accident prone because of his impulsivity. Luckily, the teacher is aware of our worries and doesn't just write us off as "overprotective parents." She noticed when Robby skinned his tongue by licking a metal fence on a very cold day. Robby has a very high pain tolerance, and the teachers need to be aware of that.

═══ ✧ ═══

The other kids call him "dummy" and "trouble maker."

═══ ✧ ═══

The sad truth is that children who present a challenge are sometimes seen as troublesome and disposable.

═══ ✧ ═══

My daughter's school is very good about working together with her to solve problem behavior. She feels validated and her sense of personal power and self-esteem is increasing.

═══ ✧ ═══

I see all the potential, the talent, the good, and the loveable. The school sees nothing positive about having to make basic, logical accommodations.

═══ ✧ ═══

Our kids have incredible coping skills to be able to go to school each day and be non-conformists in a mini-society that insists on conformity.

═══ ✧ ═══

My son spent so much time in the principal's office during the fourth grade that he lost a full grade level of reading skills. This was all hidden from me. I discovered the truth only when Joel began fifth grade.

═══ ✧ ═══

I've come into contact with many types of educational professionals, and I always appreciate it when I see a teacher or school psychologist who is committed to helping children with TS, and is willing to be flexible and creative in their approach.

═══ ✧ ═══

The experts in the field of neurology and TS in particular let us know that there is still so much we don't know about Tourette syndrome. But some teachers and counselors come off like they know it all and have *the* answers.

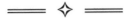

Bob told the teacher he was tired of being teased and beaten up every day at recess. The teacher said, "Go sit down." Then when Bob decided he had no alternative but retaliation, the school acted shocked at his "inappropriate behavior."

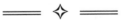

Waxing and waning of symptoms causes so much frustration at school. When tics are waning, teachers get fooled into thinking the TS is "better." Then when tics wax, teachers want to believe your child can control this—even after they've been told otherwise many times.

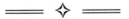

Educators often don't read material that we provide on TS. Notes about her behavior continue to come home from school, even though we've explained her problems over and over.

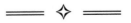

I've always tried to find at least one person in the school who is on my side.

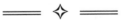

It's going real well in school. I'm very pleased with the cooperation we've received. The Early Education Special Services has been wonderful.

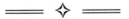

He was always class clown. He tried to camouflage his tics by doing things that were, if not acceptable, at least humorous.

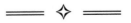

The first time anyone in school ever said anything good about my son was in fifth grade, right after his diagnosis of TS. His teacher said, "He's a neat kid. He's got a lot going for him!" That was the first time I felt my son had a chance to succeed.

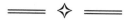

Because children with TS feel so out of control so much of the time, it's important to give them choices and "personal power." Let them have some input in their IEPs and their after-school time.

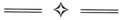

Consequences for inappropriate behavior at school do not have to be punishment, detention, loss of recess or other privileges. Instead, parents and teachers must be creative. Try role playing, or reviewing the "incident" and making plans for the next time something similar happens.

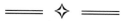

When teachers don't want to make accommodations or adaptations for your child because it encourages him to be *dependent* on others, tell them this. True *in*dependence is self-confidence and the ability to be in control of your own life. Everyone needs help from others. Help is *inter*dependence, not *de*pendence. Teachers' jobs depend on having students to help!

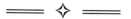

If teachers complain because your child is constantly losing control or needing to be restrained, examine the situation. What sets off these explosions? What attitudes, methods, or expectations are setting your child up for failure and frustration? The IEP obviously isn't working, so set up a new plan—devise other methods—until something does work!

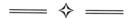

The best thing that ever happened to Kenny was to get involved in gymnastics in ninth grade. The coaches and other team members accepted him, included him, and encouraged him to be the best he could be and work as hard as he could. After working with these great people for a few months, he no longer wanted to hang around with the wild kids who had been the only ones in school to partially accept him, tics and all. He tried to straighten up and act in a way that would make his teammates proud. By the end of the school year, his "behavior" goals were taken off his IEP. By eleventh grade, he had lettered in gymnastics and received a sportsmanship award—not because of his exceptional athletic skills, but because of his enthusiasm, hard work, and helpful attitude toward the other team members. It was the proudest day of our life!

=== ✧ ===

In fourth grade, before our son was diagnosed with TS but when his behavior was probably the most "inappropriate," he started taking piano lessons. He was always fooling around on the piano and trying to play simple tunes, so we figured he was musical. His teacher thought so too, but he hated to practice. It was just one more battle to fight, and we decided it wasn't worth it. Then in sixth grade, after his TS diagnosis, our son started playing trumpet in the school band. He drove the poor teacher crazy, but she loved and encouraged him and put up with his antics during practices, which he loved. He had to practice a certain amount of time each week, and we would scrupulously record his time, including every minute he spent hitting his mouth with the mouthpiece of his horn—one of his newest tics. Now that our son's a junior in high school, his tics have subsided a lot. He gets better at the trumpet every year, and is now competing in a state-wide music contest, playing solos on his trumpet. He's always playing the piano by ear in his spare time. His music teacher was right. He had "music in him," and in spite of the TS, it's still there and going strong!

=== ✧ ===

Outline for Treatment of ADHD at Different Developmental Levels or Ages

Toddlerhood through Preschool
(mental ages 2–4)

1. Parent education regarding the disorder.

2. Parent training in the use of behavior modification through modeling, rehearsal, and correction feedback.

3. Technical assistance and consultation between parents and psychologists regarding specific problems.

4. Developmental play activities using behavior modification to forget the symptoms of the disorder. Parallel play with an adult describing appropriate behavior may be especially useful in children with language disorders.

5. A structured daily routine with clearly defined rules of conduct.

6. Direct teaching of skills necessary to be successful in school, such as sitting, listening, following directions.

7. Direct teaching of social skills through parallel play.

8. Scheduling.

9. Social skill training by rehearsal.

10. Peabody Language Kits or Flannel Board to teach interaction or turn taking.

11. Games such as "Simon Says."

Kindergarten through 3rd Grade
(mental ages 5–8)

1. Teacher education regarding the disorder

2. Teacher training in the use of behavior modification through modeling, rehearsal, and cooperative feedback.

3. Periods of work interspersed with periods of activity.

4. Positive reinforcement targeted at task completion, and elimination of task avoidance.

5. Supportive counseling if self-concept or interpersonal problems exist.

6. Training to aid in development and maintenance of peer relationships.

7. Precision teaching strategies with emphasis on mastery of basic skills.

8. Shortened schoolwork assignments if task completion is otherwise not possible. Make sure length of assignment is within child's true capability and not just teacher's guess.

9. Careful monitoring and remediation of any skill deficits that might develop.

10. Sight-word approach to reading if minor language problems are present.

11. Use of headphones or visual barriers are not helpful and may be damaging to the child's self-concept.

12. Do not assign chores or tasks that one does not expect to be completed. Encourage completion of tasks before allowing access to rewards.

4th Grade through 6th Grade
(mental ages 9–12)

1. Increased emphasis on development of compensatory skills through individual behavior therapy.

2. Self-monitoring of target behaviors.

3. Verbal mediation strategies.

4. Supportive counseling if self-concept or interpersonal problems exist.

5. Increased emphasis on the development of individual work and study skills.

6. Use of teacher-provided outline and study guides.

7. Teaching in organizational strategies such as PQRST or SQ3R (study, question, read, recite, and review).

8. If handwriting is slow or illegible, a trial of typing may be beneficial.

9. Use of study guides to help child stay focused while studying.

Adolescence/Adulthood
(mental ages 13 and older)

1. Emphasis on the development of self-reliance, good work habits, and interpersonal skills.

2. Use of daily work schedules with specific tasks to be completed at certain times.

3. Use of non-punitive, corrective feedback and supportive counseling to improve interpersonal skills.

4. Teaching in how to extract the import points from lectures and reading materials.

5. Have written material proofread by parent, peer, or teacher prior to handing it in for grading.

6. Use of memory techniques to help study for tests.

7. Use of study guides and SQ3R.

(Modified from Fisher, Burd, Kuna, and Berg, 1985)

EIGHT

$\diamondsuit$

Legal Rights
and Remedies

SONJA D. KERR, WITH DEBRA HOLTZ AND CARRIE G. MARSH*

You are probably aware that there are laws upholding the rights of people with physical and mental disabilities. For example, there are laws requiring that public places be accessible to people in wheelchairs, and laws granting children with mental and physical disabilities the right to attend school. But you may not be aware that many important disability laws also apply to children with Tourette syndrome. Because TS is a neurological handicap, all the laws that apply to children with disabilities in general also apply to your child. Some of these laws guarantee your child the right to attend school and work. Others prohibit discrimination or grant your child financial and medical assistance, if she qualifies. Still other laws can complicate long-term planning for your child's future.

As a parent, you do not need to be an expert on these laws. But understanding what your child is entitled to can help you ensure that your child receives the education, training, and special services

* Sonja Kerr received a J.D. from the Indiana University School of Law in Indianapolis. An attorney in private practice who represents children with disabilities, she serves on the advisory board for TSA Minnesota and is active in a variety of disability organizations. Debra Holtz holds a special education degree from the University of Northern Colorado and a J.D. from William Mitchell College of Law. She has worked in the field of developmental disabilities since 1979, and is currently Program Consultant in Developmental Disabilities with the state of Minnesota Department of Human Service. Carrie Marsh received a J.D. from the William Mitchell College of Law, and is a partner in the law firm of Manahan, Bluth, Green, Friedrichs & Marsh.

she needs. After all, many professionals have little or no experience in working with children with TS. At times *you* may have to tell *them* what your child needs and is entitled to under the law. You should also know enough about the law to be able to know what looks illegal and speak up for your child's rights if need be. And understanding how laws can sometimes work against families of children with disabilities can help you avoid pitfalls in estate planning.

To help you exercise your rights and fully protect your child, this chapter provides an overview of the purpose and contents of the most important federal laws, as well as information on how you can advocate for rights and services for your child. For information on state or local laws, you should contact your local Tourette Syndrome Association chapter or state Protection and Advocacy office, as listed in the Resource Guide. Your local Bar Association should be able to refer you to local lawyers who specialize in laws affecting people with disabilities. Remember, there is no substitute for consulting a knowledgeable lawyer. Although the information in this chapter is accurate and up to date, the authors are not providing legal or other professional advice.

Your Child's Right to an Education

Some children with Tourette syndrome have little or no trouble learning in the regular classroom. Many others, however, run into academic difficulties because of disruptive tics, learning disabilities, attention deficit disorders, or other symptoms. If your child has educational problems due to her TS or a related disorder, you need to learn about an important federal law: the Individuals with Disabilities Education Act (the IDEA). You may also hear this law referred to as Public Law 94–142, or by its original name, the Education for All Handicapped Children Act of 1975 (EAHCA).

The IDEA is a sweeping and complex law that ensures that every child with a disability will receive a "free appropriate public education." It does so by providing federal funds for the education of children with disabilities to every state whose special education programs meet federal standards. Currently, all states have accepted federal funding and must therefore provide a variety of approved educational services and rights to children with disabilities and their parents.

The sections below explore the major provisions of the IDEA. As you read about what the IDEA does and does not require schools to do, there are two important points to keep in mind. First, the IDEA only establishes the *minimum* requirements for special education programs. As the U.S. Supreme Court has ruled, states are required only to provide your child a program that is reasonably calculated to allow her to gain "some benefit." They do not have to provide "the best"

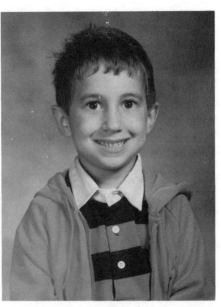

program. But states can and do create special education programs that are better than required by the IDEA. The special education director of your local school district can tell you exactly what services are available to your child.

Second, you should know that the IDEA gives parents a vital role in their child's education. In fact, when Congress first enacted P.L. 94–142, it was largely in response to parents pressuring Washington for a say in their child's education. Through this law, Congress sought to correct the traditional imbalance of power between school personnel and parents. Not only did the law specify that children with disabilities should receive certain educational services, but it also required that steps be taken to ensure parents' participation in their child's education. By law, parents must be notified if their child is being considered for special education, must be given the opportunity to help plan their child's educational program, must be notified of any changes in the program, and must be given a means of resolving disputes with the school system.* What all this means is that although the IDEA does not guarantee your child the ideal program, there are many ways you can work with the school to create a more appropriate program for her.

What the IDEA Provides

Coverage. To be eligible to receive services under the IDEA, children must have one of the "labels" that the law mentions as qualifying them to receive special educational help. Although Tourette syndrome is not one of these labels, your child may still qualify as "other health impaired"—even though she is not physically or mentally disabled in the traditional sense. If your child has learning disabilities in addition to TS, she may also qualify on the basis of being "learning disabled." Some schools suggest that children with TS be classified as "emotionally behaviorally disturbed" (EBD). Because TS is neurologically (not emotionally) based, this practice is incorrect.

Children with TS can begin to receive services as soon as they are diagnosed. All states now serve children from age three, and many are beginning to serve them from birth. Children with TS may continue to receive services through age eighteen, or longer, if the state where they live offers education services to students without disabilities who are older than eighteen.

Special Education and Related Services. If your child qualifies under the IDEA, then the school district must provide her with special education and related services. Taken together, this means extra help beyond just going to school.

Special education is instruction individually tailored to meet your child's unique learning needs. For children with TS, it can include one-to-one tutoring, modified curriculum and grading, or special classes in weak areas. For children with milder forms of TS, it can even include such accommodations as overlooking poor penmanship caused by tics or giving extra time for tests or shorter assignments.

---

* The law is undergoing change in this area. Be sure to consult a lawyer if you have questions about your rights to participate in the process.

Related services are any services your child needs to benefit from her special education. Services can include occupational therapy, counseling, personal aides, specially trained teachers, and transportation to and from school.

Least Restrictive Environment. The IDEA requires that your child receive her education in the "least restrictive environment" in which she is able to learn. The least restrictive environment is the setting that allows her to have the maximum contact possible with children in regular education programs. For children with milder TS, the least restrictive environment is often a regular classroom within a regular neighborhood school. Although they may receive help from special aides or therapists or use special equipment such as tape recorders, they still spend 100 percent of their time in a regular classroom. Other children with TS may spend part of the day in a regular classroom with nondisabled children and part of the day in a special classroom working on subjects they have trouble with be-

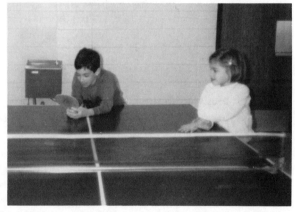

cause of learning disabilities or attention problems. A few children with TS are unable to make any academic progress within a regular school because the school district lacks the expertise to work with them. Often, these children have extremely severe physical tics that school personnel misinterpret as intentional misbehavior. In these very limited cases, the least restrictive environment might be a special education program located in a private or residential school for children with disabilities—at least until the school district acquires some expertise.

The least restrictive environment for your child depends on her *educational* needs. But you should start with the assumption that a regular classroom is right for your child, and only look into more restrictive alternatives if she runs into academic or social difficulties.

Free Appropriate Public Education. Every decision about which services your child should receive and in what setting should be made in light of the requirement that she receive a "free appropriate education." "Free" means exactly what it sounds like. Parents do not have to pay anything for their child's special education, no matter what special services she is found to need. The federal government covers any costs which exceed the school district's "average annual per student expenditure," including costs for related services such as transportation and physical, occupational, or psychological therapy.

"Appropriate" means what is educationally correct for your child's needs, so that she can learn and make reasonable progress in school. As mentioned earlier, it does not mean "best." It does not mean that your child's program must be designed to help her maximize her ability (unless your state law so provides). Instead, you and your school's staff have to jointly decide what is "appropriate."

"Public" usually means a public school, but it can also mean a private school with tuition paid for by the public school. If the public school doesn't have an appropriate program for your child, but a private school does, the public school may have to pay the costs for your child to be educated in a private setting.

Identification and Evaluation. By now it should be clear that education programs cannot be appropriate unless they are tailor-made to take into account each child's educational strengths and needs. To make sure that schools have a clear picture of children's abilities and disabilities, the IDEA requires that states have procedures for identifying and evaluating children who would benefit from special education. Under the IDEA, school districts are required to make an effort to identify all children with disabilities. But if your child has already been diagnosed with TS, you can take the first step and notify the school that your child may need special education. To set the process in motion, contact the school's special education department, explain your child's diagnosis, and request, in writing, that your child be given a special education assessment or evaluation. Although federal law does not require that a school act on your request immediately, your state law may set a specific timeline for completing an evaluation from the time it is requested by a parent.

The purpose of an evaluation is to determine your child's current level of educational performance and the areas that she needs assistance in. As Chapter 7 discusses, your child's need for special education may be evaluated in several ways. First, she may be given a variety of tests to assess her abilities in all developmental areas. In addition, she may be observed in the classroom and you may be interviewed about your child's strengths and needs. In fact, the IDEA requires that multiple procedures be used to evaluate your child. That is, the school cannot rely solely on the results of tests, for example. In addition, you have the right to be notified of the type of tests to be given, and the tests must be administered by qualified personnel. Finally, the tests must not discriminate on the basis of your child's disability or racial or cultural background.

As a parent, it is important that you make sure the assessment paints an accurate and complete picture of your child. Otherwise, the program she receives may not be appropriate, given her needs. Offer your own information or questions about your child's abilities to the evaluator. And after the evaluation, request copies of all assessment data and other information in your child's records.

If you disagree with the evaluation completed by the school district, you have the right to ask the school district to pay for an independent education evaluation. For instance, you may not agree that your child reads at a particular level, is disruptive to others, or has no strong points. You will know if it "doesn't sound like" your child.

To request an independent evaluation, write the school and ask for one. Be sure to date and keep a copy of this letter. While you wait for their response, check with doctors, the TSA, or other parents for recommendations of an evaluator. Then provide these recommendations to the school district.

The school district must pay for an independent evaluation, unless it can prove at a due process hearing that its original evaluation was appropriate. (See below for information on due process hearings.) If the district refuses, then it must establish the appropriateness of its evaluation at a hearing. Because evaluations often cost much less than formal hearings, school districts will often pay for independent evaluations in an effort to resolve disputes over assessments.

Individualized Education Program (IEP). Once a child is determined to need special education, the school district must hold a meeting to discuss the assessment results and to develop an Individualized Education Program (IEP). The IEP is a written document which describes the education a child with disabilities will receive to meet her unique needs. It specifies:

1. your child's current abilities in academic, emotional, and other areas; any health problems; and any particular problems your child is having in school;
2. long-range goals and short-term objectives for reducing the difficulties that prevent your child from performing better (a long-range goal might be: "Dan, who reads at grade 4.0, will increase his reading ability to grade 4.5 by the end of the second semester, as measured by performance in reading 4.5 grade materials." A short-term objective could be: "Dan will improve sight reading of the following words. . . ."");
3. the types of special instruction, therapy, and other assistance your child will receive; as well as where she will receive these services;
4. the projected date services will begin and their expected duration;
5. how your child's progress will be measured;
6. the extent to which your child will be able to participate in the regular classroom, and any in-class modifications that will be used;
7. whether your child will be receiving services for longer than the traditional nine-month school year (as might be necessary if the lack of a consistent program causes your child to regress, take a long time to regain skills she had in the spring, or not become as self-sufficient as she could be with a longer year);
8. for children aged sixteen or older, the assistance and services that will be provided to help them make the transition to work or post-secondary education.

Your child's IEP will be developed at a meeting, or series of meetings, attended by a school administrator, your child's regular classroom teacher, other school staff who may have evaluated or worked with your child, you, and your child, if you deem it appropriate. You may also invite other family members, a friend, doctor, social worker, advocate, lawyer, or anyone else you feel comfortable bringing to the meeting.

At an IEP meeting, your child's needs in *all* areas should be discussed. Your role is to tell the school staff who your child is and what you think she needs. Some parents take a very active role in this process, while others are content to observe and ask questions. Do what feels comfortable to you. Think of it as painting a picture of who your child is now and a futuristic picture of who your child can be. What skills does she need in order to reach the futuristic picture?

All children with Tourette syndrome have differing needs. Share what those needs might be. For example, say: "My child can't follow directions" or "My child counts ceiling tiles" or "My child hits others without planning to" or "My child swears at home, too." Then, make suggestions to help school staff deal constructively with problem behaviors. For instance, suggest: "Give my child an organizing notebook" or "If he is staring at the ceiling, remind him to look at his books" or "Tell the other kids that John doesn't mean to hit or swear."

Once your child's IEP has been designed, the school district must provide you with a copy of it, and you have a right to approve or disapprove it. If this is your child's first IEP, the school must have your written consent and must then begin providing services immediately. If this is a revision of an initial IEP, the school cannot legally change your child's program without notifying you. The school must inform you of any changes made and give you the opportunity to respond to the changes and accept or reject them. If you do object to the changes by requesting an administrative proceeding, the school district must keep your child in the program she was in when you objected. This is referred to as the "stay put" provision of the IDEA. Administrative proceedings are described in more detail below.

There is one final point about IEPs it is important to remember. As your child's strengths and needs change, so should her IEP. Consequently, the IDEA requires that children's special education programs and their progress be reviewed at least once a year; many states encourage more frequent reviews. This ensures that your child will not be "stuck" in a program that is not meeting her needs. You have a right to be notified of all meetings about your child and to participate if you wish. If you do not want to attend a meeting, the school can have one without you, provided you were told about it. If you feel additional meetings are necessary, you can request them by writing to your child's teacher, the school principal, or special education director.

Resolution of Disputes

As mentioned earlier, one of the key provisions of the IDEA is to encourage a team of people, including parents, to work together to plan a child's education program. Ideally, parents and school staff can openly discuss their concerns about a child's abilities and disabilities and jointly agree on the services and strategies that will best meet her special educational needs. Occasionally, however, disagreements arise. Examples of disputes are: 1) whether your child qualifies for services; 2) whether your child is too disruptive to be in a particular class; 3) whether your child needs occupational therapy or specific behavioral assistance. In most states, you have two options for resolving these types of disputes. You can try to resolve them through informal discussion, or you can request a formal administrative proceeding or due process hearing.

Informal Dispute Resolution. Many states give parents the opportunity to discuss disagreements with school staff in so-called *mediation* or *conciliation* settings. The format of these meetings varies from state to state. Generally, a mediation session will be hosted by someone not directly involved in the dispute. Either you or the school can request such a meeting. If you request it, do so in writing.

If you are wondering whether to participate in such a meeting, ask yourself four questions: 1) Will the meeting be moderated by an impartial third party? 2) Do you believe the disagreement can be resolved through honest discussion? 3) Are *both* you and the school interested in reaching a solution without resorting to more formal methods? 4) Is your participation truly voluntary? If the answer to each of these four questions is "yes," then by all means meet with the school staff and try to reach a solution. But if the answer to some questions is "no," do not hesitate to investigate the more formal methods of resolution discussed below. Sometimes it is helpful to discuss with an attorney or lay advocate whether you should try these informal methods or proceed to more formal means. (A lay advocate is a parent, teacher, doctor, or other individual who has considerable knowledge about the IDEA or your child. Call your TSA for help finding one.) To find out whether your district or state has an informal dispute resolution process, contact your State Department of Education.

Formal Administrative Proceedings—Due Process Hearings. The IDEA gives parents the right to formally appeal *any* decisions made by the school regarding their child's identification, evaluation, program, or placement. For example, you can challenge your school's refusal to qualify your child for services, or the types or amounts of therapy she is receiving, or the classroom setting she is in. You can set the appeals process in motion by sending a letter to the school district's Special Education Director. In the letter, explain the substance of the dispute and request a "due process hearing under the IDEA." Although it's not required, it's best to send the letter by certified mail.

The hearing must he held within thirty days from the day your school district receives your request. This hearing will give you your first opportunity to present your case before someone who does not have any stake in the outcome. An "impartial hearing officer"— someone who has not had any direct dealings with your child and does not have any professional or personal interest in the school that might cloud her objectivity—will preside over the hearing. Under the IDEA, school districts and parents have the opportunity to agree upon who the hearing officer will be; if they cannot agree, then a hearing officer may be appointed by the state education department. In either case, you may object to the hearing officer chosen if you do not believe that person is "impartial." Ultimately, the hearing officer will decide whether the school's or your arguments have more merit, so it is important that he or she be objective.

At the hearing, you can present information or "evidence" to prove that the school's decision will not give your child an appropriate education that meets her needs. Evidence may include your child's school records, independent evaluations, testimony from people such as the state TSA advocate who have special knowledge, and others. At a minimum, you should come prepared with relevant portions of your child's school history, information from her physician and other non-school care providers, a description of the school's proposed education program, and a description of the program that you feel would best meet your child's needs.

Besides presenting your own evidence, you generally have a right to review all the evidence to be presented by the school at least five days before the hearing. You can also require witnesses, including school staff, to attend and testify. You can question or cross-examine any witnesses the school district may bring. And you can ask an attorney or lay advocate to represent you at the hearing.

Where the burden of proof lies—which side must present the best information—varies from state to state. In some states, the burden is on the school district to prove that its program is appropriate. In others, the parents must prove that the school's program is inappropriate. Call your TSA to find out how it works in your state.

The hearing officer will hear both sides and must issue a decision, in writing, within forty-five days of your initial request for the hearing. If you ask for it, the school district must provide you with an electronic recording or transcript of the hearing.

If the hearing officer rules against the school, he or she will order the school district to provide whatever you requested for your child. If you prevail at the hearing, the school district must also pay your attorney's fees. This is a rather recent development, so be certain that any attorney with whom you consult is aware of the provision. You should also be aware that payment of attorney's fees might be limited or refused if you reject an offer of settlement from the school, proceed with a hearing, and then do not obtain a better result. In addition, the school district must pay for all the other costs related to the hearing, whether or not you prevail. This includes the costs of the hearing officer, the court reporter, the school's attorney, and copies of the electronic record or transcript. If teachers are called as witnesses, the school district must also pay for substitute teachers for them. Because of the possible expenses involved, many districts prefer to reach an agreement with parents without going to a hearing, unless the case is very important.

If the hearing officer rules against you, you have the right to appeal this decision. Until recently, appeals from the hearing officer were routinely heard by the State Educational Agency—the state department of education. Parents and advocates have challenged the appropriateness and fairness of permitting a state educational agency to review these decisions because that agency was not perceived as "impartial." As a result, most states are now moving to a system where the hearing officer's decision is final and appealable only to a court, or is reviewed by a truly impartial hearing review officer who is not a part of the state's educational agency. The impartial hearing review officer considers the evidence presented at the due process hearing and any additional evidence presented. Based on that evidence, the hearing review officer then issues an independent decision.

Although many parents have used due process hearings to obtain more appropriate programs for their child, it is best to think twice before embarking on a hearing. Going through a hearing can place significant emotional stresses on both your child and your family. You will have to meet with your lawyer. You may have to miss work. You will have to put your files in order and prepare what you plan to say. In some states, due process hearings are quite lengthy and very expensive, often involving attorneys for both sides. In other states, hearings are less complicated, and parents may be able to represent themselves, perhaps with the help of a lay advocate. In deciding whether to ask for a due process hearing, it is important for you to find out what hearings are generally like in your state. Ask other parents, advocates, or attorneys about the average length and cost of hearings, how often hearings are requested, and whether they think you need an attorney. Consider whether you can afford to pay attorney's fees if you lose. (You might also be able to find an attorney who will only charge you if you prevail and can recover attorney's fees.) Then weigh the importance of the issue being disputed against the emotional demands of making the request and proceeding through the hearing.

If you decide it is essential that your child receive a particular type of program or service which the school district has refused, do not be afraid to request a hearing. As mentioned above, when parents who know their rights request a hearing, schools may attempt to meet their demands rather than go to a hearing. If your dispute involves an issue that you and other parents frequently discuss, your child may need to be the "test-case" to push the issue for all children. Generally, other parents and advocates are very supportive of parents going to a hearing. In fact, some parents have said they never felt so supported as they did before, during, and after their hearing.

Civil Court Action. If you are not satisfied with the results of a due process hearing or the appeal to a hearing review officer, there are further steps you can take. You can take your appeal to a state or federal court by bringing a civil lawsuit against the school district. After reviewing the information from previous hearings and hearing additional evidence, the court must decide two questions. First, did the school district follow the procedures required under the IDEA in making the decision about the child's educational program? Second, is the educational program proposed by the school district the appropriate placement for your child? If the court rules in your favor, the school district must comply with its order.

At this stage, parents generally employ an attorney, if they have not done so already. (And once again, they may recover attorney's fees if the court decides in their favor.) Your attorney can further advise you of the specific appeal procedures from one court to the next. Basically, however, parents can appeal decisions of a court up to the highest court of the United States—the Supreme Court. Some parents have found it necessary to do so, and it is as a result of many of those cases that your child has the rights described in this chapter.

Other Federal Anti-Discrimination Laws

Rehabilitation Act of 1973

Section 504 of the Rehabilitation Act of 1973 protects the right of "an individual with handicaps" not to be discriminated against by agencies receiving federal funding, including school districts. A handicapped individual, under Section 504, is anyone having a physical or mental impairment that substantially interferes with "caring for one's self, performing manual tasks, walking, seeing, hearing, speaking, breathing, learning, and working." Someone with TS may fit this definition if her TS or associated conditions affect her in these ways. All public and private organizations receiving federal money must take action to accommodate people with disabilities so that they can "learn, work, and compete on a fair and equal basis." Agencies that don't accommodate people with disabilities can lose their federal funding.

Although Section 504 only covers discrimination in federally funded agencies, it can still be helpful to your child on a day-to-day basis. For example, if your child plays the violin well enough to belong to the orchestra at her public school, but the conductor wants to exclude her because she has loud vocal tics during concerts, you can charge the school with discrimination. Likewise, if a federally funded agency turns your child down for a summer job solely because of her TS behaviors, that is discrimination under Section 504. Because people with TS sometimes have trouble convincing agencies that they are covered under Section 504, be prepared to document that your child is disabled enough to be covered.

The Americans with Disabilities Act

In 1990, Congress passed the Americans with Disabilities Act (ADA), which many people view as an extension of Section 504. The ADA is the latest, but very natural step in the evolution of federal civil rights laws that protect people with disabilities. The ADA's purpose is simple—to eradicate discrimination in *all* aspects of life, not just in federally funded programs. It covers a large array of public and private sector activities. Under the ADA, discrimination on the basis of disability is prohibited in the following areas:

Employment. Under the ADA, a "qualified individual with a disability" is anyone who has a disability and can perform the essential functions of the job, with or without special accommodation. Basically, an employer cannot refuse to hire, train, or promote a "qualified individual" solely on the basis of Tourette syndrome or any other disability. Indeed, the employer is prohibited from asking whether a prospective employee has a disability. Furthermore, an employer is required to make modifications (accommodations) within the workplace that will enable an otherwise qualified person to perform the job. For example, if an employee with TS syndrome had trouble manually filling in forms, she would be permitted to use a typewriter instead.

Under the ADA, workers with disabilities who feel they have been discriminated against can file a complaint with the Equal Employment Opportunity Commission (EEOC). If this agency is unable to resolve the dispute, the next step is to take the employer

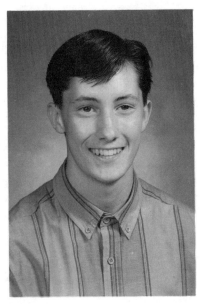

to court. During this stage, it is usually advisable to consult a lawyer with expertise in employment discrimination. Attorney fees can be recovered if the court finds in favor of the employee.

From July 1992 to July 1994, this section of the ADA applies only to employers with twenty-five or more employees. From 1994 on, it applies to employers with fifteen or more employees.

Consumer Services in Private Business. Any business that provides "public accommodations" is prohibited from discriminating against people with disabilities. That is, any facility that is open to the general public must also be open to individuals with disabilities, and under the same terms. For example, a restaurant could not seat someone with loud vocal tics in a remote corner of the room on the grounds that she might otherwise disturb other patrons. Or the managers of a movie theater or concert hall could not exclude a patron with Tourette syndrome because her tics might distract others. Unless it would impose an unreasonable cost, every store, health club, school, restaurant, hotel, motel, museum, laundry, doctor's office, dentist's office, and other business must allow people with disabilities to use their facilities on an equal footing with people without disabilities.

3. State and Local Government Services. Every service funded by state and local government must be accessible to people with disabilities.

4. Public Transportation. Under the ADA, all public transit must be accessible to people with disabilities. Buses, trains, subways, and other public conveyances must have some provision for transporting people with disabilities, and cannot refuse service on the basis of a patron's disability.

5. Telecommunication. Just like businesses in the private sector, telecommunications companies must make their services accessible to people with disabilities.

Because the ADA is so new, it will take some time to determine exactly its scope and the direction its protection will take. You should know, however, that the ADA permits a person to bring a lawsuit if she feels she has been discriminated against. It also permits recovery of attorneys' fees if the suit is successful. To keep abreast of changes in interpretation of the ADA that may affect people with TS, periodically check with your local TSA or ARC.

Government Benefits and Protection

In addition to protecting the rights of people with disabilities through the IDEA and other anti-discrimination laws, the federal government provides various programs and benefits for people with disabilities. Your child may qualify for some or all of these programs and services if she meets the eligibility requirements.

Developmental Disabilities Act of 1978

The Developmental Disabilities Assistance and Bill of Rights Act (DDA) offers a wide range of services to people with developmental disabilities. For purposes of the DDA, a developmental disability is one which occurs before age twenty-two and which limits a person's abilities to do certain activities necessary for self-sufficiency—walking, grooming, learning, earning money, and the like. Most people who are more severely affected by TS qualify for "DD" services, while people with milder symptoms do not. Different counties set different eligibility guidelines for these services. Your county Human Services agency can tell you how to find out if your child qualifies.

If your child has severe symptoms, especially symptoms that cannot be controlled by medication, there are services available under the DDA which may be necessary to your family's survival. Services include:

1. Child development (early intervention)—P.L. 94–142 now requires that eligible children receive special education services from age three. But some states try to enhance the

development and learning of children with disabilities from birth on. These states typically offer early intervention services—occupational therapy, physical therapy, speech therapy, or other specialized help designed to help minimize ' problems that would otherwise affect the child's development. If your child received a diagnosis of TS before age three, she may qualify for these services.

2. Case management—When a child with disabilities needs the services of many educational and medical professionals, a case manager helps to arrange for these services and facilitates communication between parents and the professionals. A case manager may be an educational, medical, social work, or other professional who is dedicated to your child's protection and rehabilitation.

3. Provision of services such as assistance from in-home aides, behavior specialists, or respite care workers to help your child live as independently as possible within the community.

The DDA also provides for the establishment of a Protection and Advocacy (P&A) office in each state. These P&A offices protect and advocate for the civil and legal rights of people with developmental disabilities. Many serve people with Tourette syndrome, depending upon the office's criteria. If you or your child encounter problems related to education, employment, housing, or other activities, the attorneys and advocates at your P&A agency should assist you at no cost. State P&A offices are listed in the Resource Guide at the back of the book.

Vocational Rehabilitation

Vocational Rehabilitation (VR) services are offered to all adults with disabilities in every state. Services are designed to help people with disabilities gain employment, and job training and placement assistance. VR services are supported by federal funding and are provided at no cost for those who cannot afford to pay.

If you think your child may need assistance in getting or keeping a job, begin inquiring about vocational programs when your child is still in high school so that you will have ample time to prepare for the transition from school to the workplace. The first step in obtaining services is to request a vocational needs assessment no later than age sixteen. If it is determined that your child has vocational needs, goals and objectives should be written into your child's IEP. To request services after high school, you will need to contact your state Department of Vocational Rehabilitation. Your child will be assigned a personal counselor and given an assessment, similar to that provided under the IDEA. Once her needs are determined, an Individual Written Rehabilitation Plan (IWRP) will be developed, clearly setting forth the specific services to be provided. The types of services most commonly provided are vocational counseling and guidance in selecting the most appropriate career; medical examinations and other tests which help to determine job potential; instruction and training, books, equipment, and initial set-up materials for self-employment; placement; and follow-up services to make sure the adult with Tourette syndrome obtains employment and remains satisfactorily employed.

Even though your child may qualify for vocational rehabilitation services, it is important to realize that these services may not always be available. Often vocational rehabilitation offices have long waiting lists of people who are eligible for assistance, but the funding and personnel are simply not available to satisfy everyone's needs. Services are generally doled out to the people who are judged to have the severest problems first. This makes it doubly important for you to take advantage of any vocational assistance available through the school system before your child graduates, while she is still covered by the IDEA.

Social Security Programs

Adults and children with TS can apply for and receive two types of Social Security before they are of retirement age. The benefits available are Supplemental Security Income (SSI) benefits, and Social Security Disability Income (SSDI). Both programs can provide additional income to qualified children with disabilities and their families. To qualify, your child must meet the strict requirements of the program and establish financial need. If your child is under eighteen or is living at home, need is based not only on your child's income, but also on the income and resources of you, the parents.

SSI. Supplemental Security Income is designed to provide income for people who cannot work. It is available not only to people who have worked for a period of time and paid Social Security taxes during that time, but also to people who have never worked or have worked only for a limited period of time. Adults are eligible if they can demonstrate that they are unable to engage in "substantial gainful activity" because of a disability. Children who have disabilities similar to those that prevent an adult from working can also qualify. Both children and adults with disabilities must also meet the financial need requirement set by the Department of Social Security. Since the cut-off figure changes frequently, you should contact your local Social Security office to find out what the current income requirement is. They can also advise you as to how any assets in your child's name or earnings from a part-time job can reduce her benefits.

To apply for benefits for your child, contact your local Social Security Administration Office. Your first request will most likely be denied. Many people with TS are denied benefits because the Social Security Administration is still unfamiliar with the syndrome. Ask that your doctor explain in writing that your child's symptoms are chronic and will not disappear. Have the doctor detail all areas in which TS limits your child's abilities, including speech, reading, sight, hand and arm movements, and compulsive behaviors. Be persistent in your efforts.

SSDI. Your child is eligible to receive Social Security Disability Insurance if one of her parents becomes disabled and is no longer able to work. The amount that parent and child receive is based on the number of years the parent worked before becoming disabled. A child who is disabled before the age of eighteen can also receive SSDI payments based on the amount of a retired or deceased parent's Social Security coverage. The process of applying for SSDI is the same as for SSI. Unlike SSI, however, applicants are not required to meet certain income qualifications.

Medicaid

Sometimes children with TS can qualify for Medicaid, a government-sponsored health insurance program. To be eligible, your child must qualify for SSI or have insufficient funds to pay for medical care. Usually, but not always, your child's medical needs will have to be pretty extensive for her to qualify. Medicaid can pay for medications, doctor visits, evaluations, and hospital stays. Call your local social services office to apply. Ask for a written explanation of what services are covered in your state.

Planning for the Future

Tourette syndrome is a life-long disability. But because TS symptoms may change in severity over the course of a lifetime, the needs of a person with TS are extremely difficult to predict. Most adults with TS are able to care for themselves, but some may need some assistance. For example, when medication is not effective or produces severe side effects, adults with TS may not be able to care for themselves independently. Adults with learning disabilities may have difficulty getting a job that pays enough for them to fully support themselves. And adults with echolalia or coprolalia will most likely encounter obstacles to employment, housing, and other rights that non-disabled people take for granted. (Although such discrimination is definitely illegal under the ADA, people with TS need funds to fight it.)

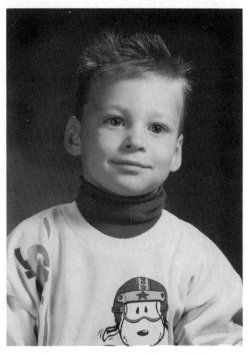

If there is a chance that your child's Tourette syndrome will prevent her from caring for all her own needs as an adult, it is important that you plan now for her future well-being. You will, of course, also want to provide monetarily for your child in the event you die before she reaches adulthood. There are, however, numerous pitfalls that parents of children with disabilities need to avoid in developing a personal estate plan.

Many of the pitfalls associated with estate planning have to do with the concepts of financial need or cost-of-care liability. As explained above, many government benefits that may be available to your child are dependent upon financial need. If you would like your child to be eligible for these benefits after you are no longer around to look after her, this means you must take care that poor estate planning does not disqualify your child from receiving government assistance. Similarly, if you think your child might need services such as in-home care or health insurance provided by the state, you must keep cost-of-care liability in mind when planning your estate.

Cost-of-care liability is a provision that enables states to require a person with disabilities to use her own funds to pay for state services if she is able to do so. States can draw upon funds owned by the person with disabilities herself as well as funds in some types of trust funds. Some states can even require parents to pay for services for adult children with disabilities. This practice may sound fair in theory. But the catch is that the funds you or your child provide are seldom used to benefit your child directly.

The section below outlines some do's and don't's of estate planning that can help you avoid the cost-of-care liability trap while ensuring that your child's needs will be adequately provided for. These strategies are provided primarily to help you evaluate the appropriateness of any estate plan you might have now or in the future. To develop an estate plan, it is of utmost importance that you seek professional legal counsel and advice from an attorney specializing in estate planning for people with disabilities. Without assistance, all that you have worked for could be lost due to the high costs of care.

Estate Planning

As mentioned above, most children with TS grow up to be self-supporting adults who are entirely capable of managing their own assets. If you are reasonably certain that your child will be able to manage on her own after your death, you can probably plan your estate much as any other family would. But if you think your child may need to rely on government benefits such as SSI, SSDI, or Medicaid once she reaches adulthood, or that she may need assistance from the state, estate planning becomes more complicated.

If you want to make sure that your child does not inherit money or property that would be subject to cost-of-care liability or jeopardize her eligibility for government benefits:

1. Be sure to leave a properly written will. If you die without a will, your estate will be distributed according to the laws of inheritance, and your child with TS and her siblings will likely share equally in your estate.
2. Don't rely on joint tenancy instead of a will. If both parents die simultaneously or if one spouse fails to execute a will after the other dies, the result can be the same as if you died without a will.
3. Don't leave property to your child with TS. Instead, leave it to siblings with the unwritten understanding that they will use it to help support their brother or sister with TS.
4. Don't create a support trust for your child with TS; the result is the same as leaving property to her.
5. Don't name your child with TS as a beneficiary in an insurance or retirement plan. Name a sibling or siblings as beneficiary instead, so they can use the funds on their sibling's behalf.
6. Don't establish a UGMA (Uniform Gifts to Minors) account for your child with TS, as these funds become her property once she reaches the age of eighteen.
7. Consider setting up a discretionary or luxury trust for your child with TS. In some states, funds left to a child with disabilities through these kinds of trusts cannot be tapped by the state for cost-of-care liability. Consult a lawyer knowledgeable about estate planning for people with disabilities to find out if this is a viable option in your state.

Be sure to tell family members about these estate planning issues. If your child has relatives who may attempt to provide monetarily for her future in their own estate plans, it is essential that they know about all the pitfalls described above. Otherwise, they may leave property to your child via a will or support trust, only to have that property disqualify your child from receiving government benefits or fall into the hands of the state.

Last, but not least, remember that proper estate planning varies for each family, and every will needs to be tailored to individual needs. To develop an effective estate plan, you must let your attorney or estate planner know what the unique needs of your family are. You should be prepared to give your estate planner the following information: 1) nature and degree of your child's disability, including educational and IQ level; 2) functional capabilities and independence; 3) any special medical needs; 4) any work or earnings history; 5) any assets your child owns; 6) any current wills or trusts that exist; 6) current and anticipated educational and living arrangements; and 7) governmental assistance programs such as SSI or SSDI in which your child presently participates or could participate in the future.

Raising a child with Tourette syndrome can be financially and emotionally exhausting. Not only do you have a child with a disability, you have a child with a disability that most people have never heard of or do not understand. This means that it may sometimes be up to you to see that your child receives the special help and benefits she is entitled to and that all her rights are respected. But there are also many professionals who can help you know and exercise your rights. Remember, learn as much as you can about the laws and programs affecting your child, consult knowledgeable professionals, and then trust your own instincts as to what is best for your child.

Advocacy

There are probably many other rights and benefits besides those discussed in this chapter that you think your child should have. Unfortunately, lawmakers are not going to pass laws granting these rights just out of the goodness of their hearts. The only way to make sure that new and improved laws get on the books is through advocacy. The only way to make sure that good laws get enforced is through advocacy. And the only way to make sure that people understand what your son or daughter needs is through advocacy.

To advocate simply means to plead another's cause. Advocacy can take many different forms. Informing teachers, doctors, and other professionals about the supports and services that your child needs is a form of advocacy. So, too, is educating strangers about appropriate ways to react to your child's TS behaviors. Writing or calling local or federal lawmakers to voice your support for legislation that would benefit your child is yet another form of advocacy. As the parent of a child with Tourette syndrome, you will likely feel compelled to get involved in at least one of these forms of advocacy sooner or later.

The Need for Advocacy

When your child was diagnosed with Tourette syndrome, you were thrust into a new world of parents who have children with special needs. You will find that there is much support and understanding from other parents who have children with disabilities. Other parents understand what you mean when you describe the frustrations and anger you have with the "system." But even though you will find much support and understanding from parents, you will also find that the 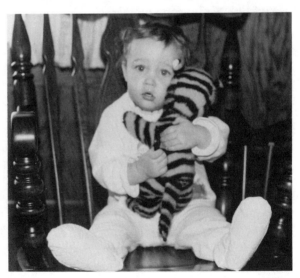 system is not so understanding, and that it can be extremely difficult for you to get the services your child needs.

Because there are so many misunderstandings about TS, there is often a greater need for advocacy than for other disabilities. Your child has a disability that seems invisible to most people. The only visible signs of her disability may be behavioral difficulties such as motor tics, swearing, spitting, or aggressive behavior. These symptoms are *not* going to be recognized by most people as a form of disability. Most people who see these behaviors are going to incorrectly assume that you have a "bad" child or that you are a "bad" parent. Neighbors may not want their children to play with your child. Strangers may make rude comments to you. Because of these and many other gross misunderstandings about Tourette syndrome, your child will probably need someone to advocate for her on a *daily* basis.

Another important reason for advocacy on behalf of children with Tourette syndrome is to ensure that good employment, housing, and training programs exist in the future. Currently, there are precious few of these programs, and long waiting lists confront people who need them. Public officials do not spontaneously decide to establish programs that meet the needs of people with disabilities. They usually must be pushed, and sometimes pushed hard. This is done by advocates working in organizations like the TSA and by advocates working on their own. But unless people fight now and fight hard for services and programs in the future, there is a great risk they won't be there when your child might need them.

Children with TS need to have someone explain the symptoms of Tourette syndrome to their teachers, relatives, and others. Someone needs to explain to teachers what support services are needed in the educational system. Someone needs to explain to doctors what is and isn't working for your child. Someone needs to explain to insurance companies that your child needs medical coverage. This section on advocacy is designed to provide you with enough information about advocacy so that you can determine what is best for your child and what kind of advocacy *you feel most comfortable doing.*

As a parent, you must decide what type of advocacy you will provide for your child. Remember, your primary role in life is not as an advocate. *First and foremost, you are your child's mother or father. First and foremost, any child with disabilities is still a child.* It is essential to remember that being a good parent simply means doing your best.

You probably did not choose to be the parent of a child with Tourette syndrome. You certainly did not choose to be an advocate for the rest of your life. Advocacy is, in the words of many parents, "thrust upon you." Remember that you are a parent first, and then an advocate, *if you choose to be.* You must find your own style and determine what kind of advocate, *if any*, you will be for your child.

Many parents feel comfortable providing individual advocacy for their son or daughter. Others feel more comfortable in requesting the assistance of a professional advocate. You should choose the role you feel most comfortable with.

Gathering Information

The underlying purpose of advocacy is usually to convince someone to do something that they would not otherwise do for your child. For example, you might want to convince the school that your child needs a peer tutor. Or you might want to change your health insurance so it covers your child's Tourette syndrome. Whatever you want to accomplish, you need facts to back up your argument. You must be prepared to show why what you are asking for is in your child's best interests, as well as why your child will suffer if you don't get your way. Typically, the more information you learn about Tourette syndrome and how it affects your child, the more comfortable you will feel about telling others what your child needs. Here are some ideas on how to gather information:

1. Read, read, read. Request information from the TSA, subscribe to their newsletter, consult the publications listed in the Reading List—read everything you can about TS.
2. Talk to other parents—in the doctor's office, at school, in support groups. Find out what has and has not worked for their children. Find one parent you can regularly call. It is helpful to be able to get support and advice from someone who knows exactly what you are going through.
3. Find out where the local advocacy agency is in your area by calling your local TSA or ARC chapter. Get on their mailing list so you can receive information on advocacy workshops, new legal findings, community resources, and the advocacy efforts of others with an interest in TS.
4. Watch your child. Learn what does and doesn't work for her by observing her.
5. Ask questions of parents, professionals, and other *adults* who have Tourette syndrome.
6. Gather more information than you think you want or think you will read. If you don't read it now, just put it away and

save it for later. It is better to have too much information available than not enough.

7. Keep copies of all your child's medical and educational records, and request written documentation of your child's needs from doctors and teachers.

Advocating in Your Child's School

As pointed out earlier in the chapter, federal law guarantees only that your child receive an "appropriate" education. It does not spell out what constitutes an appropriate education for any one child, but leaves that up to the school personnel and the parents to decide. Sometimes, teachers and parents agree on what services a child with TS should receive and where she should receive them. But more often, parents and school personnel have different ideas about what an appropriate education for a child with TS should be like. If disagreements arise, you do not have to let the school have its way; you can advocate.

Frequently, school personnel will disagree about how to handle your child's education simply because they know little or nothing about TS and how it affects your child's ability to learn. You may be able to bring them around to your way of thinking by educating them about TS. You can get literature written especially for teachers from the national TSA. Chapter 7 suggests some ways to explain TS to teachers and other school personnel.

If the professionals in your child's school are knowledgeable about TS, but still will not provide your child an education that you feel is appropriate, you may have your work cut out for you. You must find out *why* the school personnel don't want to do as you ask, and then try to counter their arguments. For example, are they refusing to provide your child with occupational therapy because of the cost involved? Then you need to gather documentation from professionals that your child's fine motor skills will continue to lag unless she receives OT. Are teachers refusing to give your child her tests orally because it takes too much of their time? Then you may need to work with them to figure out a time schedule that would be fair to your child and to them. (They can't refuse to test your child orally because of time constraints; oral testing is often necessary.)

Here are some pointers to keep in mind when advocating within the educational system:

1. Be familiar with your child's educational rights. That does *not* mean that you need to know all the laws, but before you go to an IEP or other meeting, call a local advocacy agency and ask them for a brochure on the special education laws in your state, and reread this chapter.
2. Discuss potentially troublesome issues with teachers *before* they arise at a meeting. It is often easier to resolve issues informally before a meeting.
3. Bring a notebook and take notes at meetings in case further court involvement or due process is necessary and you need to document what was said. You can also bring a tape recorder if that is easier.
4. Bring a friend or your spouse if that will make you more comfortable at the meeting.
5. Find an ally in the school system to act as a buffer between you and any angry, frustrated, or insensitive staff members. He or she may be able to provide you with inside information, calm down frustrated staff members, or assist you in indirect ways. For instance, he or she might help staff implement educational strategies in a positive way, help other staff members learn to trust and respect you, or direct you to "good people" within the system.
6 Keep a small note pad by your phone or in your briefcase at work. Whenever you discuss important issues with *any* school personnel, jot down the date and a few notes about the conversation, in case documentation becomes necessary.
7. Remember that everyone needs support, even professionals. Let your child's classroom teacher and other school personnel know that you appreciate the positive things they do. This will make it more likely that they will continue to go to bat for your child.
8. Compromise only on the small issues. Be persistent about your long-range goals, such as boosting your child's self-esteem through appropriate behavior management strategies or having an inservice on TS for school staff every year.
9. Determine what role you are comfortable with in the school system. You may decide to attend all meetings by yourself, or you may want to bring a special education advocate to

some. If you need to start a due process appeal, you may want a formal advocate or an attorney.

Advocating in the Medical System

In the educational arena, the IDEA guarantees that parents have a say in decisions made about their child's schooling. Unfortunately, there are no equivalent laws requiring professionals to work with parents in making decisions about their child's medical care. Because of the nature of Tourette syndrome, however, there are many reasons a doctor *should* consult you when treating your child. As Chapter 3 explains, the information you supply about your child's symptoms and responses to medications is invaluable in planning your child's treatment plan. Ordinarily, doctors have no problem requesting this information from parents, and parents have no problem providing it. But what happens if you would like to be more involved in your child's treatment plan? For example, what if you have read about a new medication that you think might help your child, but your doctor has never mentioned it? Or what if you think your child's medication causes too many side effects, but the doctor seems unwilling to consider a change? You can advocate for specific medical services just as you advocate for educational services. Here are some pointers to keep in mind:

1. Be informed. Read as much as you can about Tourette syndrome and the medications and treatments that have been successful. Always ask your doctor about anything you don't understand. Ask him to spell the names of medications and what the side effects of medications are.
2. Remember that there is much disagreement among physicians as to the treatment of TS. There is so much *new* information about TS that there is still much misunderstanding. Your doctor may not recommend a new treatment because he is waiting for more information about its risks and benefits, or then again he may not even be aware of the treatment. It doesn't hurt to ask what your doctor thinks.
3. If you want to discuss any aspect of your child's treatment with the doctor, try to schedule an appointment in the morning. Doctors are fresher then and less hurried. Be concise and prepared when you meet with the doctor. It helps

to come to the appointment with a written list of questions that you can check off as you ask them.

4. Ask for a second opinion if you are not satisfied with your doctor's answers.

5. Remember that you are the consumer. Switch doctors if you are not getting the help you are asking for. Ask other parents of children with TS or your local TSA for referrals to experts in the field.

Legislative and Class Advocacy

The previous sections have discussed ways that you, as a parent, can provide individual advocacy for your son or daughter. But there will also be times when the voice of one person is simply not enough. There will be times when laws need to be changed, and you may want to become part of a larger group to help change the system. Here again, as with individual advocacy, you must decide what you are comfortable with. There are many different ways to become involved in *class* advocacy—advocacy aimed at reforming the system as a whole. It may be as simple as voting for the right candidate or writing a short letter, or as complex as testifying before a legislative body or participating in a class action lawsuit.

It is extremely important to recognize the power that parents have as a large group, and to remember the changes in laws that parents have brought about. The special education laws that now *guarantee* your child's right to a free and appropriate education were a result of the efforts of organized parents. The IDEA passed in large part because parents just like you were frustrated and angry that their children with disabilities were not being served by the educational system. They joined forces with other parents and *they changed the system*. It only takes one parent to start talking, and soon you have large numbers who do make a difference. *Never underestimate your power as a parent.*

Parents of children with Tourette syndrome should feel an urgency to band together. Because of widespread misunderstandings about the disability, many issues need the immediate attention of lawmakers. As a parent, you may already recognize many of these problems. For example, some professionals continue to disagree as to whether Tourette syndrome is a mental health issue or a developmental disability or a neurological disorder. Because of this, there is no guaranteed funding stream for service. Often Human Service and other agencies won't provide funding unless they can conveniently pigeonhole a disability. And insurance companies are able to get away with paying less than they should by claiming that TS is a mental illness. Furthermore, many professionals continue to give low priority to this disability because they mistakenly believe that the incidence of TS is low. As a result, medical researchers don't put enough time into looking for better treatments, and educators don't spend enough time looking for better ways to teach children with TS. To complicate matters, because of behaviors such as tics, spitting, and swearing, children with TS are not perceived by the general public as cute children. Therefore, many people, including legislators, would rather not think about the problem.

For parents of young children with Tourette syndrome, *now* is the time to organize with other parents. *Now* is the time to demand appropriate services and better funding so that adulthood will be easier for your child.

The first step is to locate the local and national advocacy groups already in existence. The national Tourette Syndrome Association is relatively new and needs your support. There may also be a local or state TS group in your area; check the Resource Guide at the back of this book to determine if there is. If there are no local groups, you may need to gather the strength and just start one. If you do, you will be amazed by the number of people who will come out of the woodwork to join. Parents of children with TS have a desperate need to network and find others.

Reaching the Lawmakers

As a member of an advocacy group, you will be in the best position to change the system through legislative reforms and court decisions. You will also find it easier to keep abreast of any legislative issues that may affect your child. This is important because—as with individual advocacy—the key to successful legislative advocacy is to be informed and know the issues.

One of the best ways for your local TS group to find out about pertinent legislation is to have your group's name added to the mailing list of larger advocacy groups that watch the state and national legislative changes. Examples of these groups are listed in the Resource Guide at the back of the book, and include Children with Attention Deficit Disorders (CH.A.D.D.) and ARC. Most organizations of this nature develop "Action Alerts" in response to proposed legislation. These alerts will inform your group of actions that individual members should take to help get a desirable bill passed, or an undesirable bill defeated. They may, for instance, recommend that you write letters to legislators or sign petitions. These larger advocacy groups can also provide you with information sheets that describe a proposed bill and how it may affect your child.

Once you know the formal name of a bill or proposed law and how it will affect your child, the next step is to contact your legislator. There are many ways you can do this, but the simplest, most effective ways are to simply call or write your legislator.

Calling Your Legislator. Parents are often reluctant to call their legislator, fearing that their opinions couldn't possibly matter and that their phone calls would be an unwelcome intrusion. But nothing could be further from the truth. Legislators must vote on hundreds of issues each year and they simply do not have the time or the expertise to learn about each issue on which they are voting. If a bill is proposed that will affect your child, chances are very likely that your legislator knows *nothing* about TS and will need information before voting. Because your child has TS, you are an expert compared to most people. Many legislators will base a vote on as little as one or two phone calls if that is all the information they have. One phone call can make a difference.

To call your legislator, first jot down a few notes about the major points you want to make. Then when you actually talk to someone, you will know exactly what you want to say. (Don't forget to mention that you are a constituent and you do vote!) Often if a bill is coming up for a vote, a secretary or aide will answer the legislator's phone and just tally the yes and no calls. Legislators really do count these calls and listen to their constituents' opinions. So make that call and urge other parents you know to do the same thing.

Writing Your Legislator. Letters are also an extremely effective way of getting your legislator's ear. Writing is an especially good method if you have a number of facts to convey that you think might help sway your legislator's vote. Here are some guidelines to help you put your opinion in writing:

1. Keep your letter short and concise.

2. Start with a pleasant introduction, being sure to identify yourself as a parent of a child with Tourette syndrome.
3. Focus on the issues and how they affect you and your child personally.
4. Always refer to the proposed legislation by the proper bill number and title.
5. Conclude with your request or recommendation for a vote and thank the legislator for his or her time.
6. If your group organizes a letter-writing party, don't send form letters. Personalize your letters.
7. When bills pass that will help your child, write your legislators and thank them if they voted for it.

Recharging Your Batteries

Earlier chapters have emphasized how important emotional support is to coping with a wide range of issues—from adjusting to the initial diagnosis to managing your child's daily care. Support is also important when you are advocating, whether individually or in a group. You are dealing with such emotionally charged issues on such a regular basis that you need the opportunity to share what you are going through with others.

Becoming a member of an advocacy group, as suggested above, is an excellent way to find support. You can get comfort and practical advice from other parents who have experienced *the very same issues* you are facing. If you are married or have a partner, you can not only share some of the emotional burden, but also the advocacy work. You can take turns attending meetings, if possible, and also divide the advocacy work so that each of you winds up with the role you feel most comfortable with. For example, one of you may want to become the expert on medical issues related to TS, and the other may want to become the educational expert. Or, one of you may prefer to gather all the information you need to support your argument, while the other attends meetings and presents your case.

Whatever you do, don't let the need for advocacy rule your life. Recognize that it is okay to feel tired and worn out. Don't become a martyr parent. Recognize your limits and periodically refuel yourself. Even if you think you only have five extra minutes a day, don't forget about your own needs. Remember to play, sleep, love, laugh, work, and just take time for yourself. Taking a break is especially important if you are a single parent and must handle all the advocating on your own. Try to space apart educational meetings and medical appointments. If you can schedule two meetings in two weeks, rather than two meetings in one week, it may be an easier schedule for you to live with.

Finally, to keep your motivation high, periodically take stock of your accomplishments. Write down the things you have accomplished for your child. Have you helped your child's teacher *really understand* that she can't control her tics? Have you helped the doctor find a combination of medications that improves your child's tics? Have you helped to raise money for a candidate who is sensitive to the needs of children with disabilities? Make a habit of focusing on your successes, not your failures. And above all, believe in yourself.

Conclusion

There are many ways you can advocate for your son or daughter. And when you do, you are not only advocating for your child, but for all the children who will eventually be born with Tourette syndrome. Every minor, positive change that you are able to make in the system will affect thousands of other people in the future. As a parent, you are incredibly powerful and you can make a difference.

Margaret Mead said it best: "Never doubt that a small group of thoughtful, committed citizens can change the world; indeed, it's the only thing that ever does."

Parent Statements

Don't go to an IEP meeting unless you know your child's legal rights. Don't expect the school to let you know what they are. I learned everything the hard way until I met other parents of kids with TS. They are the people with real helpful information.

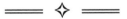

I am treated as a respected and equal member of my child's IEP team. This makes me feel "listened to" and helps me put my trust in the professionals who have such an important role in Holly's life.

━━━ ✧ ━━━

The most frustrating aspect of having a child with Tourette syndrome is dealing with the schools. They resist programming for Dan's special needs (including LD), and instead just drop him into the most handy EBD [emotional-behavioral disorder] slot they have available.

━━━ ✧ ━━━

Placing a child with TS in a class with kids with emotional and behavioral disturbances will often cause the child with TS to imitate the other children's inappropriate behavior. Children with TS usually behave more appropriately in a mainstreamed setting where there are positive role models to follow.

━━━ ✧ ━━━

Once parents learn about the laws and their child's rights, they're in a much better position to negotiate with the school.

━━━ ✧ ━━━

The ADA looks great on paper. I guess we'll just have to wait and see whether it really will help our kids.

━━━ ✧ ━━━

When I first got involved in legislative advocacy, I was amazed at the impact each individual can have on the system if he is committed to a cause.

━━━ ✧ ━━━

Get everything in writing and make copies!

━━━ ✧ ━━━

I've needed to learn advocacy for my child just like the parents of a kid with a hearing impairment need to learn sign language and the parents of a kid with cystic fibrosis need to learn pummeling. It's never accomplished once and for all; it never ends.

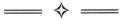

Long before I realized that I had rights (and that Kenny had rights), the only time I got any action from the school was when I said, "Well, I guess I'll just have to keep him home then." Now I know the reason that threat got results was because if I kept Kenny home from school, we would end up in court. That's the last place schools want to end up.

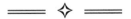

Being involved in advocacy helps reduce the feelings of powerlessness encountered when you have a child with TS. In two short years, I have made great strides in educating people in my child's world about TS.

Often the attorney can get the school to pay her fees. The first time the school procrastinates in meeting your child's needs, find an attorney who knows school law. Every bad day at school chips away at your child's self-esteem and potential.

Something that has been hard for me to accept is that an "appropriate" education does not necessarily mean "best" education. The schools are only required to go so far.

When a child with TS has problems getting an appropriate education, no one tells the parents what their legal rights are. Instead, the schools say, "We can't provide this service." And no one gives the other side—that they are required by law to provide the service. There should be an advocate at each school to give the other side.

I have been my child's advocate for four years now, and my son is now beginning to take over and learn to advocate for himself.

Through this experience, he will learn so much about people, negotiations, and feeling personal power.

═══ ✧ ═══

When we showed the school the law that they had to provide services, they wrote a nice IEP, but it was never enforced.

═══ ✧ ═══

I'd say that if the school punishes your child for his symptoms *after* you've explained to them that he can't help it, get an attorney.

═══ ✧ ═══

One thing the laws can't legislate is understanding and tolerance. I worry about this sometimes when I think about what kinds of problems my son could run into on the job.

═══ ✧ ═══

I'm tired of parent advocacy groups always saying "the parent is the best advocate." When you spend twenty-four hours a day coping with your child with TS and the rest of your family, where do you get the energy necessary to become an advocate?

═══ ✧ ═══

I wish someone had told us when our child was diagnosed that we would have to become pseudo-lawyers just to have our child's legal rights upheld.

═══ ✧ ═══

I have been very fortunate. I have not had to take our school district to a due process hearing. The right people have been in place to advocate for his special needs.

═══ ✧ ═══

Because there was no one else to advocate for my child, I fell into the role of his advocate. I have learned a lot, just by believing in my child's rights and by taking a risk to be assertive.

═══ ✧ ═══

NINE

$$\diamond$$

Living with Tourette Syndrome: "I Am Not My Tics!"

WILLIAM V. RUBIN, M.A.*

I have lived with Tourette syndrome for approximately forty years. Since the age of about six I have had a variety of head and facial tics (blinking, head shaking, nose and mouth movements); other body tics (leg and foot movements, stomach contractions, hand tightening, and arm and shoulder movements); vocalizations (sniffing, barking, grunting, and throat clearing); and rituals (checking that the coffee pot is unplugged, pushing my bed up to the wall until it feels right, feeling that I have to be places on time).

When I began having these symptoms as a child, nobody knew much about TS. I was very lucky, though, and generally had no problems in school or out in public. I was almost never teased, ridiculed, or reprimanded by classmates, teachers, parents, or other adults. Still, I often felt isolated even in a room filled with my

* William Rubin is the president and founder of Synthesis, Inc., a mental health research and consulting company, and a clinical instructor at the Wright State School of Professional Psychology in Dayton, Ohio. He worked for the Ohio Department of Mental Health in the areas of research, program evaluation, and planning for nearly ten years. He has served as both the Vice President and Director of Training, Research, and Development for the Tourette Syndrome Association of Ohio, and presently is a co-founder and staff member of the Minnesota TSA Family Camp. He earned a bachelor's degree with honors in psychology from Brandeis University and a master's degree in psychology from the University of Nebraska.

friends. I could not understand why I had to have strange "habits" and be so different from the other kids. When I was a teenager, my father and I battled for several years over my tics. Why was I making these noises to disturb everybody? I could control them for periods of time, so why did I have to make sounds at all? It must have been just to "get them." Luckily, my parents finally realized that no matter what, I could not control the symptoms, and the confrontations ended.

After high school, I attended Brandeis University, and graduated with a bachelor's degree with honors in psychology. I next enrolled in the University of Nebraska Graduate School of Psychology on a National Institute of Mental Health Fellowship in Clinical Psychology. I had completed most of my courses for the Ph.D., and was finishing up an internship in Child Clinical Psychology, when one of my colleagues agreed to help me try to reduce my tics and noises. We thought this would be good for my professional career as a psychologist. We attempted several behavioral approaches, including aversive electric shocks, before one of the psychiatric residents suggested that I try a powerful medication called Haldol™. I was told that this drug, frequently used to treat severe psychiatric disorders, had just recently begun to be used, in small doses, to treat tics. I started taking Haldol, and it reduced my symptoms by about 75 percent. Shortly afterwards, however, I decided to drop out of school as a result of unrecognized side effects of the medication. I later returned to graduate school at Case Western Reserve University, but again dropped out because of side effects such as short-term memory loss, depression, doubts about my skills, and difficulty understanding complex materials. Although some of my professors may have suspected TS, no one diagnosed me as having the disorder.

I was finally diagnosed as having Tourette syndrome at the age of thirty-five. While visiting close friends in Connecticut, I met a relative of theirs who had children with TS and was serving as the state TS coordinator. She recognized my symptoms and gave written materials to our friends, who passed them on to my wife. On our trip home, my wife showed me the information from the national TS Association. Coincidentally, at about the same time, my parents saw a television show in which neurologists described this unusual syndrome. They mentioned what they had seen to me, and several months later I went to the Cleveland Clinic pediatric neurology department for my formal diagnosis.

People frequently ask how I felt after being diagnosed. Although I firmly believe that knowing that you have TS is very important, it still takes time getting used to. For me, knowing that I had TS was a double-edged sword. On the positive side, I finally knew why I had to make the strange sounds and movements. On the negative side, however, I had to acknowledge that there was something "wrong" with me. Accepting the reality of a disabling condition doesn't mean giving up, but it does mean coming to grips with something that will probably never go away. It took me about six months to begin to work through and accept these realities.

Once I began to accept the fact of my TS, I became active in the Tourette Syndrome Association of Ohio, serving as its Vice President for four years and its first Director of Training, Research, and Development. Since 1985, I have helped the Tourette Syndrome Association of Minnesota operate the only camp for children with TS and their families in this country. I have also provided consultation to and conducted many seminars and workshops in schools, mental health facilities, correctional facilities, vocational rehabilitation offices, and homeless shelters.

Currently I am president of SYNTHESIS, INC., a private applied research and consulting organization that I founded in 1986. We conduct major policy research studies and consult with local human service boards and agencies to assist them in planning and evaluating their services.

Since my childhood, major strides have been made in understanding Tourette syndrome and in educating the community about it. Still, the condition continues to be misdiagnosed, inappropriately treated, and misunderstood by health care professionals, educators, employers, parents, and the general public. It is little wonder that children and adults with TS are themselves often misinformed. Many must face the world with only a poor sense of who they are and what they are capable of accomplishing, fewer coping strategies than they need, and a limited sense of responsibility for their own lives and the choices they can make.

Over the years, I have been very lucky in the way my family and society have responded (or in fact, not responded) to my symptoms. While I certainly have been, and continue to be, affected by my disorder, I have not suffered the great ridicule and isolation that many with TS experience. In writing this chapter, I have tried to pinpoint what it is about my experiences that has enabled me to live with Tourette syndrome. I have also drawn on the conversations and experiences I have had with several hundred children and adults with TS. This insight, I hope, will help children with Tourette syndrome and their families better understand and cope with the disorder.

What Does It "Feel" Like to Live with TS?

When I think about this question, I identify two separate types of "feelings." These are: 1) how I feel physically before, during, and after having symptoms; and 2) how I feel emotionally about what I do.

Physically, I am aware of almost every tic or sound that I make. This awareness is in the form of a feeling of "tension" in a specific

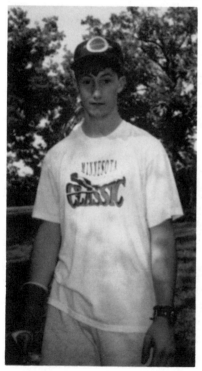

body location. It also feels as if something "is going to happen." That is, it feels as if I am going to blink or shake my head forward. Although I am aware of these events, my mind does not constantly focus on them. It's only when they are really interfering with my activities or when I am trying to suppress them that the awareness, prior to having the symptom, is heightened. For example, I play competitive volleyball and when I am very tired, I have ankle, leg, and hip tics that can slow down my movements and interfere with my jumping. Sometimes I become so conscious of these tics that I have to force myself to concentrate on the rest of the game.

From my observations, it appears that children may be less aware of their symptoms. This could be because of a real lack of awareness or because they have absolutely no explanation for why they do such strange things. As a result, they may "lie about," or deny, having done something (for example, poking at their classmate as he walks by). Some children even carry the "lie" to extremes by purposely becoming class clowns to cover up for their inability to control their behavior. (Sometimes it's more acceptable to be a "problem child" than a "crazy child.") Even though my parents noticed my tics at about the time I started school, I really don't remember being very aware of them until I reached junior high school. I can remember many times over the years when I "lied" to people about my symptoms, calling them "habits" when I really had no idea what was going on. In any event, I think most adults are aware of most of their symptoms. We are aware of them when we are having "good" days, and definitely aware of them during "bad" times.

Once I have the tic (or other symptom), there is a release of tension. It's not that it feels so good *while* I'm expressing the symptom, but that the tension is gone *after* I've expressed it. I have only mild compulsive symptoms, but I can still recognize that tension will be relieved, for instance, after I *check* to make sure the stove burners are turned off, even though I'm standing right across the kitchen and can see them.

Motor tics, vocalizations, and other behaviors can also have specific physical effects on your body. My neck muscles, for example, are always tight and stiff. For many years, I have had a head-shaking tic that is made worse by wearing dress shirts with ties, or anything up around my neck. Both my head and neck would be in pain after a day of meetings at the office. For about the last seven years, I have not worn ties or the types of shirts that increase these symptoms.

Fatigue and pain come from both the repetition and the severity of symptoms. For example, sometimes I shake my head and sniff in so many times that I give myself a headache and severe neck pains. Sometimes symptoms can even result in temporary or permanent physical damage. For example, when changing medications from Haldol to Catapres™, my symptoms got very severe for about two months. This is called a "rebound effect," and can occur after long-term use of medications like Haldol. I made such loud noises that my voice was damaged, and ten years later I still can no longer carry a tune. Children, too, can experience the rebound effect. I know some who have bitten their lips or picked at themselves until they caused infections after discontinuing medication.

When I do training workshops for parents or professionals, I always have them experience how it feels physically to have tics. If you want to get a sense of what it's like, just stand in front of a mirror and blink by squeezing your eyes shut about one hundred times.

As difficult as the physical discomfort can be to deal with, I think the most damaging part of Tourette syndrome is its emotional impact. What does it feel like emotionally to have tics or compulsions, or to make noises? It's frightening, frustrating, terribly embarrassing, and very saddening. It can make you feel about as small as you can possibly feel. We have grown up (or are growing up) doing things that we can't seem to control. They don't make sense and we don't know why we do them. Even when we have a diagnosis and intellectually know that we have a "neurotransmitter imbalance," we live every day knowing that we will always stand out. No matter where we go, some people will be looking at us, wondering, laughing.

I never know exactly how people will respond to me. The feedback can be violent (being hit, ridiculed, or kicked out of class) or very subtle (a raised eyebrow, a snicker, a waiter being distracted while taking your order). When others respond negatively, I get angry at them for their stupidity and cruelty. And then I hate myself for being so different that it makes me the target of taunting and teasing. As a result of many years of negative responses from those around us, I think most of us with TS live with an ongoing sense that we are being watched. This awareness produces a constant level of stress for us. Even though my symptoms would be considered moderate and generally not socially unacceptable, I routinely encounter the more subtle responses mentioned above. Again, if you want to experience some of the emotional feelings that your child, spouse, or friend with TS may be having, ask somebody you know to stand right in front of you and watch while you blink, or grimace, or shake your head for about one minute.

As a scientist, I have wondered whether there are ways to reduce this stress of being watched in specific situations. On several occasions, I have tried a little experiment while sitting in airport waiting areas. I closed my eyes and pretended to sleep so that I would get no visual feedback from other passengers. In fact, this strategy did make me more comfortable. I didn't really care if they were looking, or wondering, or laughing. It was like a demonstration of the old expression, "what you don't know can't hurt you." In many ways, I think coping with Tourette syndrome is being able to emotionally close your eyes for periods of time so you can get on with your life.

I am sometimes asked how it feels to know that tics, vocalizations, or other behaviors that I have annoy other people. First, it is important to recognize that your symptoms may not always be as annoying as you believe. When I think back to my childhood, I realize that one of the things that has enabled me to live with TS is that in the beginning, my parents were virtually the only ones who said anything about my tics and noises. No teachers or classmates asked me to stop making noises, twitching, or shaking my head. This was extremely unusual. But my experience has shown me that there are two factors that greatly affect others' ability to ignore my symptoms of TS: 1) their general attitude of acceptance; and 2) their getting to know me over time. In work settings, after initially being very aware of my tics, most of my co-workers hardly notice them unless I am having a "bad" period. In fact, co-workers and close friends are so at ease with my symptoms that they even remark to me about funny movements (tics) or sounds that other people may have.

Although there are obviously some symptoms that are not easily tolerated, I believe many people can adapt to many symptoms. Indeed, it is critical for parents, siblings, friends, teachers, employers, co-workers, and others to learn to ignore symptoms. Since stress exacerbates the symptoms of TS, knowing that people are listening or watching for your tics, or concentrating on holding them back, only increases stress and eventually makes the symptoms worse. When I think of the six Family Camps I have helped to run in Minnesota, I realize just how much you can accomplish when most of the people around you accept or ignore most of your symptoms (including coprolalia).

The other side of this issue, though, is that at times (and over time) some symptoms *are* annoying to others. When my wife and I go to symphony concerts, I try to suppress my tics, and I still worry about annoying other patrons who expect quiet during the performance. It is even more distressing to me that some of my tics and noises interfere with my wife's life. When I awaken (in the middle of the night or in the morning), my tics start immediately. This frequently disrupts her sleep. Or think about putting your arm around someone you love and barking in her ear. There will always be some symptoms that put stress on your relationship with your spouse, family, and friends. Sometimes you can laugh about them, sometimes you cry, and sometimes you get angry. Without apologizing for the symptoms, I think people with TS must accept responsibility for trying to reduce the effect of their symptoms on those they care about. For example, if my wife and I are watching TV and my vocal tics are very bad, I sometimes leave the room and watch TV in the bedroom.

Many people with TS can suppress symptoms for varying lengths of time. How successfully they can do so usually depends on the seriousness of their disorder, the symptom, and the specific situation. For example, I can usually suppress symptoms better when my wife and I go to a movie than when I go to watch a football or basketball game. My love of sports and the excitement of the game make my tics and noises worse. At the same time, with everybody else shouting and jumping around at the game, who cares?

On the other hand, when we go to movies or concerts, it takes tremendous energy for me to be both quiet and still. Withholding symptoms is like repeatedly trying to hold your breath for as long as you can, then quietly getting a breath, and then holding your breath again. At the end of a two-hour movie or a concert, not only am I physically tired, *but my tics come out even more intensively on the way home.* Trying to suppress tics and other symptoms also requires that you focus part of your mind on that effort. If you try holding your breath, you will find that after a while you start thinking about your chest or mouth or head. You must split your concentration between what is going on around you and the portion of your body (or mind if you have obsessive thoughts) that you are trying to control. Having to divide your attention like this can certainly affect your ability to study or perform other complex tasks. That's why I believe we must expect the symptoms to occur and learn to adapt to many of them.

I don't know any parent who doesn't feel guilty for having *expected* his or her child to stop having tics, and I think most of us have felt at some time or another that we should be able to stop. But for a number of reasons I feel that *expecting* individuals with TS to suppress symptoms is both unrealistic and harmful. As described above, holding back symptoms may take considerable physical and mental energy. This adds to the difficulty the person may already have in learning, taking care of his day-to-day needs, or interacting with others. I have emphasized the word "expecting" because those of us with TS will try to suppress our own symptoms anyway. We are just like anybody else. We don't want to look funny, disturb others, or be ridiculed or thrown out of movies or school. We want our parents, friends, and spouses to love us, so we don't want to do things that irritate them. But when I feel that somebody expects me to suppress my tics, I feel they are really saying that I'm not OK with them. This heightens the already difficult emotions (anger, shame, etc.) I have toward my tics. Likewise, when people with TS themselves feel that they ought to suppress all their symptoms so as not to bother others, we are saying to ourselves that we are not OK with ourselves.

What I am really trying to say is "WE ARE NOT OUR TOURETTE SYNDROME." Some "experts" have attempted to fuse us together with our disorder—to make the symptoms seem a part of our personalities—of who we feel we are. Some even use the term "Touretter" to describe us. I do not believe this is fair. The symptoms I have are not part of "me." In fact, most symptoms of Tourette syndrome make little sense to those of us who have them or to others—especially when viewed in the context of the rest of our lives. Take, for example, an eight-year-old boy who is having unusual sexual obsessions about members of his family. They frighten him because they are not part of who he feels he is. Or consider the professional photographer whose head, arm, and body movements increase when he is excited by a beautiful landscape and therefore interfere with his efforts to capture the scene on film. I sincerely believe that the more we can learn to view our symptoms as "add-ons" to whomever we really are, the better we will be able to go on with our lives.

How Can We Live with TS?

I think one of the most important factors in being able to live with TS is developing the strength from within to go out and take on the world. Over the years, I have met some remarkable people with serious symptoms of TS or other disabling conditions who go

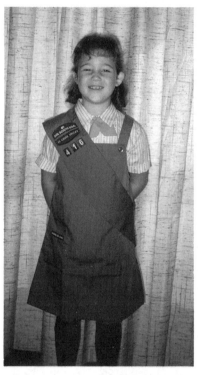

out day after day and live their lives. For example, I have a friend with cerebral palsy who uses enormous physical energy just to go from his office to the rest room. Another friend with TS must allow himself at least two hours to dress because of his compulsions. A young woman I know attends college while experiencing very severe full-body tics and coprolalia.

This strength from within must first come partly from the support of others. As we are growing up, we all develop a feeling of whether we can master our environment. We get a feeling that we are OK and that although we may not always succeed, we can still go on with our lives. I really can't say enough about how much my family and friends have con-

tributed to my own feelings about myself. Their love and support never wavered, even in the face of my "mystifying" behaviors. *They looked right past my tics to the person I really was becoming, and responded to that person.* This even included punishing that person when he did something wrong. My parents never seemed to let my symptoms come between them, and they have both been there for me throughout my life. My brother and our friends never let my symptoms get in the way, either. They never even mentioned the movements and noises I made. Although I believe that people with TS, their parents, siblings, spouses, and friends must be able to talk comfortably about TS, I do not feel it needs to become a regular topic of conversation. To allow it to do so only focuses attention and effort away from the rest of our lives. Today, growing up seems very different for most of the children with Tourette syndrome I have met. Much more emphasis is placed on appearance, and fitting in seems even more important. However, once teenagers with TS begin to feel more comfortable with themselves, they still become more eager and able to make friends. They may have fewer friends than some other children, but they start doing and experiencing the same things that other teens do. They play sports or play in the band; they have girlfriends and boyfriends; they like (and are liked by) some of their teachers, and don't like (and are not liked by) others; they want to learn to drive; they don't always do what adults want them to do, and so forth.

In order to learn to live with Tourette syndrome, I think we must all learn to live—period. That is, we must focus on things we would do if we did not have TS, and figure out ways to accomplish those things. During our Family Camp each summer, we video tape many activities. When I go back and look at the tapes, I see members of twenty-five to thirty families running around, doing arts and crafts, eating, swimming, playing volleyball, and generally having a good time—just like any other family. I even see some kids fighting, pushing, or teasing, just like other kids. I am not trying to minimize the problems that some symptoms can cause, but I am trying to emphasize that we can become so focused on those symptoms that we forget that we are very much like other families or individuals. Families talk about not being able to go out and do things together. Adults with TS complain that their options are limited. Many people, however, have the same fears that we do. For example, how many people do you know who are afraid to go for a job interview— and not just because they have Tourette syndrome? If we learn to perform well in a job interview, we will learn how to handle or discuss our symptoms with our new employer. Or, if we can figure out how any three children and their parents can take a two-week vacation together in their mini van without killing each other, we can figure out how to do it when one of the children has TS.

There is, of course, no way to totally ignore the many additional problems TS creates for us. But the more we can try to live our lives as others do, the better we will be able to handle the special burdens placed on us by the symptoms of TS.

Coping Strategies

Part of this learning to live as others do is developing coping strategies. Although everybody develops them, people with TS must learn how to handle more unusual and difficult situations than most individuals need to. I certainly don't claim to have all the answers about how to cope with Tourette syndrome, but I feel very strongly that each of us with TS must develop our own sets of coping mechanisms to enable us to deal with other people and situations, and to live meaningful lives. I believe that learning these things is important because the world doesn't really change very quickly. That is, attitudes toward people with TS and other disabling conditions change slowly, so we must learn to live in a society that—while not specifically "against us"—is certainly not actively "for us." Parents and others can really help us by being supportive as we try out these coping skills.

There is no way to describe how to cope with every different situation people with TS may face. But, I'd like to discuss at least a few of the ways that I try to make my life easier and, I hope, more productive.

First, it's important to understand that the goal of my coping strategies is to be able to live my life as normally as possible. Most of my strategies involve how I try to cope with:

1. Being out in public;
2. Interacting with people who do not know me well (students, employees, acquaintances);
3. Relating to people very close to me;
4. Accomplishing specific tasks (work, school assignments, sports, etc.).

As explained below, my coping strategies for each of these situations are rooted in "non-confrontation" and on presenting an image of competence.

Being Out in Public

If I am out in public and become aware that others are staring or laughing at me behind my back, I attempt to ignore them, and go on as if nothing were wrong. I usually don't try to confront people unless they directly interfere with what I'm doing. Rather, I try to show my "competence." For example, if I'm in a department store and a clerk notices my tics, I don't walk away or confront him by asking what he is staring at. Instead, I ask the clerk about something I am interested in purchasing. Or, if I'm ready to buy something, I do it with my charge card. This says to the clerk that while I may do some "funny" things, I am competent enough to be able to buy something, or earn enough to have a charge card at the store. That is, I'm not so different from their other customers (maybe I'm even a *better* customer). A child could use the same tactics. Since many adults "expect" inappropriate behavior from children, he could ask a question *politely* about an item in the store, pick something off the floor that another customer had dropped, purchase the item he came for, or just slowly leave the store.

I've also found that speaking to others first is a way of putting them at ease about my various symptoms. It's also more difficult to laugh at, be afraid of, or make fun of someone with whom you've just had a brief but pleasant conversation about the basketball game last night, the math exam you had yesterday, how bad yesterday's school lunch was, the weather, or how crowded the stores are today.

Sometimes when people are really unpleasant, it's difficult to just ignore them or disarm them by having a chat. I know teenagers who have had to fight their way off the school yard each day until the other children finally stopped teasing them. I know other adults whose symptoms are much more serious than mine, who must sometimes respond to others' comments, threats, or insults. Sometimes you can do this by walking up to your tormentors and quickly informing them about TS (before you duck); sometimes you just walk away; and sometimes you fight verbally or physically. There is no simple rule about how to cope with people who continue to ridicule or threaten you. I think it is very important, though, for children with TS to tell their parents when they are being confronted or harassed. They must work together to develop strategies to resolve the issue.

In general, I do not believe that people with TS should avoid going places or doing things just because their symptoms might mildly disturb or annoy others. When I choose to avoid situations, it is for only one of two reasons:

1. *I* am likely to be uncomfortable in the situation or with the way people may respond, or
2. My symptoms are *so severe or disruptive* that it's not fair to others for me to be there.

Places I would not generally visit for the first reason include bars where I know the patrons' response to my tics might make me uncomfortable. My wife and I also generally avoid going out to dinner or to evening movies when I am very tired after a long week at the office, because crowds make my symptoms worse, and trying to control them would make me very uncomfortable.

Places that should be avoided for the second reason depend on the symptoms an individual has that might be considered very inappropriate for a particular situation. For example, if someone has a compulsion to break drinking glasses or dinnerware, going to a fine restaurant would only cause him trouble. Or if one's coprolalia could not be controlled, going to the theater or a school play might be too disruptive for actors and audience members. On the other hand, I know of children with coprolalia who can attend church regularly because the members of the congregation know and accept their symptoms. You just have to use your judgement in deciding how disruptive is *too* disruptive. There are no hard and fast rules for determining whether or not a situation should be avoided.

Dealing with Acquaintances at Work, School, and in the Community

As I indicated earlier, I had an easier (but not easy) time than most children growing up with Tourette syndrome. That is, I was almost never teased, ridiculed, isolated, or rejected by my playmates, classmates, or teachers. I think this was partly due to luck, partly to the times, and partly to the way my family and I coped with the strange behaviors I was exhibiting. Not knowing that I had TS, and finally accepting that no matter what, it didn't seem as if I could stop the symptoms, my family and I went back to trying to live our lives.

One of the most valuable things my family did, I believe, was to "model" for others how I should be treated. That is, my family made it clear that they saw me as a valued and "OK" child, and this helped others to see me the same way. Even if others weren't sure about me, my family established the expectations for others' behavior toward me. For example, when I was a child, we used to go regularly to a dinner buffet at an older hotel near our house. While hotel staff and other patrons must certainly have noticed my symptoms, nothing was ever said to me. If anything was ever said to my parents, I don't know. However, I do know that we ate at this restaurant for many years, and I was always treated with courtesy and friendliness.

In establishing expectations, what family members and friends *don't* do is often as important as what they do. For example, if my brother had laughed at me or teased me or told our playmates that I was weird, I could have easily been more isolated. Instead, he was one of my best friends. If my aunt had told my parents that they could come for dinner if I would try to be more quiet and still, I would have become even more self-conscious about being in social settings. If my wife had asked me to please try to stop the "twitching" when we were out on a date, I most certainly would never have felt comfortable dating or in other close personal relationships. Although I definitely recognize that in all of these examples, members of my family may sometimes have been annoyed or embarrassed, or have thought I was weird, they seldom, if ever, let me know.

The expectations my family set for themselves and others—coupled with their consistent emotional support—played a critical role in teaching me how to cope with classmates, roommates, teammates, employers, co-workers, clients, and employees. And today, I follow my family's lead and try not to let the focus of any relationship be upon my Tourette syndrome. For example, I've often been asked what you should say about your TS in an interview. Clearly, federal law prohibits potential employers from asking about disabling conditions except in specific situations. The chances are, however, that the employer will witness some of our symptoms during the interview. In contrast to someone in a wheelchair, we have symptoms that appear much more bizarre. We may be seen as emotionally unstable, nervous, "high" on drugs. Consequently, I believe it is important to mention TS in an interview. I don't, however, do this the moment I walk in. I try to work it into the interview at an appropriate place that makes me look good. For example, if I were applying for an entry-level position and I was asked about my organizational skills, I might describe my volunteer work with the Tourette Syndrome Association, scheduling appearances at health fairs. I would then take the opportunity to mention what TS is and that I have it. Again, my whole focus is on demonstrating competence, understanding and acceptance of my TS, and an openness about it.

Of course, when in the interview you talk about your TS depends on the severity of your symptoms and on how well you can control them in the interview. I haven't gotten every job I've applied for using this approach. Indeed, I've been turned down because of my TS. But many times over I have found that these strategies are successful in disarming and reassuring others.

Children and their parents can use basically the same approach when trying out for a youth baseball league, applying for ballet school, and the like. That is, they can concentrate on showing and talking about their skills and interests, and then work in a mention of TS—perhaps by talking about medication or that their eyes are OK and that the blinking is caused by Tourette syndrome.

In the long run, the best strategy is to demonstrate the relationship and interaction you expect from others. When I interview new staff people for my company, I only mention my TS if the subject comes up naturally. I tell them about it after I've hired them, but again this occurs during our normal interactions. Once again I try to say, "I am not my TS."

Relating to People Very Close to You

Family members, spouses, girl friends, boy friends, and others who are close to us should be the easiest for us to get along with. Yet sometimes I think they're the hardest. This is because these are the people we care most about; the people who care most about us; the people we want to please the most; and the people (aside from ourselves) whose lives are most seriously disrupted by our symptoms.

I believe that coping involves beginning to share, with those close to us, how we feel about our symptoms. Sharing our feelings about TS is like sharing feelings about other very important aspects of our lives. Our ability to share and the way we do it depends not only on how old we are, but on the

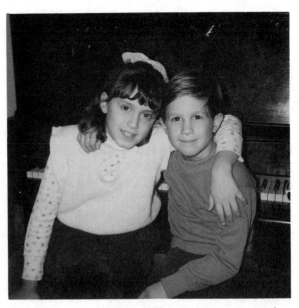

relationship we have with our parents, siblings, spouse, or other important people in our lives. This means, for example, that children of different ages will understand information about TS differently, express their feelings differently, and relate to their parents differently. There is almost no way for an elementary school child to come to grips with the concept of a "neurological disorder." He must first be assured that he won't die from it, that others can't catch it, that his parents know it is frightening for him, and that his parents will try to protect him from doing anything *too* strange or "crazy."

For many of the children with TS I have met, their symptoms have become so much a focus of their family's life that I think it is important not to talk so much about the disorder at first and not to *push* them to share their feelings. Rather, parents, siblings, and other relatives need to demonstrate their understanding of how difficult it must be to live with TS and acknowledge that the child has legitimate feelings about what is happening to him. For example, your child should not always have to tell you how hurt he was by a problem that developed in school because he could not "keep his hands to himself." All you might need to do is put your hand on your child's shoulder and say, "I know you're trying really hard, and it's frustrating when the other students can't seem to understand that you can't stop doing certain things." Over time, this acknowledgement of a child's feelings will help him learn to share them more directly with parents and others.

Coping also involves beginning to understand how our symptoms affect others. It involves understanding that parents, siblings, and spouses are human too . . . that they occasionally need "their space" and distance from us . . . that they sometimes get tired of having to deal with our symptoms (at home or in public) . . . that they get beaten down by schools, human service systems, employers, and neighbors as they try to help us learn to cope. Understanding and working through these situations is very painful but essential.

Naturally, people who live together have some conflicts. Yet what is so difficult for those of us with TS is that some of these conflicts are caused by things we can't control. This puts us at risk of losing those we love because of something we can't change. For example, some children with TS have compulsions to repeat or question what others say—over and over, *ad infinitum*, again and again. Parents, siblings, and others can become quite frustrated with this repetition, even when they know it is part of the TS. In my own life, conflicts arise because I wake up frequently in the middle of the night. If I cannot get back to sleep quickly, my tics begin and these noises and body movements awaken my wife. At times, neither of us gets a good night's sleep for several days, which certainly can lead to tension.

Again, I think coping must start with openness and sharing. If the caring is there, and families are willing to work hard together, the coping will follow.

Accomplishing Tasks

Developing coping strategies to accomplish work, school, or other projects means beginning to take control of our lives. Although we cannot totally control our symptoms, we *can* take steps to help reduce their impact on our lives. We can use our minds to figure out how best to get things accomplished. Because my Tourette syndrome was undiagnosed for many years, many of my coping strategies just seemed to develop naturally. For example, we all know that fatigue makes TS symptoms increase. I have always been an early riser, so in college I found myself doing most of my studying in the morning and early afternoon. Whenever possible, I also scheduled classes during the morning. Even after a late night of partying on the weekend, I would get up at 7 a.m. to study while my dormmates slept. I tended to visit the library at off hours when there were fewer people to disturb, because trying to withhold my tics made reading and concentrating very difficult.

After college, I continued to adjust my schedule to my tics. For instance, when I began reviewing research for the Ohio Department of Mental Health, I would get to work at 7 a.m. I seldom reviewed a grant after 2 p.m. because I knew my tics would be worse and disrupt my ability to concentrate on the technical material.

Another coping strategy that I stumbled upon before I knew I had TS was to participate regularly in sports and physical exercise. I discovered that my ability to cope with my TS, as well as the many stresses of everyday life, was enhanced by taking part in these activities. One reason is that being quiet and still is extremely difficult for people with TS, but TS symptoms seem to be reduced when the body is in motion. I have found that when I participate in sports in which there is more continuous activity (racquetball, volleyball, weight training, swimming), I have fewer tics than when I play sports in which there is more time between activities (for example, softball, baseball, golf).

Physical activities help with coping in other ways, too. First, sports and other physical activities such as dance and karate can give children with TS an opportunity to succeed through hard work. This does not mean that every child must be a "star," but that they can see progress and a temporary reduction of symptoms. (It is important to remember that when fatigue sets in after the activity, the symptoms will likely be worse for a time.) In addition, team sports and other physical activities offer opportunities for children and their families to be with other children and families. This gives parents a chance to "model" how others should view and treat their child. Parents can also explain TS to others (when needed), have fun with their children, or just cheer them on. Finally, not only are exercise and sports good for anyone's overall health, but they are an enjoyable way to reduce stress.

Of course, developing coping strategies for getting things accomplished involves more than managing our tics and other symptoms. It also requires that each of us look carefully at how our symptoms affect our ability to do essential tasks, and then accept responsibility for making the adjustments needed to accomplish our goals. It is equally important to develop the ability to make legitimate demands on others to accept us and make accommodations that enable us to succeed. For example, an employee with TS and his boss might mutually adjust a work schedule to enable the employee to work a shift when his symptoms would be less disruptive. Or even more important, the employee might share information about TS with co-workers while supervisors and management "model" an attitude of acceptance. This is the balancing act of accepting responsibility for our symptoms, while refusing to be limited or defined by them.

When we are children, this responsibility falls on our parents, but as we become teenagers, we must learn to play a much larger role in this process. This role becomes especially important when an education plan is being developed. In my experience, developing a successful plan rests on getting a clear picture of the child's tics, noises, and behaviors; understanding how they are affecting his school performance or behavior; and figuring out what specifically will help him. The more input the child himself can give about these issues, the better. For example, suppose that a student is not getting his homework assignments completed. We really must determine: whether attention problems are causing him to miss the assignments, or whether arm and head tics prevent him from writing down the assignment fast enough, or whether vocal tics prevent him from hearing the assignment. Have medication side effects caused short-term memory loss, or has fatigue made his tics get so severe that he can't complete his homework at night? Has that fatigue caused poor handwriting which always results in a failing grade, so he has decided just not to do the work, or is he such a good student that the class bully steals his homework every day and threatens a beating if he tells? Any of these may be the problem. We must, however, understand what is really going on before we can devise a strategy to cope with the situation.

Because of the fluctuating nature of Tourette syndrome, we must also recognize that what works sometimes might not work as well another time. At times, my tics and other symptoms are somewhat reduced, and then they begin to get worse for no apparent reason. This is known as "waxing and waning." Fatigue can also trigger some of my more disruptive symptoms. For example, after several long days at the office followed by late nights of sports and limited sleep, I get mouth and stomach movements that can make eating very difficult. Some of my leg and head movements can affect my sports activities, and it's very frustrating to be playing volleyball well one week and not nearly as well the next. These are times when I must keep doing most of the things I normally do, but be willing to accept a somewhat lower level of performance. These are times when I have to remember that nobody performs at their highest level all the time, and that people who don't have TS also perform inconsistently, although for different reasons.

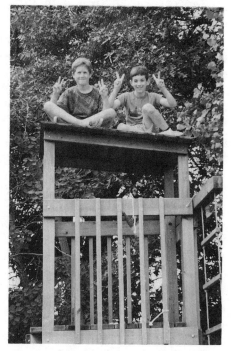

As individuals and families coping with TS, we must really try to understand the condition. We must seek out accurate information. We must ask questions. And we must learn to trust and use our own observations and judgement about our symptoms.

Keeping Your Perspective

I think finally that one of the most important ways to cope with Tourette syndrome is to cultivate a sense of humor about it. Being able to laugh about TS with loved ones can really help.

All of us can think of humorous stories about our symptoms and others' reactions to them. For example, whenever I come home from work, I purposely make some noise like singing, whistling, or calling to my wife to make sure she knows I'm home and doesn't think I'm a burglar. Every once in a while, she teasingly reminds me that she always knows where I am in the house. After all, what kind of burglar comes into a house grunting, sniffing, and clearing his throat?

Or how about the time my then three-year-old niece first started to notice that Uncle Bill made some funny noises and faces? She wasn't sure what I was doing, so she stared at me. My brother and sister-in-law tried to explain TS to her and told her not to stare. For the rest of the weekend, she very pointedly walked around without even *looking at me.*

One of the funniest episodes of all occurred during the planning meeting for adults with TS that was held at the TSA National Conference in November of 1989. Twenty competent, bright, motivated individuals, including professionals, managers, students, and administrators, all with motor tics and vocalizations, were gathered in a small meeting room. Suddenly, several individuals with coprolalia began responding to each others' statements. Others in the group goaded them on. Raucous laughter filled the room. We spent a very productive two days identifying issues for adults with TS, but most importantly, shared many good, long-needed laughs.

If people with Tourette syndrome and their families can occasionally laugh at their symptoms, they can definitely see themselves as distinct from their TS. This, as I pointed out earlier, is the key to coping and to beginning to take control of those portions of your life over which you have control. That TS affects our lives every day is inescapable. That having to live with it and adapt to it helps shape the person we become is also undeniable. That it defines who we are, however, is a terrible falsehood. Living with TS is not easy living, but we have much more to offer the world than our sounds, tics, compulsions, and other strange behaviors. "WE ARE NOT OUR TOURETTE SYNDROME," and as families, we must work together to let others know that this is true.

Personal Statements

I didn't even know I had TS until I was eleven. Life was really hard before my tics were diagnosed. The kids at school would tease me. They decided to torment me because they didn't know about my problem. When I *was* diagnosed, the school nurse talked to them and *then* they understood.

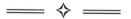

I've met a lot of friends at a camp for kids with TS that I go to one week out of the year. Camp is a place for your family to learn about Tourette syndrome, and a place for kids to have fun.

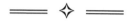

Several of the kids at school teased me by imitating my tic. Kids on the bus called my name so I would turn around and they could see my face as I made the bizarre movement. I was a constant source of frustration to my teacher because she couldn't tolerate my tics; I really felt that she hated me for them. My father was sure that I was doing it on purpose—for attention or just to bug him. My mother was concerned that it was something she had done wrong as a parent. I didn't know why I was doing it, but the constant scrutiny put a tremendous amount of pressure on me. Unable to express myself, I felt totally responsible for the discomfort everyone was feeling.

I was about seven when I had the first vocal tic I can clearly recall. It was a guttural, grunt-like noise. My parents used to hassle me constantly about it and tried to make me stop because they thought I did it to annoy them. When they did, I used to think, "But I really need to do this now; I can't stop." That thought scared me because I knew that I should be able to control it.

At school I was placed in the hall for being noisy and disruptive, so then I learned to suppress my tics as much as possible. I really wanted to please the teacher.

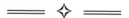

My grandmother told me that making noises wasn't something a good girl did and that I was disappointing her. That really upset me, so I used to leave when I needed to tic because I wanted her

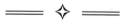

approval. Even to this day, I feel uncomfortable having tics in front of her.

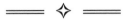

I tried to tell people that I couldn't help it, but I got so much backlash when I did that I stopped. Because they felt I could stop it, and I felt I couldn't, I thought I was going crazy. I felt as though any day someone would see how really messed up I was and then I would really get into trouble.

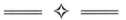

When I was ten, I saw William Shatner make a public service announcement about TS. I was all alone watching TV, and when he started to list some symptoms, I knew that was what I had. I got so scared that I ran up to my room and just lay on the bed in the dark until Dad came home from work. I told him I felt sick, but I really thought that I had a bizarre disease and I would be dead at any moment.

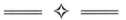

In junior high, I started a very noticeable neck tic. The kids really picked up on it and started teasing me about it. I was really upset, especially when my friends started joining in. I didn't know how to deal with them, so I withdrew. I began carrying a book with me at all times so that if I got to class early, I could just read instead of talking to anybody. Finally I went back to my friends and asked them to help me. I figured if I was punished every time I had a tic, they would stop, so I asked my friends if they could please hit me as hard as possible in the back of my head when I threw my head back. None of them would do it. That made me feel worse, because I felt they didn't care enough to help me stop doing these weird things.

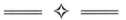

Most people think I'm a jerk, but I'm really not. I'm always quiet and they think I'm dull. But I'm not anything like that. I'm tough because I don't let things get to me. I'm hardworking. Once I get started on something, I keep going. I'm alert and observant. I see everything that's going on.

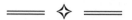

As far back as first grade, I can recall knowing I was different from the other kids, but not being able to place my finger on what it was. The other children used to tease me then, but even so, I really don't think I knew exactly what was different. I just can remember knowing I didn't fit in as well as everyone else.

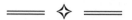

Sometime during the third grade, the blinking started. I remember blinking so hard that my eyes would water like a dam had burst. But even though I continued to blink and have other minor tics, I don't remember it bothering me socially. Socially, I was accepted, and although I was a fairly hyper child, I didn't cause problems for my teachers.

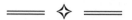

In junior high, my symptoms changed. I began making high-pitched sounds that I could keep under control when I was conscious of them. I remember comparing myself to our German Shepherd, in that we both made high-pitched whining sounds. However, no one in my family or at school compared me to the dog or made fun of my tics.

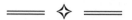

I started dating in about ninth grade. Outside of the normal nervousness that teenagers have about first dates, I had no worries about my tics, for two reasons. First, my tics weren't that severe. Although occasionally the twitching became a little excessive, it was always controllable when I was conscious of it. The second reason was the sense of humor that I was either born with or brought up with or both. The ability to laugh at myself, not take myself too seriously, helped me deal with my tics.

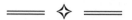

Sports always made me feel good mentally. Although I was small, I always hustled. The open court or field was a place where I could relax the conscious effort to suppress my audible tics. I still use sports to allow the noises or tics to do their things.

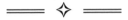

When I was thirty, I was diagnosed by my sister as having Tourette syndrome after she read an article in a women's magazine about tics.

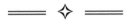

My biggest hope is that I will be the end of the line for TS in my family, and, of course, that the ultimate cure will pop up anytime. In the meantime, I try to keep my sense of humor.

═══ ✧ ═══

GLOSSARY

Absence (petit mal) seizure—Type of seizure characterized by brief loss of consciousness, usually for not more than ten seconds.

Adaptive behavior—The ability to adjust to new environments, tasks, objects, and people, and to apply new skills to those new situations.

Advocacy—Supporting or promoting a cause. Speaking out.

Advocacy groups—Organizations that work to protect the rights and opportunities of handicapped children and their parents.

Affect—An emotion.

Affective disorder—A mental disorder involving the emotions; includes depression and bi-polar disorder (manic depression).

Akathisia—A feeling of inner restlessness which is relieved by moving about. A common side effect of neuroleptic medication.

Anafranil. *See* Clomipramine.

Anticonvulsant—A drug used to control seizures. Even though all seizures are not convulsions, this term is commonly used.

Applied behavior analysis—A method of teaching designed to change behavior in a precisely measurable and accountable manner. Also called **behavior modification.**

Assessment—Process to determine a child's strengths and weaknesses. Includes testing and observations performed by a team of professionals and parents. Usually used to determine special education needs. Term is used interchangeably with **evaluation.**

Associated behaviors—The spectrum of behaviors often seen in association with Tourette syndrome; includes OCD, ADHD, impulsivity, and aggression.

Ataxic—Having unbalanced, jerky movements.

Attention—The ability to concentrate on a task.

Attention deficit disorder (ADD)—A condition beginning early in life which is characterized by inattention and impulsive behavior.

Attention deficit hyperactivity disorder (ADHD)—Attention deficit disorder accompanied by hyperactivity.

Attention span—The amount of time one is able to concentrate on a task. Also called attending in special education jargon.

Auditory—Relating to the ability to hear.

Auditory sequential memory—Ability to hear and repeat a sequence of words or numbers.

Babbling—The sound a baby makes when he combines a vowel and consonant and repeats them over and over again (e.g., ba-ba-ba, ga-ga-ga).

Basal ganglia—Part of the brain that some researchers believe could be location of abnormalities which cause tics.

Behavior modification. *See* Applied behavior analysis.

Behavioral dysinhibition—The inability to control inappropriate behavior because of neurological impairment.

Beneficiary—The person indicated in a trust or insurance policy to receive any payments that become due.

Biofeedback therapy—Use of biofeedback machine to teach oneself relaxation of muscles.

Bi-polar disorder—Another name for manic-depression, a disorder involving extreme ups and downs in mood.

Blood level—The amount of medication in someone's blood; determined by taken a blood sample.

Bradycardia—Very slow heart rate.

Brain stem—Portion of the brain between the cerebellum and spinal cord.

Bruxism—Grinding of teeth repeatedly.

Busipirone—A drug used as an adjunct to tic medications, often used to treat anxiety or OCD in people with TS.

Carbamazepine—An antiepileptic (seizure medication).

Case manager—The person responsible for coordinating services and information from members of interdisciplinary team.

CAT scan (CT scan)—Computerized axial tomography. A test involving X-raying the brain to find any possible malformations.

Catapres. *See* Clonidine.

Cause-and-effect—The concept that actions create reactions.

Central nervous system—The brain and spinal cord. The part of the nervous system primarily involved in voluntary movement and thought processes.

Cerebellum—Part of the brain that helps coordinate muscle activity and control balance.

Cerebrum—The largest part of the brain, located in the upper part of the head. Believed to control intellectual functions such as thinking, remembering, learning.

Childhood schizophrenia—A major psychiatric disorder, probably with multiple causes. Symptoms include disturbances in form and content of thought, perception, emotions, sense of self, volition, relationship to the external world, and psychomotor behavior. Childhood schizophrenia is very rare.

Chorea—Abrupt, quick, jerky movements of the head, neck, arms, or legs.

Chromosomes—Microscopic, rod-shaped bodies in cells which contain genetic material.

Chronic—Long-lasting.

Chronic tic disorder—A tic disorder involving the presence of motor or vocal tics—but not both—for over one year.

Clomipramine—An antidepressant medication used in Tourette syndrome to treat symptoms of OCD.

Clonic seizures—Seizures that affect the whole brain, causing a series of muscle contractions and relaxations.

Clonidine—A high blood pressure medication used in treatment of TS. It can be helpful in controlling tics and ADHD symptoms.

Cognition—The ability to know and understand the environment.

Cognitive dulling—A common side effect of neuroleptic drugs; involves short-term memory loss and slowed thinking.

Co-morbid condition—Medical term meaning a medical condition that occurs along with another medical condition, although one condition does not directly cause the other.

Compensatory skill—A skill used in place of another skill that an individual is unable to perform. For instance, a compensatory skill for someone who is unable to speak might be sign language.

Competitive employment—Jobs which pay workers at least minimum wage to produce valued goods or services, and which are performed in settings that include nondisabled workers.

Complex-partial seizure—Type of seizure that occurs in the temporal lobe of the brain and causes loss of consciousness.

Compulsion—The feeling of being compelled or forced to do a behavior, even though the person experiencing the compulsion does not want to do it. For example, evening things up, washing hands, cleaning.

Congenital—relating to a condition that exists at birth.

Consciousness—The state of awareness.

Convulsion—Involuntary contractions of the muscles. A seizure.

Cost-of-care liability—The right of a state providing care to a handicapped person to charge for the care and to collect from the handicapped person's assets.

Cytogeneticist—A doctor or professional who studies chromosomes and genes and their effect on heredity.

Depression—Disorder producing depressed mood, appetite changes, sleep changes, and sometimes suicidal thinking. Can have a neurochemical basis and can often be treated with medication.

Desipramine—A tricyclic antidepressant used in the treatment of ADHD associated with TS.

Development—The process of growth and learning during which a child acquires skills and abilities.

Developmental disability—A handicap or impairment originating before the age of eighteen which may be expected to continue indefinitely and which constitutes a substantial disability.

Developmental milestone—A developmental goal such as sitting or using two-word phrases that functions as a measurement of developmental progress over time.

Developmentally delayed—Having development that is slower than normal.

Diagnostic and Statistical Manual of Mental Disorders (DSM III-R)—A manual published by the American Psychiatric Association (APA) which describes all of the diagnostic criteria and the systematic descriptions of various mental disorders.

Discretionary trust—A trust in which the trustee (the person responsible for governing the trust) has the authority to use or not use the trust funds for any purpose, as long as funds are expended only for the beneficiary.

Disinherit—To deprive someone of an inheritance. Parents of handicapped children may do this to prevent the state from imposing cost-of-care liability on their child's assets.

Dispute resolution procedures—The procedure established by law and regulation for the fair resolution of disputes regarding a child's special education.

Dopamine—One of the neurotransmitters (brain chemicals) involved in motor and vocal tics.

Drug vacation—Time off of any medication, usually in summer months. Suggested for children on certain medications.

DSM III-R. *See* Diagnostic and Statistical Manual of Mental Disorders.

Due process hearing—Part of the procedures established to protect the rights of parents and special-needs children during disputes under Public Law 94–142. These are hearings before an impartial person to review the identification, evaluation, placement, and services by a handicapped child's educational agency.

Dysarthria—Impaired articulation due to problems in muscle control.

Dysinhibition of aggression—Inability to control aggressive behavior, as a result of neurological impairment.

Dyskinesia—A general term for involuntary movements.

Dyslexia—One type of learning disability that affects reading ability.

Dyspraxia—Difficulty planning movements or putting them into sequence.

Early development—Development during the first three years of life.

Early intervention—The specialized way of interacting with infants to minimize the effects of conditions that can delay early development.

Echolalia—A parrot-like repetition of phrases or words just heard (immediate echolalia), or heard hours, days, weeks, or even months ago (delayed echolalia).

Education for All Handicapped Children Act—Former name of Public Law 94–142. *See* IDEA.

EEG. *See* Electroencephalogram.

Electroencephalogram (EEG)—The machine and test used to determine levels of electrical discharge from nerve cells.

Emotional lability—Instability of expression of emotions. For example, having a "short fuse," being quick to anger. Common in people with TS.

Enzyme—A secretion from cells that changes chemicals in other body substances.

Epilepsy—A recurrent condition caused by abnormal electrical discharges in the brain that causes seizures.

Estate planning—Formal, written arrangements for handling the possessions and assets of people after they have died.

Etiology—The study of the cause of disease.

Evaluation. *See* Assessment.

Expressive language—The ability to use gestures, words, and written symbols to communicate.

Extinction—A procedure in which reinforcement of a previously reinforced behavior is withheld.

Extrapyramidal effects—Side effects of neuroleptic medications. Examples are bradykinesia, akathisia, and dystonia.

Febrile seizures—Seizures that are associated with fever.

Fine motor—Relating to the use of the small muscles of the body, such as those in the hands, feet, fingers, and toes.

Fluoxetine—An antidepressant used in TS to treat OCD and depression.

Fluphenazine—A neuroleptic drug used in treating TS. It is a dopamine blocker and may help reduce tics.

Focal motor seizure—Jerking of a few muscle groups without an initial loss of consciousness.

Generalization—Transferring a skill taught in one place, or with one person, to other places and people.

Genes—Material within the chromosomes that determines specific traits, such as hair and eye color and stature.

Genetic—Pertaining to a trait determined by the genes; inherited.

Graduated guidance—Systematically and gradually reducing the amount of physical guidance used.

Grand mal seizure. *See* Tonic clonic seizure.

Gross motor—Relating to the use of the large muscles of the body.

Haldol. *See* Haloperidol.

Half life—The time it takes a drug to decrease in potency in the blood by fifty percent.

Haloperidol—A neuroleptic medication used in treating the tics of TS.

Handicapped—Refers to people who have some sort of disability, including physical disabilities, mental retardation, sensory impairments, behavioral disorders, learning disabilities, and multiple handicaps.

Hyperactivity—A specific nervous-system-based difficulty which makes it hard for a person to control muscle (motor) behavior.

IDEA—The federal law that guarantees all handicapped children the right to a free appropriate public education. It is Public Law 94–142.

Identification—The determination that a child should be evaluated as a possible candidate for special education services.

IEP—Individualized Education Program. The written plan that describes what services the local education agency has promised to provide your child.

IFSP—Individualized Family Service Plan. The written document that describes what services a child will receive through his early intervention program.

Imitation—The ability to observe the actions of others and to copy them in one's own actions. Also known as **modeling.**

Impulsive—Lacking impulse control; prone to "acting without thinking."

Infantile myoclonic seizures—Seizures that cause sudden, brief, involuntary muscle contractions involving one or several muscle groups.

Inhibition—The ability to inhibit or stop messages sent by the brain to other parts of the body.

Input—Information that a person receives through any of the senses (vision, hearing, touch, feeling, smell) that helps that person develop new skills.

Insistence on sameness—A tendency to become upset when familiar routines are changed.

Integration. *See* Mainstreaming.

Interdisciplinary team—A team of professionals who evaluate your child and then develop a comprehensive summary report of his or her strengths and needs.

Interpretive—The sessions during which parents and teachers review and discuss the results of a child's evaluation.

Intracranial—Within the skull.

Intractable—Difficult to control, treat, or cure.

Involuntary movements—Uncontrolled movements, such as tics.

I.Q. (Intelligence Quotient)—A measure of cognitive ability based on specifically designed standardized tests.

Language—The expression and understanding of human communication.

Learning disability—Difficulty processing certain types of information in a child of normal intelligence.

Least restrictive environment—The requirement under Public Law 94–142 that children receiving special education must be made a part of a regular school to the fullest extent possible. Included in the law as a way of ending the traditional practice of isolating children with disabilities.

Limbic system—Seen as "emotional center" of the brain. Studied in TS research.

Lithium—Medication used to treat manic depression, which is sometimes a co-morbid condition to TS.

Local Education Agency (LEA)—The agency responsible for providing educational services on the local (city, county, and school district) level.

Luxury trust—A trust that describes the kind of allowable expenses in a way that excludes the cost of care in state-funded programs in order to avoid cost-of-care liability.

Magnetic Resonance Imaging (MRI)—A type of computerized brain scan.

Mainstreaming—The practice of involving handicapped children in regular school and preschool environments. Also called integration.

Medicaid—A joint state and federal program that offers medical assistance to people who are entitled to receive Supplementary Security Income.

Medicare—A federal program that provides payments for medical care to people who are receiving Social Security payments.

Mental retardation—Below normal mental function. Children who are mentally retarded learn more slowly than other children, but "mental retardation" itself does not indicate a specific level of mental ability. The level of mental function may not be identifiable until a much later age.

Metabolism—The chemical and physical changes in human cells that provide energy.

Methylphenidate—A stimulant drug often prescribed for ADHD; can cause increase in tics of TS.

Modeling. *See* Imitation.

Motor—Relating to the ability to move oneself.

Motor patterns—The ways in which the body and limbs work to make sequenced movements.

Motor planning—The ability to think through and carry out a physical task.

MRI. *See* Magnetic Resonance Imaging.

Multidisciplinary team. *See* Interdisciplinary team.

Multihandicapped—Having more than one handicap.

Neuroleptic—Medicine which produces symptoms resembling those of diseases of the nervous system.

Neurological impairment—Dysfunction of neurological functions in the brain.

Neurologist—A physician specializing in medical problems associated with the brain and spinal cord.

Neuromotor—Involving both the nerves and muscles.

Neurons—Nerve cells in the brain.

Neuropsychiatric disorder—A behavioral disorder which is poised between mind and body, influenced by environmental and internal neurological factors.

Neurotransmitter—The chemical substance between nerve cells in the brain which allows the transmission of an impulse from one nerve to another.

Norepinephrine—One of the brain's neurotransmitters involved in formation and function of dopamine and serotonin. Can be regulated by clonidine.

Norpramine. *See* Desipramine.

Obsessions—Recurring thoughts that often will not go away until a compulsion is performed.

Obsessive Compulsive Behavior (OCB)—Having symptoms of obsessional thinking and compulsive behavior.

Obsessive Compulsive Disorder (OCD)—As classified in the DSM, a disorder involving obsessive compulsive behavior which severely interferes with life functions.

OCB. *See* Obsessive Compulsive Behavior.

Occupational therapist (O.T.)—A therapist who specializes in improving the development of fine motor and adaptive skills. May also be qualified to work on sensory integration problems.

OCD. *See* Obsessive Compulsive Disorder.

OHI. *See* Other Health Impaired.

Oral motor—Relating to the movement of muscles in and around the mouth.

Oral tactile defensiveness—An over-sensitivity to touch around the mouth.

Orap. *See* Pimozide.

Other Health Impaired—A classification within special education law detailing criteria under which children can qualify for special education services. Tourette syndrome falls under the OHI category in federal law.

Parallel play—One or more people playing alongside, but not together, with one another.

Parent-professional partnership—The teaming of parents and teachers (or doctors, nurses, or other professionals) to work together to facilitate the development of babies and children with special needs.

Partial seizure—Type of seizure in which the abnormal discharge takes place in one specific part of the brain. A focal or local seizure.

Peabody Language Kit—A series of language stimulation exercises available commercially.

Perseveration—Repetitive movement or speech that is thought to be created by the person's own inner preoccupations.

PET scan. *See* Position Emission Tomography.

Pharmacotherapy—The use of medications in treating a disorder.

Physical therapist (P.T.)—A therapist who works with motor skills.

Pimozide—A neuroleptic drug used to help reduce tics of TS.

Placement—The selection of the educational program for a child who needs special education programs.

Polypharmacy—Use of more than one medication in treating a condition; common in TS.

Position Emission Tomography (PET scan)—Test that identifies metabolic activity.

Prognosis—A prediction about the likely course of a disease or condition in an individual.

Prolixin. *See* Fluphenazine.

Prompt—Input that encourages a child to perform a movement or activity. *See* Cue.

Prozac. *See* Fluoxetine.

Pseudoephedrine—Over-the-counter medication commonly used for colds, flu, and allergy symptoms. Can exacerbate tics of TS. Sold under brand name Sudafed.

Psychomotor (complex partial) seizures—Seizures which cause decreased alertness and changes in behavior.

Public Law 94–142. *See* IDEA.

Punishment—A consequence that is applied following a behavior to reduce the probability of that behavior occurring again. Punishment can be very mild (a frown or scolding), more moderate (a brief time-out), or very severe (electric shock to reduce life-threatening behavior).

Receptive language—The ability to understand spoken and written communication as well as gestures.

Rehearsal—Practicing a desired behavior with a child in preparation for him to do it on his own.

Reinforcement—Providing a pleasant consequence (positive reinforcement) or removing an unpleasant consequence (negative reinforcement) after a behavior in order to increase or maintain that behavior.

Related services—Services that enable a child to benefit from special education. Related services include speech, occupational, and physical therapies, as well as transportation.

Remission—A complete absence of symptoms for a period of months to years. Sometimes occurs in TS.

Respite care—Skilled adult- or child-care and supervision that can be provided in your home or the home of a care-provider. Respite care may be available for several hours per week or for overnight stays.

Ritalin. *See* Methylphenidate.

School phobia—Fear or avoidance of school attendance. Seen often in children with TS, it can be a side effect of neuroleptic medications, or a result of harassment or ridicule at school.

Screening test—A test given to groups of children to sort out those who need further evaluation.

SEA—The State Education Agency.

Secure employment—Vocational training that prepares adults with disabilities to enter the work force. The training is designed specifically to teach the skills needed to survive and succeed in supported or competitive employment situations.

Sedation—Sleepiness; common side effect of some TS medications.

Seizure—Involuntary movement or changes in consciousness or behavior brought on by abnormal electrical discharges in nerve cells in the brain.

Self-help—Relating to the ability to take care of one's self, through such skills as eating, dressing, bathing, and cleaning.

Self-injurious behaviors (SIB)—Behaviors that result in self-inflicted injuries—for example, biting, head banging, picking scabs, cutting self.

Sensory ability—The ability to process sensations, such as touch, sound, light, smell, and movement.

Sensory impairments—Problems handling information relayed to the brain from the senses.

Sensory integration therapy—Treatment aimed at improving the way the brain processes and organizes sensations.

Sensory seizures—Seizures that produce dizziness or disturbances in vision, hearing, taste, smell, or other senses.

Sensory tics—Tics that produce disturbances in vision, hearing, taste, smell, or other senses.

Serotonin—One of the brain's neurotransmitters, believed by some researchers to be involved in depression and OCD.

Serum blood levels—The level of medications in the blood. Used to monitor drug therapy in the control of seizures or other conditions.

Sheltered employment—Employment in work settings where all workers have disabilities, are continually supervised, and are paid less than minimum wage. There is no expectation for workers to move on to more independent, integrated employment.

Side effects—Secondary, unwanted effects of using a medication.

Sight word approach—A method of reading in which the child says what he sees rather than sounding out words.

Simple partial seizure—A seizure that remains in one part of the brain and causes no loss of consciousness.

Single Photon Emission Computed Tomography—Device which measures brain function through blood flow and glucose metabolism.

Social ability—The ability to function in groups and to interact with people.

Special education—Specialized instruction based on educational disabilities determined by a team evaluation. It must be precisely matched to educational needs and adapted to the child's learning style.

Special needs—Needs generated by a person's handicap.

SPECT. *See* Single Photon Emission Computed Tomography.

Speech/language pathologist—A therapist who works to improve speech and language skills, as well as to improve oral motor abilities.

SQ3R—Study, Question, Read, Recite, Review; a educational method designed to help students learn and remember material.

S.S.D.I.—Social Security Disability Insurance. This money has been paid into the Social Security system through payroll deductions on earnings. Disabled workers are entitled to these benefits. People who become disabled before the age of twenty-two may collect S.S.D.I. under a parent's account, if the parent is retired, disabled, or deceased.

S.S.I.—Supplemental Security Income is available for low-income people who are disabled, blind, or aged. S.S.I. is based on need, not on past earnings.

Steady state—This term describes the drug level in the blood once it has reached a therapeutic level. Daily doses of medication maintain this level.

Stimulant—A psychotropic drug such as Ritalin and Dexedrine often used to control hyperactivity in children.

Stimulus—A physical object or environmental event that *may* have an effect upon the behavior of a person. Some stimuli are internal (earache pain), while others are external (a smile from a loved one).

Supported employment—Paid employment for people with developmental disabilities for whom competitive employment at or above minimum wage is unlikely. Employment is supported by any activity—a job coach, for example—designed to keep the worker employed.

Support trust—A trust that requires that funds be expended to pay for the beneficiary's expenses of living, including housing, food, and transportation.

Symptomatic—Having a cause that is identified.

Tactile—Relating to touch.

Tactile defensiveness—Abnormal sensitivity to touch.

Tardive dyskinesia—Involuntary movements of the mouth, tongue, and lips can occur and may be associated with choreo-athetoid (purposeless, quick, jerky movements that occur suddenly) movements of the trunk and limbs. Some medications prescribed for Tourette syndrome can contribute to the development of this condition.

Therapeutic blood level—For any given individual, each drug has a level at which it is most effective. The therapeutic blood level refers to the amount of a medication within the blood that provides the most effective results.

Therapist—A trained professional who works to overcome the effects of developmental problems.

Tic—An involuntary movement (motor tic) or involuntary vocalization (vocal tic).

Titrate—To increase the dose of medication slowly over time until the optimum level is achieved.

Tonic clonic (grand mal) seizure—A type of seizure which causes a sudden loss of consciousness followed immediately by a generalized convulsion in which extremeties become stiff, then jerk rhythmically.

Tourette syndrome—A chronic, physical disorder of the brain which causes both motor tics and vocal tics, and begins before the age of twenty-one.

Tricyclic antidepressant—Antidepressants such as desipramine and imipramine, sometimes used in treatment of TS.

Uniform Gifts to Minors Act (UGMA)—A law that governs gifts to minors. Under the UGMA, gifts become the property of the minor at age eighteen or twenty-one.

Vestibular—Pertaining to the sensory system located in the inner ear that allows that body to maintain balance and enjoyably participate in movement such as swinging and roughhousing.

Visual motor—The skill required to carry out a task such as putting a puzzle piece into a puzzle or a key into a keyhole.

Vocational training—Training for a job. Learning skills to perform in the workplace.

Waxing and waning—A naturally occurring rising and falling of severity and frequency of tics.

READING LIST

This Reading List is intended to help parents learn more about the topics discussed in each chapter of the book. It includes books specific to Tourette syndrome, obsessive compulsive disorder, and attention deficit hyperactivity disorder, as well as more general resources for raising a child with a disability. Because periodicals often offer the most up-to-date information on TS and related subjects, a list of helpful newsletters and magazines is also included at the end of the section.

Much of the current reading material on TS is in the form of pamphlets and videos published by the Tourette Syndrome Association (TSA). We cannot list all TSA publications here, but we encourage you to contact the TSA at 1–800–237–0717 or write to TSA at 42–40 Bell Blvd., Bayside, NY 11361–2861. Ask for the "Catalog of Publications and Films." There is a pamphlet to answer questions on almost any aspect of Tourette syndrome. Also check with your local TSA chapter, as listed in the Resource Guide, for any articles or pamphlets they may have. Other useful publications on your particular interest area may be available from your local library or bookstore, as well as from parent groups listed in the Resource Guide.

Foreword

Tourette Syndrome Association. Offers a free article on how Jim Eisenreich coped with Tourette syndrome. For a copy, send a self-addressed, stamped envelope to: Tourette Syndrome Association, Attn.: Eisenreich article, 42–40 Bell Blvd., Bayside, NY 11361.

Chapter 1

Barkley, Russell. *Attention Deficit Hyperactivity Disorders: A Handbook for Diagnosis and Treatment.* New York: Guilford Press, 1990. This book discusses ADHD symptoms, behavior management strategies, and family issues.

Baton Rouge TS Support Group. *Toughing Out Tourette's.* Baton Rouge, LA: Baton Rouge Tourette's Support Group, 1989. Compiled by the Baton Rouge Tourette's support group, this book is a collection of articles on all aspects of TS, and how it affects daily life.

Bruun, R., D. Cohen, and J. Leckman. "Guide to Diagnosis and Treatment of TS." New York: Tourette Syndrome Association, 1989. Covers symptoms, pharmacology, differential diagnosis, clinical assessment. Good resource to give physicians.

Buehrens, Adam. *Hi, I'm Adam*. Duarte, CA: Hope Press, 1991. Written by a child with TS, this book discusses, from a child's viewpoint, how it feels to have TS, getting a diagnosis, medications, school problems, etc. It is written for children aged 4–14, and offers support and encouragement to children with TS.

Buehrens, C. and A. Buehrens. *Adam and the Magic Marble*. Duarte, CA: Hope Press, 1991. Written and illustrated by a boy with TS and his mother, this book is about two boys with TS and a magic marble. It is for all ages and all readers, whether they have a disability or not.

Cohen, D.J., R.D. Bruun, and J.F. Leckman, eds. *Tourette's Syndrome and Tic Disorders: Clinical Understanding and Treatment*. New York: Wiley, 1988. A professional text presenting current research and thinking in Tourette syndrome. It thoroughly covers diagnostic criteria for TS and explains associated behaviors, family and school issues, and pharmacology. Very useful in educating professionals, but it may be too technical for some parents.

Comings, David. *Tourette Syndrome and Human Behavior*. Duarte, CA: Hope Press, 1990. Written for both the lay reader and the health or educational professional, this book covers a broad spectrum of disorders, and their possible relation to TS. It also gives very readable information on medication, helpful diagrams of the neurological systems, and neurotransmitter interactions.

Hughes, Susan. *Ryan - A Mother's Story of Her Hyperactive/Tourette Syndrome Child*. Duarte, CA: Hope Press, 1990. The mother of a child with TS tells of her struggle with understanding her child's unusual behaviors, of getting a diagnosis, and struggling with her own feelings. Supportive and encouraging, especially for parents of a child with TS and ADHD.

Jenike, M.A., L. Baer, and N.E. Minichiello, eds. *Obsessive Compulsive Disorders: Theory and Management*. Littleton, MA: PSG Publishing Co., 1989. A thoughtful and informative book on obsessive compulsive disorder, with one chapter devoted to TS.

Moore, Cory. *A Reader's Guide for Parents of Children with Mental Physical, or Emotional Disabilities*. Rockville, MD: Woodbine House, 1990. A comprehensive, annotated reading list for parents on all subjects related to developmental disabilities. A valuable resource.

Rapoport, Judith. *The Boy Who Couldn't Stop Washing: The Experience and Treatment of Obsessive Compulsive Disorder*. New York: Plume Books, 1990. Written for the lay reader, this book explores obsessive compulsive disorder, including current research into the neurological basis of the disorder and current treatment options. It offers an understanding view to parents of children with obsessive compulsive disorder, which often accompanies TS.

Chapter 2

Kushner, H.S. *When Bad Things Happen to Good People.* New York: Avon, 1981. A biographical account of a rabbi and his family following the death of their son from a rare disease. A moving and compassionate work, helpful for anyone coming to grips with strong emotions.

Melton, David. *Promises to Keep: A Handbook for Parents of Learning Disabled, Brain Injured, and Other Exceptional Children.* New York: Franklin Watts, 1984. A good general guide to raising and caring for children with special needs.

Murphy, Albert T. *Special Children, Special Parents: Personal Issues with Handicapped Children.* Englewood Cliffs, NJ: Prentice Hall, 1981. A look into the emotions of parents of children with disabilities. Includes many statements from parents.

Perske, Robert. *Hope for Families: New Directions for Parents of Persons with Retardation or Other Disabilities.* Nashville, Abingdon Press, 1981. A compassionate and philosophical book for parents about adjusting to life with a child with a disability.

Chapter 3

Cohen, D.J., R.D. Bruun, and J.F. Leckman, eds. *Tourette's Syndrome and Tic Disorders: Clinical Understanding and Treatment.* New York: Wiley, 1988. Discusses pharmacotherapy in Tourette syndrome, and also clinical care of TS patients. For professionals.

Comings, David. *Tourette Syndrome and Human Behavior.* Duarte, CA: Hope Press, 1990. Includes very readable information on medication, helpful diagrams of the neurological systems, and information on neurotransmitter interactions.

Tourette Syndrome Association. Offers many pamphlets on medical issues in Tourette Syndrome. You can get a list of these by calling 1–800–237–0717 and requesting the "Catalog of Publications and Films."

Chapter 4

Bruun, R. and K. Rickler. "Tourette Syndrome and Behavior." New York: Tourette Syndrome Association, 1991. The most current thought on behavior problems frequently associated with TS. Also includes practical behavior management ideas for parents.

Budd, Linda. *Living with the Active Alert Child: Ground Breaking Strategies for Parents.* New York: Prentice Hall, 1990. Although this book does not specifically address Tourette syndrome, parenting strategies suggested are pro-active and focus on meeting the needs of children who may provide more of a challenge than the average child. It is encouraging and uplifting reading. Many practical ideas included.

Fontenelle, Don H. *How to Live with Your Children.* Tucson: Fischer Books, 1989. Dr. Fontenell has much experience with Tourette Syndrome. He discusses the disorder and treatment in a book written for parents.

Fowler, Mary Cahill. *Maybe You Know My Kid.* New York: Birch Lane Press, 1990. This informative book looks at ADHD from a parent's viewpoint, and discusses difficulties in receiving a diagnosis, tips for management, and support for families with a child with the disorder.

Garber, S., M. Daniels Garber, and R. Freedman Spizman. *If Your Child Is Hyperactive, Inattentive, Impulsive and Distractible.* New York: Villard Books, 1990. This parents' guide offers many practical strategies for behavior management which would apply to many children with Tourette syndrome.

Nelson, Jane. *Positive Discipline.* New York: Ballantine Books, 1987. This book offers fresh, positive behavior management strategies for parents and schools. Although not designed specifically for families with TS, techniques are helpful in working with behavioral issues in all children. It is especially helpful for families dealing with behavioral difficulties such as children with TS often have.

Chapter 5

Berne, P. and L. Savary. *Building Self Esteem in Children.* New York: The Continuum Publishing Co., 1989. This book offers very practical tips for building self-esteem in children. Very useful for parents of a child with TS.

Christopher, William and Barbara. *Mixed Blessings.* Nashville: Abingdon Press, 1989. A moving personal account about raising a child with autism. Many of their experiences are similar to those of families raising children with more severe TS.

Clark, Jean Illsley. *Self Esteem: A Family Affair.* New York: Winston Press, 1978. Written for parents, this book guides families to building self-esteem of members. This book would be quite helpful for a family with a child with TS. It is written in workbook form.

Featherstone, Helen. *A Difference in the Family: Life with a Disabled Child.* New York: Penguin, 1982. A very compassionate account of one family's journey on the road to acceptance of their child's severe disabilities. Highly recommended.

Moss, Deborah. *Shelly, The Hyperactive Turtle.* Rockville, MD: Woodbine House, 1989. This is a children's book about Shelley and his family. In recounting how Shelly's family copes with the many challenges of hyperactivity, it explains hyperactivity to children. It is positive and realistic. Helpful to children with TS and ADHD.

Meyer, Donald J., Patricia Vadasy, and Rebecca R. Fewell. *Living with a Brother or Sister with Special Needs: A Book for Sibs.* Seattle: University of Washington Press, 1985. Written for siblings, this book provides general information on disabilities and suggests strategies for dealing with emotions and solving common problems.

Chapter 6

Ayres, A. Jean. *Sensory Integration and the Child.* Los Angeles: Western Psychological Services, 1979. This book addresses a topic which is of interest to many parents of children with TS. It offers a look at sensory integration aimed at helping the child achieve more in school and at home.

Brodzinsky, D., A. Gormly, and S.R. Ambron. *Lifespan Human Development.* New York: Holt, Rinehart and Winston, 1987. This book describes the basics of normal human development throughout a lifetime. It would be useful to those who wish to review the fundamentals of human growth.

Chapter 7

Anderson, Winifred, Stephen Chitwood, and Deirdre Hayden. *Negotiating the Special Education Maze: A Guide for Parents and Teachers.* Rockville, MD: Woodbine House, 1989. A step-by-step guide through the special eduction process. Helpful to parents in ensuring that their children receive appropriate special education services under P.L. 94–142.

Shore, Kenneth. *The Special Education Handbook.* New York: Teachers College Press, 1986. Excellent book for parents written by a school psychologist. Clearly explains the special education process.

Silver, A. and R. Hagin. *Disorders of Learning in Childhood.* New York: Wiley, 1990. A professional text presenting current research and thinking on learning disorders. Included is a chapter on Tourette syndrome, which offers case studies and focuses on learning problems in TS. May be too technical for some parents.

Silver, Larry B. *The Misunderstood Child: A Guide for Parents of Learning Disabled Children.* New York: McGraw-Hill, 1984. This understanding guide is intended to help parents become "an informed consumer" and "an assertive advocate" for a child with learning disabilities. It includes suggestions for dealing with schools, and tips about techniques and approaches for parents to use at home.

Taylor, John F. *Helping Your Hyperactive Child.* Rocklin, CA: Prima Publishing and Communication, 1990. This book offers a comprehensive look at ADHD and how it affects all aspects of family life. Offers many helpful suggestions for dealing with ADHD.

Wender, Paul. *The Hyperactive Child, Adolescent, and Adult: Attention Deficit Disorder through the Lifespan.* New York: Oxford University Press, 1987. A guide for parents of children with ADHD, this book extends what has been learned about the disorder into adulthood.

Chapter 8

Apolloni, Tony and Thomas P. Cooke. *A New Look at Guardianship: Protective Services that Support Personalized Living.* Baltimore: Paul H. Brookes, 1984. This book reviews options for providing future support for people with handicaps.

Biklen, Douglas. *Let Our Children Go: An Organizing Manual for Advocates and Parents.* Syracuse, NY: Human Policy Press, 1974. A handbook for organizing a grassroots campaign to improve the treatment and education of children with special needs. Although written before the passage of P.L. 94–142, much of the advice is still useful.

Budoff, Milton and Alan Orenstein. *Due Process in Special Education: On Going to a Hearing.* Cambridge, MA: Brookline Books, 1988. A thorough examination of due process procedures in special education.

Des Jardins, Charlotte. *How to Organize an Effective Parent/Advocacy Group and Move Bureaucracies.* Chicago: Coordinating Council for Handicapped Children (20 E. Jackson Blvd., Room 900, Chicago, IL 60604), 1980. A handbook on organizing parent advocacy groups and working for change in educational services for children with disabilities.

Des Jardins, Charlotte. *How to Get Services By Being Assertive.* Chicago: Coordinating Council for Handicapped Children (20 E. Jackson Blvd., Room 900, Chicago, IL 60604), 1985. A handbook for preparing to advocate for your child or any child with a disability. Very useful for parents, even just as help getting through an IEP meeting.

Chapter 9

Buehrens, Adam. *Hi, I'm Adam.* Duarte, CA: Hope Press, 1991. Written by a child with TS, this book discusses from a child's viewpoint what it's like to have TS. It is written for children ages 4–14, and offers support and encouragement.

Tourette Syndrome Association. Has pamphlets written by people with Tourette syndrome. They address issues such as a teenager's viewpoint or a lifetime of coping without a diagnosis. Call 1–800–237–0717 for more information.

Newsletters and Magazines

CH.A.D.D.ER. CH.A.D.D. (Children with Attention Deficit Disorders), Suite 185, 1859 N. Pine Island Rd., Plantation, FL 33322 (305–587–3700). Bi-annual publication dedicated to furthering information on attention deficit disorders. Articles for parents and professionals dealing with ADD.

Challenge: A Newsletter on ADHD. Challenge, Inc., 42 Way to the River, West Knobbier, MA 01985.

Disabled USA. President's Committee on Employment of the Handicapped, 1111 20th St. NW, 6th floor, Washington, DC 20036. Reports progress in opportunities for people with disabilities and developments in rehabilitation employment.

Especially Grandparents. King County ARC, 2230 Eighth Ave., Seattle, WA 98121. A quarterly newsletter that contains articles on topics of concern to grandparents of special-needs children, designed to help them cope with the special challenges facing them.

Exceptional Parent. 1170 Commonwealth Ave., Boston, MA 02134 (617–730–5800). Magazine for parents of children with disabilities. Includes personal accounts, articles on daily care and educational and legal issues, and resources for parents of children with special needs.

Newsbriefs. Association for Children and Adults with Learning Disabilities, 4156 Library Rd., Pittsburgh, PA 15234 (412–341–1515). Published six times annually, this newsletter covers current developments in the field of learning disabilities.

Newsletter. NICHCY, Box 1492, Washington, DC 20013. A quarterly newsletter on issues of importance to people living or working with children with special needs. Free subscription.

OCD Newsletter. OC (Obsessive Compulsive) Foundation, P.O. Box 9573, New Haven, CT 06535 (203–772–0565). This newsletter is published five times a year to expand research, understanding, and treatment of obsessive compulsive disorder.

OSERS News in Print. Office of Special Education and Rehabilitative Services, 330 C St. SW, 3018 Switzer Bldg., Washington, DC 20202. Newsletter reporting federal activities that affect people with disabilities.

Pacesetter Newsletter. Parent Advocacy Coalition for Educational Rights (PACER), 4826 Chicago Ave., Minneapolis, MN 55417. A quarterly newsletter for parents interested in special education issues. PACER also offers a range of information sheets, pamphlets, and books for parents of children with disabilities. Request a publications catalog.

Sibling Information Network Newsletter. Connecticut's University Affiliated Program, School of Education, the University of Connecticut, Box U–64, Room 227, Storrs, CT 06268. Covers research and literature reviews, meetings, family relationships, and other information of interest to siblings.

Tourette Syndrome Association, Inc. Newsletter. Tourette Syndrome Association, 42–40 Bell Blvd., Bayside, NY 11361. This newsletter is published bi-annually and includes up-to-date information about TS research and TSA organization happenings.

RESOURCE GUIDE

National Organizations

The national organizations listed below provide a variety of services that may be of help in meeting the needs of people with Tourette syndrome and their families. For more information about any of these organizations, call or write them and request an information packet.

American Association of University Affiliated Programs for Persons with Developmental Disabilities (AAUAP)
8630 Fenton St., Suite 410
Silver Spring, MD 20910
(301) 588–8252
A network of university-based and university-affiliated centers that diagnose and treat people with developmental disabilities such as Tourette syndrome. Consult the Local Organizations list for the AAUAP nearest you.

ARC
500 E. Border St., Suite 300
Arlington, TX 76010
(817) 261–6003
ARC, formerly known as the Association for Retarded Citizens, is a non-profit association committed to helping individuals with developmental disabilities achieve full participation in the community through support and advocacy. See the Local Organizations for the address of your state chapter.

The Association for Persons with Severe Handicaps (TASH)
7010 Roosevelt Way, NE
Seattle, WA 98115
(206) 523–8446
Professional/parent organization that uses legal and educational advocacy to work for a dignified lifestyle for all people with severe handicaps. Publishes a newsletter and a professional journal.

Association for the Care of Children's Health (ACCH)
7910 Woodmont Ave., Suite 300
Bethesda, MD 20814
(301) 654–6549
An organization dedicated to the well-being of chronically ill children and children with special needs, ACCH publishes a newsletter and a variety of booklets addressing the concerns of parents of children with disabilities.

Children with Attention Deficit Disorders (CH.A.D.D.)
1859 N. Pine Island Rd.
Suite 185
Plantation, FL 33322
(305) 587–3700
A non-profit organization that provides information and support to parents who have children with attention deficit disorders. Chapters of Ch.A.D.D. have been formed or are being formed in many states; contact the national organization for the location nearest you.

City of Hope National Medical Center
Department of Medical Genetics
Duarte, CA 91010
(818) 359–8111, ext. 2631
Provides treatment of children with TS. Also can provide information and support for families coping with TS. Support groups sponsored by the center are being formed in various locations. Contact Dr. David E. Momings, M.D., for information.

Disability Rights Education and Defense Fund, Inc.
2212 Sixth St.
Berkeley, CA 94710
(415) 644–2555
Conducts educational programs aimed at furthering the civil rights and liberties of people with disabilities. Distributes publications about the rights of children with special needs to a free, appropriate public education.

Kids on the Block
9385 C Gerwig Lane
Columbia, MD 21046
(410) 290–9095; (800) 368–KIDS
This is a performing arts puppet show that gears its shows to school-aged children. The puppets have a variety of handicaps. KIDS performs in 49 states.

Learning Disabilities Association of America (LDAA)
4156 Library Rd.
Pittsburgh, PA 15234
(412) 340–1515
This organization offers membership to parents and professionals and is a national association with both state and local chapters. It can provide information on educational programs for students with LDs and on legislative issues, and offers publications on a variety of issues related to learning disabilities. Consult the Local Organizations list for the chapter nearest you.

Mental Health Law Project
1101 15th St., NW, Suite 1212
Washington, DC 20005
(202) 467–5730
A public interest law firm which conducts test cases to defend the rights of people with mental disabilities. Can provide information about the Americans with Disabilities Act (ADA).

National Association of Protection and Advocacy Systems
900 2nd St., NE, Suite 211
Washington, DC 20002
(202) 408–9514
A legal organization established to protect the rights of people with disabilities. It can supply information about education, health, residential, social, and legal services available for children with TS.

National Center for Hyperactive Children
5535 Balboa Blvd., Suite 215
Encino, CA 91316
(818) 986–0514; (818) 780–9819
A non-profit research and treatment center for hyperactive and learning disabled children.

National Center for Youth with Disabilities
University of Minnesota
Box 721—UMHC
Harvard St. at East River Rd.
Minneapolis, MN 55455
(612) 626–2825; (800) 333–NCYD
Distributes information to individuals or programs working with adolescents with a chronic illness or disability. Operates a computerized network of information on research, legislation, programs and projects, and training or education materials relevant to adolescents with disabilities. Also publishes monographs and newsletters on adolescent issues.

National Coalition for Research in Neurological Disorders
3050 K Street, NW, Suite 310
Washington, DC 20007
(202) 293–4543
A coalition of professional and voluntary health organizations encouraging research into disorders of the brain, spinal cord, and peripheral nervous system.

National Foundation of Dentistry for the Handicapped
1600 Stout St., Suite 1420
Denver, CO 80202
(303) 573–0264
Offers publications on dental care for people with disabilities and makes referrals to dentists with expertise in treating children and adults with disabilities.

National Information Center for Children and Youth with Disabilities (NICHCY)
BOX 1492
Washington, DC 20013
(202) 884–8200; (800) 695–0285
NICHCY was established to provide practical advice on locating educational programs and other kinds of special services for children and adolescents with disabilities. NICHCY produces fact sheets on a variety of disabilities, information packets, and "State Sheets" which list each state's resources for people with disabilities. Parents can call or send in requests for free information.

National Institute of Neurological Disorders & Stroke (NINDS)
9000 Rockville Pike
Bethesda, MD 20892
(301) 496–5751
A national organization which funds research on neurological disorders, including TS. Offers information and publications on causes, treatment, diagnosis of neurological disorders.

National Organization for Rare Disorders (NORD)
P.O. Box 8923
New Fairfield, CT 06812
(203) 746–6518; (800) 999–6673
A national data bank of information on rare disorders. They can provide information on TS, an organization resource list, and a reading list.

National Organization on Disability (NOD)
910 16th St., NW, Suite 600
Washington, D.C. 20006
(202) 293–5960; (800) 248–ABLE
An independent federal agency which operates a national data bank of information on disabilities and related issues.

National Rehabilitation Information Center (NARIC)
8455 Colesville Rd., Suite 935
Silver Spring, MD 20910–3319
(301) 588–9284; (800) 34–NARIC
Can perform computer searches and provide research reports on any subject related to the rehabilitation or employment of people with disabilities. Nominal charge for database searches.

Obsessive Compulsive Foundation
P.O. Box 9673
New Haven, CT 06535
(203) 772–0565
A national foundation which provides information and support to people with OCD. Foundation programs include education, research, a newsletter, and support groups. Local chapter information is available by calling this number.

Office of Civil Rights
U.S. Department of Education
The Office of Civil Rights maintains ten regional technical assistance offices which can answer questions on the legal interpretation of the ADA, IDEA, and other laws upholding the rights of people with disabilities.

Region I: (Connecticut, Maine, Massachusetts, New Hampshire, Rhode Island, Vermont)
U.S. Department of Education
Office for Civil Rights
J.W. McCormack Post Office and Courthouse Building, Room 222, 01–0061
Boston, MA 02109–4557
(617) 2233–9662; (617) 223–9695 (TDD)

Region II: (New Jersey, New York, Puerto Rico, Virgin Islands)
U.S. Department of Education
Office for Civil Rights
26 Federal Plaza, 33rd Floor, Room 330130, 02–1010
New York, NY 10278–0082
(212) 264–4633; (212) 264–9464 (TDD)

Region III: (Delaware, District of Columbia, Maryland, Pennsylvania, Virginia, West Virginia)
U.S. Department of Education
Office for Civil Rights
3535 Market St., Room 6300, 03–2010
Philadelphia, PA 19104–3326
(512) 596–6772; (215) 596–6794 (TDD)

Region IV: (Alabama, Florida, Georgia, Kentucky, Mississippi, North Carolina, South Carolina, Tennessee)
U.S. Department of Education
Office for Civil Rights
101 Marietta Tower, 27th Floor, Suite 2702
P.O. Box 1705, 04–3010
Atlanta, GA 30310–1705
(404) 331–2954; (404) 331–7816 (TDD)

Region V: (Illinois, Indiana, Michigan, Minnesota, Ohio, Wisconsin)
U.S. Department of Education
Office for Civil Rights
401 South State Street, Room 700C, 05–4010
Chicago, IL 60606–1202
(312) 886–3456; (312) 353–2541 (TDD)

Region VI: (Arkansas, Louisiana, New Mexico, Oklahoma, Texas)
U.S. Department of Education
Office for Civil Rights
1200 Main Tower Building, Suite 2260, 06–5010
Dallas, TX 75202–9998
(214) 767–3959; (214) 767–3639 (TDD)

Region VII: (Iowa, Kansas, Missouri, Nebraska)
U.S. Department of Education
Office for Civil Rights
10220 N. Executive Hills Blvd., 8th Floor
P.O. Box 901381, 07–6010
Kansas City, MO 64190–1381
(816) 891–8026

Region VIII: (Colorado, Montana, North Dakota, South Dakota, Utah, Wyoming)
U.S. Department of Education
Office for Civil Rights
Federal Office Building
1961 Stout Street, Room 342, 08–7010
Denver, CO 80294–3608
(303) 884–5695; (303) 884–3417 (TDD)

Region IX: (Arizona, California, Hawaii, Nevada, Guam, Trust Territory of Pacific Islands, American Somoa)
U.S. Department of Education
Office for Civil Rights
221 Main Street, 10th Floor, Suite 1020, 09–8010
San Francisco, CA 94105–1925
(415) 227–8040; (415) 227–8124 (TDD)

Region X: (Alaska, Idaho, Oregon, Washington)
U.S. Department of Education
Office for Civil Rights
915 Second Ave., Room 3310, 10–9010
Seattle, WA 98174–1099
(206) 442–1636; (206) 442–4542 (TDD)

Orton Dyslexia Society
8600 LaSalle Rd.
Chester Bldg., Suite 382
Baltimore, MD 21204
(800) ABC–D123
A non-profit organization which focuses on continuing research on dyslexia, and on increasing public awareness about dyslexia.

Random House Audio Books
(800) 733–3000; (301) 296–0232 (in MD)
Recorded Books
(800) 638–1304
Recording for the Blind
(800) 221–4492; (609) 452–0606 (in NJ)
Audio books are helpful for people with eye, face, or other tics that make reading difficult. They may also be helpful for people with learning disabilities.

Sibling Information Network
1776 Ellington Rd.
S. Windsor, CT 06074
(203) 648–1205

A clearinghouse of information on people with disabilities and their families with a concentration on siblings. Publishes a quarterly newsletter containing reviews, resource information, and discussions of family issues.

Siblings for Significant Change
105 E. 22nd St.
New York, NY 10010
(212) 420–0430
A sibling membership organization that provides information and referral services, workshops, and conferences to increase public awareness of the needs of children with disabilities and their families.

Special Education Software Center
(800) 426–2133
The center can help parents, teachers, or administrators track down software to aid children with special needs. The center has a database full of information on software for children with disabilities and will search its database for a listing of the most helpful items and send a free printout to you.

STOMP (Specialized Training of Military Parents)
East Coast Office:
Georgia/ARC
1851 Ram Runway, Suite 104
College Park, GA 30337
(401) 767–2258
Coordinator: Kathy Mitten
West Coast Office:
12208 Pacific Highway, SW
Tacoma, WA 98499
(206) 588–1741
Program Manager: Heather Hebdon
STOMP assists military families stationed in the U.S. or overseas.

Tourette Syndrome Association (TSA)
42–40 Bell Blvd.
Bayside, NY 11361
(718) 224–2999; (800) 237–0717
This association organizes workshops and symposiums for scientists, clinicians, and others working in the field of Tourette syndrome. It also operates NASRET, National Service Response Team. NASRET provides information on health insurance for individuals with TS, employers who hire workers with TS, and physicians, clinics, social workers, school personnel, and attorneys and advocates in each state who have experience working with people with TS. Additionally, TSA organizes and assists local chapters and support groups throughout the U.S. and provides resource information such as pamphlets, films, and videotapes. Contact TSA for the name and phone number of the chapter leader nearest you.

Local Organizations

The following list contains addresses, phone numbers, and names of contact people for public and private agencies in each state that provide assistance to people with special needs and their families. We wish to thank the National Information Center for Children and Youth with Disabilities (NICHCY) for providing much of this information, and the Tourette Syndrome Association for supplying a list of local chapters as of January, 1992.

Below are brief descriptions of the types of organizations this list includes:

Tourette Syndrome Association chapters are state or local affiliates of the national Tourette Syndrome Association. Your local TSA is the best resource in helping you find which other listed organizations are especially sensitive to the needs of people with TS in your area. Local chapters of TSA can help you find support groups, conferences, inservices, physicians, etc. State chapters establish support groups in local communities throughout their states. Because the presidents of local chapters change fairly often, addresses and phone numbers are *not* given below. Call the national TSA at (800) 237–0717 for the name and phone number of the current president of the chapter nearest you.

Obsessive Compulsive Foundation (OC Foundation) chapters provide literature, support groups, and treatment information on OCD. They also support research on OCD. For information on more recently formed chapters, call the national office at (203) 772–0565.

Association for Children and Adults with Learning Disabilities (ACLD) chapters are local affiliates of the national organization that provides support and education to parents of children with LD. They can also direct parents to numerous resources in their areas.

The State Department of Education is the agency responsible for providing education to school-aged children, including special education services to children with Tourette Syndrome.

The State Vocational Rehabilitation Agency provides medical, therapeutic, educational, counseling, training and other services needed to prepare people for work. The state agency will refer you to the local office nearest you.

The Developmental Disabilities Council provides funding for direct services for people with developmental disabilities. Most provide services such as diagnosis, evaluation, information and referral, social services, group homes, advocacy, and protection. Remember, however, that not all states recognize Tourette syndrome as a developmental disability. To find out what, if any, developmental disability services your state offers for children with TS, contact your state D.D. council.

The Protection and Advocacy (P&A) Agency is a legal organization established to protect the rights of people with disabilities. It can supply information about the educational, health, residential, social, and legal services available for children with Tourette Syndrome.

American Association of University Affiliated Programs (AAUAP) are federally funded centers that offer diagnostic and treatment services to parents of children with special needs.

Parent Programs include privately and publicly funded groups that offer support, information, and referral services to parents of children with special needs.

ARC chapters help to promote goal of the national ARC to bring people with developmental disabilities into full participation in their communities. They often offer, or can help parents locate, advocacy services, respite care, and support groups.

Alabama

TSA—Alabama Chapter
(serves entire state)
For current phone number,
contact national TSA

Alabama Association for Children and Adults
with Learning Disabilities (ACLD)
P.O. Box 11588
Montgomery, AL 36111
(205) 277–9151

Contact: Suzanne Fornaro, President

Special Education
50 N. Ripley St.
Montgomery, AL 36130
(205) 242–8114

Contact: Bill East, Director

Division of Rehabilitation & Crippled
Children's Services
Department of Education
P.O. Box 11586

2129 E. South Blvd.
Montgomery, AL 36111
(205) 281–8780
Contact: Lamona Lucas, Director

Department of Mental Health & Mental Retardation
200 Interstate Park Dr.
Montgomery, AL 36193
(205) 271–9208
Contact: J. Michael Horsley, Commissioner

Alabama Developmental Disabilities Planning Council
P.O. Box 3710
Montgomery, AL 36193–5001
(205) 271–9278
Contact: Joan Hannah, Director

Alabama Developmental Disabilities Advocacy Program
P.O. Box 870395
The University of Alabama
Tuscaloosa, AL 35487–0395
(205) 348–4928
Contact: Rueben Cook, Director

Sparks Center for Developmental & Learning Disorders
University of Alabama at Birmingham
1720 Seventh Ave., South
Birmingham, AL 35233
(205) 934–5471
Contact: Dr. Gary Myers, Director

Special Education Action Committee (SEAC)
P.O. Box 161274
Mobile, AL 36616–2274
(205)478–1208; (800)222–7322 (in AL)
Contact: Carol Blades, Dir.

ARC of Alabama
444 S. Decatur
Montgomery, AL 36104
(205) 262–7688
Contact: Douglas Sandford, Executive Director

Alaska

Alaska Tourette Syndrome Association
9440 Chenega Dr.
Anchorage, AK 99507
(907) 333–0969; (907) 337–1583
Contact: Becky Aftreth

Alaska Association for Children and Adults with Learning Disabilities (ACLD)
108 W. Cook Ave.
Anchorage, AK 99051
(907) 279–1662
Contact: Mavis Hancock

Office of Special Services
Department of Education
Pouch F
Juneau, AK 99811
(907) 465–2970
Contact: William S. Mulnix, Director

Office of Special Services & Supplemental Programs (Ages 3–5)
Dept. of Education
P.O. Box F
Juneau, AK 99811
(907) 456–2970

Division of Vocational Rehabilitation
Dept. of Education
Pouch F, Mail Stop 0581
State Office Bldg.
Juneau, AK 99811
(907) 456–2814
Contact: Keith Anderson, Director

Developmental Disabilities Planning Council
600 University Ave., Suite B
Fairbanks, AK 99709–3651
(907) 479–6507
Contact: Dorothy Turan, Director

Advocacy Services of Alaska
325 E. Third Ave., 2nd Floor
Anchorage, AK 99501
Contact: David Maltman, Director

Alaska Parent Coalition
7530 Blackberry
Anchorage, AK 99502

Special Education Parent Team
210 Ferry Way, Ste. 200
Juneay, AK 99801
(907) 586–6806
Contact: Linda Griffith

Alaska ARC
2211–A Arca Dr.
Anchorage, AK 99506
(907) 277–6677
Contact: Mary Jane Starlings

Alaska Management Technologies
2900 Boniface Pkwy., Ste. 100
Anchorage, AK 99504
(907) 536–6373

Arizona

Arizona Tourette Syndrome Association Contact
342 W. Shaw Butte Dr.
Phoenix, AZ 85029
(602) 993–1573
Contact: Dan Willets

Arizona Association for Children and Adults
  with Learning Disabilities (ACLD)
11225 E. Stetson Place
Tuscon, AZ 85794
(602) 993–3942
Contact: Shirley Hilts-Scott, President

Arizona ACLD—State Office
815 E. Camelback Rd.
Suite 108
Phoenix, AZ 85014
(602) 230–7188 or 230–7194

CHADD of Flagstaff
Flagstaff, AZ
(602) 774–6364
Contact: Tina Appelton, Parent Coordinator

Special Education
Dept. of Education
1535 W. Jefferson
Phoenix, AZ 85007–3280
(602) 542–3183
Contact: Kay Lund, Asst. Commissioner

Rehabilitation Services Bureau
Department of Economic Security
1300 W. Washington St.
Phoenix, AZ 85007
(602) 524–3332
Contact: James Griffith, Administrator

Div. of Dev. Disabilities
Dept. of Economic Security
P.O. Box 6123
Phoenix, AZ 85005
(602) 258–0419
Contact: Lyn Rucker, Asst. Director

Program for Youths & Adolescents
Division of Behavioral Health Services
Department of Health Services
411 N. 24th St.
Phoenix, AZ 85008
(602) 220–6478
Contact: Stephen Perkins, Coordinator

Governor's Council on Developmental Disabilities
1717 W. Jefferson
P.O. Box 6123
Phoenix, AZ 85005
(602) 255–4049
Contact: Rita Charron, Dir.

Arizona Center for Law in the Public Interest
363 N. First Ave., Suite 100
Phoenix, AZ 85003
(602) 252–4904
Contact: Tom Berning, Staff Attorney

Pilot Parent Partnerships
2150 E. Highland Ave., #105
Phoenix, AZ 85016
(602) 468–3001
Contact: Mary Slaughter, Exec. Dir.

ARC
5610 S. Central
Phoenix, AZ 85040
(602) 243–1787

Arkansas

TSA—Arkansas Chapter
(serves entire state)
For current phone number,
contact national TSA

Association for Children and Adults with
  Learning Disabilities (ACLD)
P.O. Box 705
Hope, AR 71801
(501) 777–5572
Contact: Sue Bruner, President

Association for Child and Adults with Learn-
  ing Disabilities (ACLD)
State Office
P.O. Box 7316
Little Rock, AR 72217
(501) 666–8777
Contact: Lynn Frost

Special Education Section
Department of Education
Education Building, Room 105–C
Little Rock, AR 72201
(501) 682–4221
Contact: Dr. Diane Sydoriak, Associate Direc-
  tor

Special Education Section (Ages 3–5)
Department of Education
4 Capital Mall, Room 105–C
Little Rock, AR 72201
(501) 682–4222
Contact: Mary Kay McKinney, Coordinator

Division of Rehabilitation Services
Department of Human Services
P.O. Box 3781
7th & Main Sts.
Little Rock, AR 72203
(501) 682–6708
Contact: Bobby Simpson, Deputy Director

Governor's Developmental Disabilities Planning Council
4815 W. Markham St.
Little Rock, AR 72201
(501) 661–2589
Contact: Orson Berry, Director

Advocacy Services, Inc.
1120 Marshall St., Ste. 311
Little Rock, AR 72202
(501) 324–9215
Contact: Nan Ellen East, Exec. Director

Arkansas Disability Coalition
10002 W. Markham, Ste. B–7
Little Rock, AR 72205
(501) 221–1330
Contact: Bonnie Johnson, Director

FOCUS, Inc.
2917 King St. Suite C
Jonesboro, AR 72401
(501) 953–2750
Contact: Barbara Semrau

Parent-to-Parent
Union Station Square, Ste. 350
Little Rock, AR 72201
(501) 375–4464
Contact: Brenda Reed, Coordinator

ARC
Union Station Square, Ste. 406
Little Rock, AR 72201
(501) 375–4464
Contact: Nancy Sullivan, Exec. Director

California

TSA—Northern California Chapter
(serves Eureka, Fresno, Marysville, North Redding, Bay, Oakland, Sacramento, Salinas, San Francisco, San Jose, and Stockton)
For current phone number,
contact national TSA

TSA—Southern California Chapter
(serves Alhambra, Bakersfield, Englewood, Long Beach, Los Angeles, Oxnard, Pasadena, Santa Ana, San Bernardino, San Diego, Van Nuys, and Wojave)
For current phone number,
contact national TSA

Tourette Syndrome Clinic
Department of Medical Genetics
City of Hope National Medical Center
Duarte, CA 91010
(818) 359–8111, ext. 2631; (818) 357–7624
Contact: David Comings, MD

Association for Children with Learning Disabilities—California (ACLD)
5290 Mt. Ariane Ct.
San Diego, CA 92111
(619) 565–8937
Contact: Mary Ann Golembesky, President

Association for Children and Adults with Learning Disabilities (ACLD)
State Office
17 Buena Vista Ave.
Mill Valley, CA 94941
(415) 383–5242

Special Education Division
California Department of Education
721 Capitol Mall
Sacramento, CA 94244–2720
(916) 323–4768
Contact: Patrick Campbell, Director

Department of Rehabilitation
Health & Welfare Agency
830 K Street Mall
Sacramento, CA 95814
(916) 445–3971
Contact: P. Ceilio Fontanoza, Dir.

Department of Developmental Services
Health & Welfare Agency
1600 9th St. NW, 2nd Floor
Sacramento, CA 95814
(916) 323–3131
Contact: Gary Macomber, Director

State Council on Dev. Disabilities
200 O St., Room 100
Sacramento, CA 95814
(916) 322–8481
Contact: James Bellotti, Exec. Dir

Client Assistance Program
830 K Street Mall, Room 220
Sacramento, CA 95814
(916) 322–5066
Contact: Director

California Protection & Advocacy, Inc.
2131 Capital Ave.
Sacramento, CA 95816
(916) 447–3324; (800) 952–5746
Contact: Albert Zonca, Exec. Director

Center for Child Development & Developmental Disorders
University Affiliated Training Programs
Children's Hospital of Los Angeles
4650 Sunset Blvd.
Los Angeles, CA 90027
(213) 669–2151
Contact: Dr. Wylda Hammond, Director

Team of Advocates for Special Kids (TASK)
100 W. Cerritos Ave.
Anaheim, CA 92805
(714) 533–TASK
Contact: Joan Tellefson

Parents Helping Parents
535 Race St., Ste. 220
San Jose, CA 95126
(408) 288–5010

DREDF
2212 6th St.
Berkley, CA 94710
(415) 644–2555

Disabilities Services Matrix
P.O. Box 6541
San Rafael, CA 94903
(415) 499–3877
Contact: Joan Kilburn

ARC
120 I St., 2nd Fl.
Sacramento, CA 95814
(916) 522–6619
Contact: Frederic Hougardy, Exec. Director

Colorado

TSA—Colorado Chapter
(serves entire state)
For current phone number,
contact national TSA

Colorado Association for Children with Learning Disabilities (ACLD)
1835 Cherry
Denver, CO 80220
(303) 973–3134
Contact: Liz Hesse, President

State Office ACLD
P.O. Box 32188
Aurora, CO 80041
(303) 973–3134

Special Education Services Unit
Dept. of Education
201 E. Colfax Ave.
Denver, CO 80203
(303) 866–6694
Contact: Dr. Brian McNulty, Dir.

Special Education Division (Ages 3–5)
Dept. of Education
201 E. Colfax Ave.
Denver, CO 80203
(303) 866–6710
Contact: Elizabeth Soper, Coordinator

Division of Rehabilitation
Dept. of Social Services
1575 Sherman St., 4th Fl.
Denver, CO 80203
(303) 866–5196

Division for Developmental Disabilities
3824 W. Princeton Circle

Denver, CO 80236
(303) 762–4560
Contact: Director

Colorado Dev. Disabilities Council
777 Grant St., Ste. 410
Denver, CO 80203–3528
(303) 894–2345
Contact: Paula Kubicz, Dir.

The Legal Center
455 Sherman St., Ste. 130
Denver, CO 80203
(303) 722–0300
Contact: Mary Ann Harvey

Parents Education & Assistance for Kids (PEAK)
6055 Lehman Dr., Ste. 101
Colorado Springs, CO 80918
(719) 531–9400
Contact: Judy Martz or Barbara Buswell, Directors

ARC
4155 E. Jewell Ave., No. 916
Denver, CO 80222
(303) 756–7234
Contact: Jeffrey Strully, Exec. Dir.

Connecticut

TSA—Connecticut Chapter
(serves entire state)
For current phone number,
contact national TSA

Association for Children with Learning Disabilities (ACLD)
27 Brainard Rd.
W. Hartford, CT 06117
(203) 233–6191
Contact: Ann Seigel, President

ACLD State Office
139 N. Main St.
Boatner Bldg.
W. Hartford, CT 06107
(203) 236–3953

Bureau of Special Educ. & Pupil Personnel Svcs.
Dept. of Education
25 Industrial Park Rd.
Middletown, CT 06457
(203) 638–4265
Contact: Tom B. Gillung, Bureau Chief

Early Childhood Unit (Ages 3–5)
Division of Curriculum and Professional Development
Dept. of Education
P.O. Box 2219

Hartford, CT 06145
(203) 566–5670
Contact: Kay Halverson, Coordinator

Div. of Rehabilitation Services
Board of Education
10 Griffin Rd. North
Windsor, CT 06195
Contact: Marilyn Cambell, Division Dir.

Department of Children and Youth Services
170 Sigourney St.
Hartford, CT 06115
(203) 566–8614
Contact: Judy Jacobs

Developmental Disabilities Council
90 Pitkin St.
East Hartford, CT 06108
(203) 725–3829
Contact: Edward Preneta

Office of Protection & Advocacy for Handicapped & DD Persons
60 Weston St.
Hartford, CT 06120–1551
(203) 297–4300; (800) 842–7303 (in CT)
Contact: Eliot J. Dober, Exec. Dir.

Connecticut's University Affiliated Program on Developmental Disabilities
991 Main St.
East Hartford, CT 06108
(203) 282–7050
Contact: Director

Connecticut Parent Advocacy Center
P.O. Box 579
East Lyme, CT 06333
(203) 739–3089
Contact: Nancy Prescott, Director

Parent-to-Parent
Department of Pediatrics
University of Connecticut
The Exchange
Farmington, CT 06032
(203) 674–1485; (203) 951–0045
Contact: Molly P. Cole

ARC
1030 New Britain Ave., Ste. 102B
West Harford, CT 06110
(203) 953–8335
Contact: Margaret Dignoti, Exec. Director

Delaware

Tourette Syndrome Association
Delaware Contact
Rt. 1, Box 186–1
Hartley, DE 19953

(302) 492–8140
Contact: Pam Thompson

Delaware Association for Children with Learning Disabilities (ACLD)
177 E. Sutton Pl.
Wilmington, DE 19810
(302) 994–0707
Contact: Janet Walton, President

ACLD
State Office of New Castle Co.
P.O. Box 577
Bear, DE 19701
(302) 994–0707

Exceptional Children/Special Programs Division
Department of Public Instruction
P.O. Box 1402
Dover, DE 19903
(302) 739–5471
Contact: Dr. Carl Haltom, Director

Division of Vocational Rehabilitation.
Department of Labor
321 E. 11th St.
Wilmington, DE 19801
(302) 577–2850
Contact: Anthony Sokolowski, Director

Developmental Disabilities Council
156 S. State St.
P.O. Box 1401
Dover, DE 19903
(302) 736–4456
Contact: James Linehan

Disabilities Law Program
144 E. Market St.
Georgetown, DE 19947
(302) 856–0038
Contact: Christine Long, Administrator

ARC
240 N. James St., Ste B–2
Wilmington, DE 19804
(302) 994–9400
Contact: David Richard, Exec. Director

District of Columbia

TSA—Greater Washington Chapter
(serves Maryland, Virgina, and D.C.)
For current phone number,
contact national TSA

District of Columbia Association for Children with Learning Disabilities (ACLD)
1648 NW Hobart St.
Washington, DC 20009
(202) 462–0495
Contact: Alan Ponze, President

ACLD State Office
P.O. Box 6350
Washington, DC 20015

Division of Special Education
D.C. Public Schools
10th and H Sts., NW
Washington, DC 20001
(202) 724-4018
Contact: David Burkett, Asst. Superintendent

Vocational Rehab. Services Administration
Department of Human Resources
605 G. St., NW, No. 1101
Washington, DC 20001
(202) 727-3227
Contact: Administrator

Child/Youth Services Administration
DC Commission on Mental Health Services
1120 19th St., NW, No. 700
Washington, DC 20036
(202) 673-7784
Contact: Deputy Commissioner

Developmental Disabilities Planning Council
801 N. Capitol, NE
Washington, DC 20001
(202) 724-5696
Contact: Executive Director

Information, Protection and Advocacy Center
  for Handicapped Individuals
300 I St., NE, Suite 202
Washington, DC 20002
(202) 547-8081
Contact: Executive Director

ARC
900 Varnum St., NE
Washington, DC 20017
(202) 636-2950
Contact: Shirley Wade

Florida

TSA—Florida Chapter
(serves entire state)
For current phone number,
contact national TSA

Florida ACLD
7016 N. Donald Ave.
Tampa, FL 33614
(813) 637-8957
Contact: Arnold Stark, President

ACLD
State Office
331 East Henry St.
Punta Gorda, FL 33950

(904) 488-1570
Contact: Cheryl Kron, Exec. Secretary

Bureau of Education for Exceptional Children
Department of Education
325 W. Gaines St., No. 614
Tallahassee, FL 32399
(904) 488-1570
Contact: Chief

Division of Vocational Rehabilitation
Department of Labor and Employment
  Security
1709-A Mahan Dr.
Tallahassee, FL 32399
(904) 488-6210
Contact: Calvin Melton, Director

Developmental Services Program Office
Department of Health & Rehabilitative Ser-
  vices
1311 Winewood Blvd.
Building 5, Room 215
Tallahassee, FL 32301
(904) 488-4257
Contact: Kingsley Ross, Director

Mental Health Services, Children's Program
Alcohol, Drug Abuse, and Mental Health
  Program Office
1317 Winewood Blvd.
Tallahassee, FL 32301
(904) 487-2415
Contact: Deon Hardy, Administrator

Florida Developmental Disabilities Planning
  Council
820 E. Park Ave., No. I-100
Tallahassee, FL 32301
(904) 488-4180
Contact: Joseph Krieger, Exec. Director

Advocacy Center for Persons with Disabilities
2661 Executive Center Circle, W.
Suite 100
Tallahassee, FL 32301
(904) 488-9071
Contact: Jonathan Rossman, Director

Parent Education Network of FL (PEN)
1211 Tech Blvd., Ste. 105
Tampa, FL 33619-7833
(813) 623-4088; (800) 825-5736
Contact: Janet Jacoby, Project Manager

Parent to Parent of Florida
3500 E. Fletcher Ave., Ste. 225
Tampa, FL 33612
813/974-5001
Contact: Susan Duwa

ARC
411 E. College Ave.
Tallahassee, FL 32301
(904) 681-1931
Contact: Chris Schuh

Georgia

TSA of Georgia, Inc.
(serves entire state)
For current phone number,
contact national TSA

Georgia ACLD
3160 Northside Pkwy, NW
Atlanta, GA 30327
(404) 633-5332
Contact: Jane Blalock

ACLD State Office
P.O. Box 29492
Atlanta, GA 30359
(404) 656-2425
Contact: Michele Hardin, Secretary

Program for Exceptional Students
Department of Education
1970 Twin Towers East
Atlanta, GA 30334
(404) 656-2425
Contact: Dr. Joan A. Jordan, Director

Division of Rehabilitation Services
Department of Human Resources
878 Peachtree St., NE, Rm. 706
Atlanta, GA 30309
(404) 894-6670
Contact: Director

Georgia Council on Developmental Disabilities
878 Peachtree St., NE
Atlanta, GA 30309-3917
(404) 894-5790
Contact: Zebe Schmitt, Director

Georgia Advocacy Office, Inc.
Suite 811
1708 Peachtree St., NW, No. 505
Atlanta, GA 30309
(404) 885-1447; (800) 537-4538
Contact: Pat Powell, Exec. Director

University Affiliated Program of Georgia
570 Aderhold Hall
Athens, GA 30602
(404) 542-1685
Contact: Dr. Richard Talbott, Exec. Director

Parents Educating Parents (PEP)
Georgia ARC
1851 Ram Runway, Suite 104

College Park, GA 30337
(404) 761-2745
Contact: Director

ARC of Georgia
1851 Ram Runway, Suite 104
College Park, GA 30337
(404) 761-3150

Hawaii

Tourette Syndrome Association Contact
Protection & Advocacy Agency of Hawaii
P.O. Box 15504
Honolulu, HI 96830-5504
Contact: Patty M. Henderson

Hawaii ACLD
1st Hawaiian Bank,
P.O. Box 3200
Honolulu, HI 96847
(808) 525-7098 (w)
(808) 955-7760 (h)
Contact: Michael Roeder, President

Hawaii State Office ACLD
200 N. Vineyard Blvd.
Suite 103
Honolulu, HI 96817
(808) 988-4962 (h)
(808) 536-9684 (w)
Contact: Mrs. Ivalee Sinclar, Exec. Director

Special Education Section
Department of Education
3430 Leahi Ave.
Honolulu, HI 96815
(808) 737-3720
Contact: Margaret Donovan, Administrator

Division of Vocational Rehab.
Department of Human Services
1000 Bishop St., No. 615
Honolulu, HI 96813
(808) 548-4769
Contact: Toshio Nishioka, Administrator

Child and Adolescent Mental Health Division
3627 Kilauea Ave, Suite 101
Honolulu, HI 96816
(808) 548-3906
Contact: Marvin Mathews, Dir.

State Planning Council on Developmental Disabilities
501 Ala Moana Blvd., No. 200
Honolulu, HI 96813
(808) 548-8482
Contact: Director

Protection and Advocacy Agency
1580 Makaloa St., Suite 1060
Honolulu, HI 96814

(808) 949–2992
Contact: Patty Henderson, Exec. Director

Special Parent Information Network
335 Merchant St., Rm. 353
Honolulu, HI 96813
(808) 548–2648
Contact: Exec. Director

Idaho

Idaho ACLD
4610–A Jackson Place
Mtn. Home AFB, ID 83648
(208) 832–4218
Contact: Nora Kretschmer

Special Education Division
Department of Education
Len B. Jordan Building
650 W. State St.
Boise, ID 83720–0001
(208) 334–3940
Contact: Director

Special Education Division (Ages 3–5)
Department of Education
Len B. Jordan Building
650 W. State St.
Boise, ID 83720–0001
(208) 334–3940

Division of Vocational Rehab.
State Board of Vocational Rehab.
650 W. State St.
Boise, ID 83720
(208) 334–3390
Contact: George Pelletier, Administrator

Bureau of Developmental Disabilities
Division of Community Rehab.
Department of Health and Welfare
450 W. State, 7th Floor
Boise, ID 83720
(208) 334–5531
Contact: Paul Swatsenbarg, Chief

Idaho State Council on Developmental Disabilities
280 N. 8th St., No. 208
Boise, ID 83720
(208) 334–2178
Contact: John D. Watts

Idaho Parents Unlimited (IPUL)
1365 N. Orchard, #107
Boise, ID 83706
(208) 377–8049
Contact: Martha Gilgen

Illinois

TSA, Inc. of Illinois
(serves entire state)
For current phone number,
contact national TSA

Illinois ACLD
19525 W. Washington
Grayslake, IL 60030
(312) 223–6681, ext. 220
Contact: Kathy Gemple, President

Illinois ACLD
P.O. Box A–3239
Chicago, IL 60690
(312) 663–9535
Contact: Mary Cotter

ACLD State Office
400 E. Sibley Blvd.
Room 111
Harvey, IL 60426
(708) 210–3532

Department of Special Education
State Board of Education
100 N. First St.
Springfield, IL 62777
(217) 782–6601
Contact: Gail Liberman

Department of Special Education (Ages 3–5)
State Board of Education
100 N. First St.
Springfield, IL 62777
(217) 524–4835
Contact: Sandra Crews, Education Specialist

Dept. of Rehabilitation Services
State Board of Vocational Rehabilitation
623 E. Adams St.
P.O. Box 19429
Springfield, IL 62794
Contact: Philip Bradley, Director

Department of Mental Health and Developmental Disabilities
402 Stratton Office Building
Springfield, IL 62706
(217) 782–7395
Contact: William Murphy, Deputy Director

Institute for Juvenile Research
907 S. Wolcott
Chicago, IL 60612
(312) 996–1733
Contact: Lee Combrinck-Graham, Director

Illinois Council on DD
State of IL Center
100 W. Randolph 10–601
Chicago, IL 60601

(312) 814–2080
Contact: Cathy Ficker Terrill, Dir.

Protection and Advocacy
11 E. Adams, No. 1200
Chicago, IL 60603
(312) 341–0022
Contact: Zena Naiditch, Director

University Affiliated Facility for Developmental Disabilities
University of Illinois at Chicago
1640 W. Roosevelt Rd.
Chicago, IL 60608
(312) 413–1647
Contact: Dr. David Braddock, Director

Coordinating Council for Handicapped Children
20 E. Jackson Blvd., Room 900
Chicago, IL 60604
(312) 939–3513
Contact: Charlotte Des Jardins

Designs for Change
220 S. State St., Room 1900
Chicago IL 60604
(312) 922–0317
Contact: Donald Moore, Director

Direction Service of Illinois
730 E. Vine, Room 107
Springfield, IL 62703
(217) 523–1232; (800) 634–8540 (in IL)
Contact: Merle Wallace

ARC of Illinois
600 S. Federal St., Ste 303
Chicago, IL 60605
(312) 922–6932
Contact: Exec. Director

Indiana

Indianapolis/Central TSA Contact
Carole Bremer
1017 Oakwood Trl.
Indianapolis, IN 46260
(317) 253–8333

Indianapolis Area TSA Contact
Mary Zierdt
Riley Hospital, Room N–102
702 Barnhill Dr.
Indianapolis, IN 46202–5200
(317) 274–8747

Southbend Area TSA Contact
Kathy Heinrich
1737 Caroline
South Bend, IN 46613
(219) 234–0671

Indiana Association for Children and Adults with Learning Disabilities (ACLD)
7367 East 16th St.
Indianapolis, IN 46219
(317) 357–8268
Contact: Barbara Uhrig, President

Division of Special Education
Department of Education
State House, Room 229
Indianapolis, IN 46204
(317) 232–0570
Contact: Paul Ash, Director

Department of Human Services (Vocational Rehabilitation)
P.O. Box 7083
Indianapolis, IN 46207
(317) 232–1147
Contact: Director

Division of Developmental Disabilities
Dept. of Mental Health
117 E. Washington St.
Indianapolis, IN 46204–3647
Contact: Director

Governor's Planning Council on DD
143 W. Market St., Ste. 404
Indianapolis, IN 46204
317/232–7770
Contact: Suellen Jackson-Boner, Dir.

Indiana Advocacy Services
850 N. Meridian St., Suite 2–C
Indianapolis, IN 46204
(317) 232–1150; (800) 622–4845
Contact: Mary Lou Haynes, Exec. Director

Task Force on Education for the Handicapped, Inc.
833 Northside Blvd.
Building 1, Rear
South Bend, IN 46617
(219) 234–7101
Contact: Richard Burden, Director

Indiana Parent Information Network
2107 E. 65th St
Indianapolis, IN 46220
(317) 257–8683
Contact: Executive Director

Iowa

Tourette Syndrome Association
2101 O Avenue, NW
Cedar Rapids, IA 52405
(319) 396–0210
Contact: Gladys Zobac, Area Representative

Tourette Syndrome Association
112 SE Leach

Des Moines, IA 50315
(515) 285–2274
Contact: Sylvia Speak, Area Rep.

LDA of Iowa
2819 48th St.
Des Moines, IA 50310
(515) 277–4266
Contact: Winifred Carr, President

Special Education Division
Department of Public Instruction
Grimes State Office Building
Des Moines, IA 50319
(515) 281–3176
Contact: Frank Vance, Director

Division of Vocational Rehabilitation Services
Department of Public Instruction
510 E. 12th St.
Des Moines, IA 50319
(515) 281–4348
Contact: Jerry Starkweather, Administrator

Governors Planning Council for Developmental Disabilities
Department of Human Services
Hoover Building, 5th Floor
Des Moines, IA 50319
(515) 281–3758
Contact: Karon Perlowski, Director

Iowa Protection and Advocacy Services, Inc.
3015 Merle Hay Rd., Suite 6
Des Moines, IA 50310
(515) 278–2502
Contact: Mervin L. Roth, Director

Iowa University Affiliated Facility
Division of Developmental Disabilities
University Hospital School
The University of Iowa
Iowa City, IA 52242
(319) 353–6390
Contact: Dr. Alfred Healy, Director

Client Assistance Program
2920 30th St.
Des Moines, IA 50310
(515) 274–1448
Contact: Evelyne Villines, Director

Iowa Exceptional Parent Center
33 N. 12th St.
P.O. Box 1151
Fort Dodge, IA 50501
Contact: Carla Lawson, Director

Parent-to-Parent
Iowa Exceptional Parent Center
33 N. 12th St.

P.O. Box 1151
Fort Dodge, IA 50501

ARC of Iowa
715 W. Locust
Des Moines, IA 50309
(515) 283–2358
Contact: Mary Etta Lane, Exec. Director

Kansas

TSA—Central Kansas Chapter
(serves Colby, Dodge City, Hays, Hutchinson, Salina, and Wichita)
For current phone number,
contact national TSA

TSA—Kansas City Chapter
(serves Topeka and Kansas City)
For current phone number,
contact national TSA

Kansas Association for Children with Learning Disabilities
6535 Maple
Mission, KS 66202
(913) 362–9535
Contact: Ela Shacklett

Special Education
Department of Education
120 E. 10th St.
Topeka, KS 66612
(913) 296–4945
Contact: Director

Special Education Administration (Ages 3–5)
Department of Education
120 E. 10th St.
Topeka, KS 66612
(913) 296–7454
Contact: Carol Dermyer

Rehabilitation Services
Department of Social and Rehabilitation Services
300 SW Oakley, 1st Floor
Topeka, KS 66606
(913) 296–3911
Contact: Gabriel Faimon, Commissioner

Child & Adolescent Mental Health Programs
506 N. State Office Building
Topeka, KS 66612
(913) 296–1808
Contact: Director

Kansas Planning Council on Developmental Disabilities
State Office Building
300 SW Oakley, 1st Fl.
Topeka, KS 66606

(913) 296–2608
Contact: John Kelly, Exec. Director

Kansas Advocacy and Protection Services
513 Leavenworth St., Suite 2
Manhatten, KS 66502
(913) 776–1541; (800) 432–8276
Contact: Joan Strickler, Director

Kansas University Affiliated Faculty
Children's Rehabilitation Unit
Kansas University Medical Center
39th & Rainbow Blvd.
Kansas City, KS 66103
(913) 588–5900
Contact: Dr. Joseph Hollowell, Director

Kansas University Affiliated Faculty
348 Haworth Hall
University of Kansas
Lawrence, KS 66045
(913) 864–4950
Contact: Jean Ann Summers, Director

Families Together, Inc.
3601 SW 29th St., No. 127
Topeka, KS 66604
(913) 267–6343
Contact: Patricia Gerdel, Dir.

Client Assistance Program
Biddle Building, 2nd Floor
2700 W. 6th St.
Topeka, KS 66606
913/296–1491
Contact: Susan Tabor

ARC of Kansas
P.O. Box 676
Hays, KS 67601

Kentucky

TSA—Kentucky Chapter
(serves entire state)
For current phone number,
contact national TSA

Association for Children with Learning Disabilities
Box 13 B
Battletown, KY 40104
(502) 497–4643
Contact: Debbie Troutman, President

ACLD State Office
2232 Alta Ave
Louisville, KY 40205
(501) 451–8001
Contact: Catherine Senn

Office of Education for Exceptional Children
Dept. of Education

Capitol Plaza Tower, 8th Floor
Frankfort, KY 40601
(502) 564–4970
Contact: Director

Office of Education for Exceptional Children
(Ages 3–5)
Capitol Plaza Tower, 8th Floor
Frankfort, KY 40601
(502) 564–4970
Contact: Betty Bright, Branch Manager

Office of Vocational Rehab.
Dept. of Education
Capitol Plaza Tower, 9th Floor
Frankfort, KY 40601
(502) 564–4566
Contact: Caroll Burchett

Children & Youth Services Branch
Department for Mental Health & Mental Retardation Services
275 E. Main Street, 1st Floor East
Frankfort, KY 40621
(502) 564–7610
Contact: Manager

Kentucky Developmental Disabilities Planning Council
Bureau of Health Services
275 E. Main St.
Frankfort, KY 40621
(502) 564–7842
Contact: Director

Office for Public Advocacy
Division for Protection & Advocacy
1264 Louisville Rd.
Frankfort, KY 40601
(502) 564–2967; (800) 373–2988
Contact: Gayla O. Peach, Director

Interdisciplinary Human Development Institute
University Affiliated Facility
University of Kentucky
114 Porter Building
730 South Limestone
Lexington, KY 40506–0205
(606) 257–1714
Contact: Dr. Melton Martinson, Dir.

Kentucky Special Parent Involvement Network
318 W. Kentucky St.
Louisville, KY 40203
Contact: Paulette Logsdon, Dir.

Directions Service Center
Blue Grass Area Chapter
1450 Newton Pike
Lexington, KY 40511

(606) 233–9370
Contact: Jenny Mayberry, Director

Client Assistance Program
Capitol Plaza Tower
Frankfort, KY 40601
(502) 564–8035
Contact: Sharon S. Fields, Director

ARC of Kentucky
833 E. Main
Frankfort, KY 40601
(502) 875–5225
Contact: Patty Dempsey, Exec. Dir.

Louisiana

Association for Children with Learning Disabilities (ACLD)
8602 Hollow Bluff Dr.
Haughton, LA 71037
(318) 949–2302
Contact: Jo Linn Burt

Special Education Services
Department of Education
P.O. Box 94064, 9th Floor
Baton Rouge, LA 70864–9064
(504) 342–3633
Contact: Director

Division of Vocational Rehabilitation
Office of Human Development
1755 Florida Blvd.
P.O. Box 94371
Baton Rouge, LA 70804
(504) 342–2285
Contact: Alton Toms, Director

Office of Mental Health
Department of Health and Human Resources
P.O. Box 4049, 655 N. 5th St.
Baton Rouge, LA 70821
(504) 342–2548
Contact: Director

State Planning Council on DD
P.O. Box 3455
Baton Rouge, LA 70821
(504) 342–6804
Contact: Anne L. Farber, Exec. Officer

Advocacy Center for the Elderly & Disabled
210 O'Keefe, Ste. 700
New Orleans, LA 70112
504/522–2337; 800/662–7705 (in LA)
Contact: Exec. Dir.

Project PROMPT
United Cerebral Palsy of Greater New Orleans
1500 Edwards Ave., Suite O
Harahan, LA 70123

(504) 734–7736
Contact: Sharon Duda, Director

Parent Linc
200 Henry Clay Ave.
New Orleans, LA 70118
(504) 896–9268
Contact: John Hill

ARC of Louisiana
721 Government St., No. 102
Baton Rouge, LA 70802
(504) 383–0742
Contact: Pat Davies, Executive Director

Maine

TSA—Maine Chapter
(serves entire state)
For current phone number,
contact national TSA

LDA of Maine
Bessey Ridge Road
Albion, ME 04901
(207) 437–9245
Contact: Harrison Sylvester, President

Division of Special Education
Department of Education & Cultural Services
State House, Station 23
Augusta, ME 04333
(207) 289–5953
Contact: David N. Stockford, Director

Bureau of Rehabilitation Services
32 Winthrop St.
Augusta, ME 04330
(207) 289–2266
Contact: Pamela Tetley, Director

Department of Mental Health & Mental Retardation
411 State Officers Bldg.
Station 40
Augusta, ME 04333
(207) 289–4223
Contact: Commissioner

Bureau of Children with Special Needs
Department of Mental Health & Mental Retardation
411 State Office Bldg., Room 424
Augusta, ME 04333
(207) 289–4250
Contact: Robert Durgan, Director

Developmental Disabilities Council
Nash Bldg, STA 139
Capitol & State Sts.
Augusta, ME 04330
(207) 289–4213
Contact: Peter Stowell, Exec. Dir.

Maine Advocacy Services
One Grand View Place, Ste. 1
P.O. Box 445
Winthrop, ME 04364
207/377–6202; 800/452–1948
Contact: Laura Petovello, Exec. Dir.

University Affiliated Handicapped Children's
Program
Eastern Maine Medical Center
417 State St., Box 17
Bangor, ME 04401
(207) 945–7572
Contact: Dr. James Hirschfeld, Dir.

Special-Needs Parent Information Network
(SPIN)
P.O. Box 2067
Augusta, ME 04338
(207) 582–2504; (800) 325–0220 (in ME)
Contact: Deborah Guimont, Director

Maryland

TSA—Greater Washington Chapter
(serves Maryland, Virgina, and D.C.)
For current phone number,
contact national TSA

Association for Children with Learning Disabilities
2919 Georgia Ave.
Baltimore, MD 21227
(410) 636–3852
Contact: Kathy Spittel, President

ACLD State Office
320 Maryland National Bank Building
Baltimore, MD 21202

Division of Special Education
Department of Education
200 W. Baltimore St.
Baltimore, MD 21201
(410) 333–2490
Contact: Richard Steinke, Director

Program Development & Assistance Branch
(Ages 3–5)
Division of Special Education
200 W. Baltimore St.
Baltimore, MD 21201
(410) 333–2495
Contact: Sheila Draper, Chief

Division of Vocational Rehabilitation
Department of Education
2301 Argonne Dr.
Baltimore, MD 21218
(410) 554–3000
Contact: James Jeffers

Developmental Disabilities Administration
Department of Health & Mental Hygiene
201 W. Preston St.
4th Floor, O'Connor Building
Baltimore, MD 21201
(410) 225–5600
Contact: Lois Meszaros, Director

Maryland Developmental Disabilities Planning Council
300 W. Lexington St.
Baltimore, MD 21201
(410) 333–3688
Contact: Director

Maryland Disability Law Center
2510 St. Paul St.
Baltimore, MD 21202
(410) 333–7600
Contact: Steve Ney, Director

Kennedy Institute
707 North Broadway
Baltimore, MD 21205
(410) 550–9000
Contact: Dr. Gary Goldstein, President

Client Assistance
Maryland State Department of Education
Division of Vocational Rehabilitation
501 St. Paul St.
Baltimore MD 21202
(410) 333–2713
Contact: Sharon Julius

Parent Support Network
Infants & Toddlers Program
118 N. Howard, Suite 608
Baltimore, MD 21201
(410) 225–4190
Contact: Carol Ann Baglin, Director

ARC of Maryland
6810 Deerpath Rd., No. 310
Baltimore, MD 21227
(410) 379–0400
Contact: Director

Massachusetts

TSA—Greater Boston Chapter
(serves Boston, Brockton, Buzzards Bay, and
Middlesex—Essex)
For current phone number,
contact national TSA

Tourette Syndrome Association
Western MA Chapter
87 Old Farm Rd.
Chicopee, MA 01020
(413) 533–6695
Contact: Paul LeMay, President

Association for Children with Learning Disabilities
37 Sleigh Rd.
Chelmsford, MA 01824
(508) 256–9598
Contact: Gordon Estabrooks, President

ACLD State Office
P.O. Box 28
West Newton, MA 02165
(617) 891–5009

Division of Special Education
Department of Education
1385 Hancock St., 3rd Fl.
Quincy, MA 02169–5183
(617) 770–7468
Contact: Mary Beth Fafard, Dir.

Early Childhood Special Education (Ages 3–5)
Department of Education
1385 Hancock St.
Quincy, MA 02169
(617) 770–7476
Contact: Elizabeth Shaefer, Director

Mass. Rehab. Commission
Fort Point Place
27–43 Wormwood St.
Boston, MA 02210
617/727–2172
Contact: Elmer C. Bartels, Commissioner

Child-Adolescent Services
Department of Mental Health
24 Farnsworth St.
Boston, MA 02210
(617) 727–5600
Contact: Joan Mikula, Asst. Commissioner

Mass. Developmental Disabilities Planning Council
600 Washington St., Rm. 670
Boston, MA 02111–1704
(617) 727–6374
Contact: Director

Disability Law Center
11 Beacon St., Suite 925
Boston, MA 02108
(617) 723–8455
Contact: Richard Howard, Executive Director

Shriver Center University Affiliated Facility
200 Trapelo Rd.
Waltham, MA 02254
(617) 642–0001
Contact: Dr. Philip Reilly, Director

Federation for Children with Special Needs
95 Berkeley St.
Boston, MA 02116

(617) 482–2915; (800) 331–0688 (in MA)
Contact: Artie Higgins, Director

Parent-to-Parent
1249 Boylston St.
Boston, MA 02215
(617) 266–4520
Contact: Cindy Politch, Parent Support Coordinator

Client Assistance Program
Mass. Office of Handicapped Affairs
One Ashburton Place, Room 303
Boston, MA 02108
(617) 727–7440
Contact: Director

ARC of Massachusetts
217 South St.
Waltham, MA 02154
(617) 891–6270

Michigan

TSA—Central Michigan Chapter
(serves Flint, Lansing, and Saginaw)
For current phone number,
contact national TSA

TSA—Metropolitan Detroit Chapter
(serves Detroit, Jackson, Kalamazoo, and Royal Oak)
For current phone number,
contact national TSA

TSA—Grand Rapids Chapter
(serves Gaylord, Grand Rapids, Iron Mountain, and Traverse City)
For current phone number,
contact national TSA

Association for Children with Learning Disabilities (ACLD)
8123 E. 9 Mile Road
Big Rapids, MI 49307
(616)796–8968
Contact: Patricia Gawne, President

Michigan ACLD
P.O. Box 12336
Lansing, MI 48901
(517) 485–8160

Special Education Services
Michigan Dept. of Education
P.O. Box 30008
Lansing, MI 48909
(517) 373–9433
Contact: Director

Special Education Services (Ages 3–5)
Michigan Dept. of Education
P.O. Box 30008

Lansing, MI 48909
(517) 373–8215
Contact: Jan Baxter, Supervisor

Bureau of Rehabilitation
Department of Education
101 Pine St., 4th floor
P.O. Box 30010
Lansing, MI 48909
(517) 373–3391
Contact: Peter Griswald, Director

Michigan Developmental Disabilities Council
Lewis Cass Building, 6th Floor
Lansing, MI 48926
(517) 373–0341
Contact: Elizabeth Ferguson, Exec. Director

Michigan Protection and Advocacy Service
109 W. Michigan, Ste. 900
Lansing, MI 48933
(517) 487–1755
Contact Elizabeth Bauer, Exec. Director

University Affiliated Facility
Developmental Disabilities Institute
Wayne State University
6001 Cass Ave.
Detroit, MI 48202
(313) 577–2654
Contact: Director

Citizens Alliance to Uphold Special Education
(CAUSE)
313 S. Washington Square, Lower Level
Lansing, MI 48933
(517) 485–4084; (800) 221–9105
Contact: Cheryl Chilcote, Exec. Director

Parents are Experts
17000 W. 8 Mile Road, Suite 380
Southfield, MI 48075
(313) 557–5070
Contact: Edith Sharp, Coordinator

Peer Support Project
530 W. Ionia St., Ste. C
Lansing, MI 48933
517/487–9260
Contact: Mary Marin

ARC of Michigan
313 S. Washington, Suite 200
Lansing, MI 48933
(517) 487–5426
Contact: Marjorie Mitchell, Exec. Director

Minnesota

TSA—Minnesota Chapter
(serves entire state)
For current phone number,
contact national TSA

Minnesota Association for Children with
Learning Disabilities (ACLD)
541 Southwood Dr.
Bloomington, MN 55437
(612) 831–1131
Contact: Burt Seeker

ACLD State Office
1821 University Ave.
Room 494–N
St. Paul, MN 55104
(612) 646–6136
Contact: Kathleen Heikkila, Exec. Director

Special Education Section
Department of Education
812 Capitol Square Bldg.
550 Cedar St.
St. Paul, MN 55101–2233
(612) 296–1793
Contact: Director

Division of Vocational Rehabilitation
Department of Jobs and Training
390 N. Robert St., 5th Floor
St. Paul, MN 55101
(612) 296–2962
Contact: Assistant Commissioner

Division for Persons with Developmental Disabilities
444 Lafayette Rd.
St. Paul, MN 55155
(612) 297–0307
Contact: Shirley Schue, Director

Governor's Planning Council on Developmental Disabilities
658 Cedar St., Room 300
St. Paul, MN 55155
(612) 296–4018
Contact: Colleen Wieck, Exec. Director

Minnesota Disability Law Center
222 Grain Exchange BUilding
323 Fourth Ave, South
Minneapolis, MN 55415
(512) 332–7301
Contact: Steve Scott, Director

University Affiliated Program on Developmental Disabilities
University of Minnesota
6 Patte Hall
Minneapolis, MN 55455
(612) 624–4848
Contact: Robert Bruininks, Director

Parent Advocacy Coalition for Education
Rights (PACER)
4826 Chicago Ave., South
Minneapolis, MN 55417–1055

(612) 827–2966; (800) 53–PACER (in MN)
Contact: Marge Goldberg or Paula Goldberg,
  Directors

Pilot Parents
201 Ordean Building
Duluth, MN 55802
(218) 726–4745
Contact: Lynne Frigaard

ARC of Minnesota
3225 Lyndale Ave., South
Minneapolis, MN 55408
(612) 827–5641
Contact: Sue Abnerholden, Exec. Director

Mississippi

Tourette Syndrome Association Contact
Ernest Tullar
181 Rodenberg Ave.
Biloxi, MS 39532
(601) 374–3103 (H)
(601) 864–2961(W)

LDA of Mississippi
Rt. 2, Box 110
Minter City, MS 38944
(601) 658–4635 (H)
(601) 453–3600 (W)
Contact: Sandra Britt, President

LDA State Office
P.O. Box 9387
Jackson, MS 39206
(601) 982–2812

Bureau of Special Services
Department of Education
P.O. Box 771
Jackson, MS 39205–0771
(601) 359–3490
Contact: Director

Department of Vocational Services
P.O. Box 1698
Jackson, MS 39205
(601) 354–6825
Contact: Morris Selby, Director

Miss. Dev. Dis. Planning Council
1101 Robert E. Lee Bldg.
Jackson, MS 39201
691/359–1290
Contact: Ed C. Bell, Director

Mississippi Protection and Advocacy System
  for Developmentally Disabled, Inc.
4793 E. McWille Dr.
Jackson, MS 39206
(601) 981–8207
Contact: Rebecca Floyd, Exec. Director

Mississippi University Affiliated Program
University of Southern Mississippi
Southern Station, Box 5163
Hattiesburg, MS 34906–5163
(601) 266–5163
Contact: Dr. Robert Campbell, Director

Easter Seals Society
3226 N. State St.
Jackson, MS 39216
(601) 982–7051
Contact: Director

Mississippi Parent Network
425 Louisa St.
Pearl, MS 39208
(601) 932–7743
Contact: Kathy Odle-Pounds

ARC of Mississippi
2727 Old Canton Rd., Ste. 173
Jackson, MS 39216
(601) 362–4830
Contact: Linda Bond, Director

Missouri

TSA—Greater St. Louis Chapter
(serves Cape Girardeau, Flat River, Mid-Mis-
  souri Facility, Poplar Bluff, Rolla, Sedalia,
  St. Louis, and Springfield)
For current phone number,
contact national TSA

TSA—Kansas City, KS Chapter
(serves Kansas City, St. Joseph, Chillicothe,
  and Harrisonville)
For current phone number,
contact national TSA

LDA of Missouri
6153 Holmes
Kansas City, MO 64110
(816) 363–5844
Contact: Pat Horacek, President

LDA State Office
P.O. Box 3302
1918 E. Meadowmere, #10
Springfield, MO 65808
(417) 864–5110
Contact: Eleanore Scherff

Division of Special Education
Department of Elementary and Secondary
  Education
P.O. Box 480
Jefferson City, MO 65102
(314) 751–2965
Contact: Dr. John Heskett, Coordinator

Division of Special Education
Department of Elementary and Secondary
Education (Ages 3–5)
P.O. Box 480
Jefferson City, MO 65102
(314) 751–0185
Contact: Melody Friedeback, Assistant Director

Division of Vocational Rehabilitation
Department of Education
2401 E. McCarty St.
Jefferson City, MO 65101
(314) 751–3251
Contact: Don L. Gann, Assistant Commissioner

Children and Youth Services
Department of Mental Health
P.O. Box 687
Jefferson City, MO 65102
(314) 751–9482
Contact: Director

Missouri Planning Council for Dev. Disailities
P.O. Box 687
Jefferson City, MO 65102
(314) 751–4054
Contact: Kay Conklin, Coordinator

Missouri Protection and Advocacy Services
925 S. Country Club Dr., Unit B–1
Jefferson City, MO 65109
(314) 893–3333; (800) 392–8667
Contact: Cynthia Schloss, Director

University Affiliated Program for Developmental Disabilities
University of Missouri at Kansas City
Institute for Human Development
2220 Holmes St.
Kansas City, MO 64108
(816) 276–1770
Contact: Dr. Carl Calkins, Director

Missouri Parents Act (MPACT)
1722 W. South Glenstone, Ste. 125
Springfield, MO 65804
(417) 882–7434
Contact: Pat Jones, Director

Missouri Parents Act (MPACT)
625 Euclid, Room 225
St. Louis, MO 63108
Contact: Margaret Taber, Director

Montana

Tourette Syndrome Association Montana Contacts
Paulette & Kieth Iverson

117 30th Street West
Billings, MT 59102
(406) 652–1883

Montana Association for Children with Learning Disabilities (ACLD)
2535 35th St., SE
Harve, MT 59501
(406) 265–5633
Contact: Maureen Ferrell, President

Special Education Division
Office of Public Instruction
State Capitol, Rm. 106
Helena, MT 59602
(406) 444–4429
Contact: Robert Runkel, Director of Special Ecucation

Department of Education Services (Ages 3–5)
Office of Public Instruction
State Capitol
Helena, MT 59602
(406) 444–4428
Contact: Marilyn Pearson

Rehabilitation Services Division
Department of Social and Rehabilitation Services
P.O. Box 4210
Helena, MT 59601
(406) 444–2590

Division of Developmental Disabilities
Department of Social and Rehabilitation Services
P.O. Box 4210
111 Sanders, Room 202
Helena, MT 59604
(406) 444–2995
Contact: Director

Developmental Disabilities Planning Council
111 N. Last Chance Gulch
Arcade Bldg., Unit C
Helena, MT 59601
(406) 444–1334
Contact: Greg Olson, Director

Montana Advocacy Program
1410 8th Ave.
Helena, MT 59601
(406) 444–3889; (800) 245–4743
Contact: Kris Bakula, Exec. Dir.

Montana Center for Handicapped Children
Eastern Montana College
1500 N. 30th St.
Billings, MT 59101–0298
(604) 657–2312
Contact: Dr. Michael Hagen, Dir.

Montana University Affiliated Programs
33 Corbin Hall
University of Montana
Missoula, MT 59812
(406) 343–5467
Contact: Dr. Richard Offner, Director

Parents, Let's Unite for Kids
Eastern Montana Collge
1500 N. 30th St.
Billings, MT 59101–0298
(406) 657–2055
Contact: Katherine Kelker, Dir.

Parent-to-Parent
Parents, Let's Unite for Kids
Eastern Montana College
1500 N. 30th St.
Billings, MT 59101–0298

ARC of Montana
7 Willowbend Dr.
Billings, MT 59102
(406) 656–9549
Contact: Leona Neufeld, President

Nebraska

TSA—Nebraska Chapter
(serves entire state)
For current phone number,
contact national TSA

Association for Children with Learning Disabilities (ACLD)
5835 Corby
Omaha, NE 68104
(402) 599–2409 (H)
(712) 328–8400 (W)

Special Education Branch
Department of Education
Box 94987
301 Centennial Mall South
Lincoln, NE 68509
(402) 471–2471
Contact: Gary M. Sherman, Director

Special Education Section (Ages 3–5)
Department of Education
P.O. Box 94987
Lincoln, NE 68509
(402) 471–2471

Jan Thelen, Coordinator
Division of Rehabilitation Services
Department of Education
P.O. Box 94987
301 Centennial Mall, 6th Floor
Lincoln, NE 68509

(402) 471–2961
Contact: Jason Andrew, Assistant Commissioner

Dept. of Health/Dev. Disabilities
P.O. Box 95007
Lincoln, NE 68509
(402) 471–2330
Contact: Mary Gordon, Director

Nebraska Advocacy Services
522 Lincoln Center Bulding
215 Centennial Mall South
Lincoln, NE 68508
(402) 474–3183
Contact: Timothy Shaw, Exec. Dir.

Pilot Parents
3610 Dodge St.
Omaha, NE 68131
402/346–5220
Contact: Arretta Johnson, Coordinator

ARC of Nebraska
521 S. 14th St., Ste. 211
Lincoln, NE 68508
(402) 475–4407
Contact: Ginger Clubine, Exec. Director

Nevada

Tourette Sydrome Assoc.
2301 Pommel Ave.
Las Vegas, NV 89119
(702) 736–8841
Contact: Elizabeth McKenna

Special Education
Department of Education
400 W. King St./Capitol Complex
Carson City, NV 89710
(702) 687–3140
Contact: Director

Special Education Branch (Ages 3–5)
Department of Education
400 W. King St./Capitol Complex
Carson City, NV 89710
(702) 885–3140
Contact: Coordinator

Rehabilitation Division
Department of Human Resources
State Capitol Complex
505 E. King St.
Carson City, NV 98710
(702) 687–4440
Contact: Delbert Frost, Administrator

Northern Nevada Children and Adolescents
Mental Health Programs
Child & Adolescent Services
2655 Enterprise Road

Reno, NV 89512
(702) 789–0300
Contact: Wilford W. Beck

Developmental Disablities Council
505 E. King St. Room 502
Carson City, NV 89710–0001
(702) 687–4452
Contact: Director

Office of Protection and Advocacy
2105 Capurro Way, Suite B
Sparks, NV 89431
(702) 789–0233; (800) 992–5715
Contact: Holli Elder, Project Director

Project ASSIST: A Direction of Service
 Nevada
CHANCE Parent Project
Box 70247
Reno, NV 89570
(702) 747–0669; (800) 522–0066

ARC of Nevada
680 S. Bailey St.
Fallon, NV 89406
(702) 423–4760
Contact: Frank Weinrauch, Exec. Dir.

New Hampshire

TSA New Hampshire Chapter
(serves entire state)
For current phone number,
contact national TSA

New Hampshire Association for Children with
 Learning Disabilities (ACLD)
20 Wedgewood Dr.
Concord, NH 03307
(603) 224–5872
Contact: Lisa Gray, Pesident

Special Education Bureau
Department of Education
101 Pleasant St.
Concord, NH 03301–3860
(603) 271–3741
Contact: Robert Kennedy, Director

Division of Mental Health and Developmental
 Services
Dept. of Health and Welfare
State Office Park South
105 Pleasant St
Concord, NH 03301
(603) 271–5013
Contact: Richard Lepore, Assistant Divisional
 Director

Philbrook Center for Children and Youth
121 S. Fruit St.
Concord, NH 03301
(603) 224–6531, ext. 2365
Contact: Wm. Wheeler, Superintendent

New Hampshire Developmental Disabilities
 Council
Concord Center
10 Ferry St.
Concord, NH 03301–5022
(603) 271–3236
Contact: Director

Disabilities Rights Center
P.O. Box 19
Concord, NH 03302–0019
(603) 228–0432
Contact: Donna Woodfin, Director

Parent Information Center
155 Manchester St.
P.O. Box 1422
Concord, NH 03302–1422
(603) 224–6299
Contact: Judith Raskin, Director

ARC of New Hampshire
10 Ferry St., Box 4
The Concord Center
Concord, NH 03301
(602) 228–9092
Contact: Christine Nicolleta

New Jersey

TSA of New Jersey, Inc.
(serves entire state)
For current phone number,
contact national TSA

Association for Children with Learning Disabilities (ACLD)
305 North Lancaster Ave.
Margate, NJ 08402
(609)823–5608
Contact: Ronee Groff, President

ACLD State OFfice
640 Ocean Ave.
West End, NJ 07740
(201) 229–1919

Division of Special Education
Department of Education
225 W. State St., CN 500
Trenton, NJ 08625
(609) 633–6833
Contact: Jeffrey Osowski, Director

Div. of Vocational Rehabilitation
Dept. of Labor and Industry
1005 Labor and Industry Building, CN 398
John Fitch Plaza
Trenton, NJ 08625
(609) 292–5987
Contact: Director

Div. of Developmental Disabilities
Department of Human Services
2–98 E. State St., CN 726
Trenton, NJ 08625
(609) 292–7260

Contact: Director
Bureau of Children's Services
Division of Mental Health and Hospitals
Capital Ctr., CN 727
Trenton, NJ 008625
(609) 777–0702
Contact: Joyce B. Wale, Chief

New Jersey Developmental Disability Council
108–110 N. Broadway St., CN 700
Trenton, NJ 08625
(609) 292–3745
Contact: Director

Department of Public Advocate
Office of Advocacy for the Dev. Disabled
Hughes Justice Complex, CN 850
Trenton, NJ 08625
(609) 292–1750; (800) 792–8600
Contact: Sara Mitchell, Dir.

University Affiliated Facility
University of Medicine and Dentistry of New
    Jersey
Robert W. Johnson Medical School
675 Hoes Lane
Piscataway, NJ 08854–5635
(201) 463–4447
Contact: Dr. Deborah Spitalnick, Director

Statewide Parent Advocacy Network (SPAN)
516 N. Ave., East
Westfield, NJ 07090
(201) 654–7726
Contact: Diana Cuthbertson, Exec. Director

New Jersey Self-Help Clearinghouse
St. Clare-Riverside Medical Center
Pocono Road
Denville, NJ 07834
(201) 625–9565; (800) 367–6274 (in NJ)
Contact: Edward Madara, Director

ARC of New Jersey
985 Livingston Ave.
North Brunswick, NJ 08902
(201) 246–2525
Contact: John Scagnelli, Exec. Director

New Mexico

Tourette Syndrome Association Contact
Reta and Duane Roth
3301 Montreal, NE
Albuquerque, NM 87111
(505) 291–8591

New Mexico ACLD
824 Vassar Dr.
Albuquerque, NM 87106
(505) 255–9324
Contact: Marjorie McCament

Special Education Unit
Department of Education
Education Building
300 Don Gasper Ave.
Santa Fe, NM 87501–2786
(505) 827–6541
Contact: Jim Newby, Director

Special Education Unit (Ages 3–5)
Department of Education
Education Building
300 Dan Gasper Ave
Santa FE, NM 87501–2786
(505) 827–6541
Contact: Diana Turner, Coordinator

Division of Vocational Rehab.
Dept. of Education
604 W. San Mateo
Santa Fe, NM 87503
(505) 827–3511
Contact: Ross Sweat, Director

Community Programs
Department of Health and the Environment
1190 St. Francis Dr.
Santa Fe, NM 87503
(505) 827–2573
Contact: Steve Dossey, Chief

New Mexico DD Planning Council
2025 Pacheco St., Ste. 200–B
Santa Fe, NM 87505
(505) 827–2707
Contact: Chris Isengard, Dir.

Protection & Advocacy System
1720 Louisiana Blvd., NE, Ste. 204
Albuquerque, NM 87110
(505) 256–3100; (800) 432–4682 (in NM)
Contact James Jackson, Exec. Dir.

Education for Parents of Indian Children with
    Special Needs (EPICS Project)
P.O. Box 788
Bernalilo, NM 87004
(505) 867–3396
Contact: Director

Parents Reaching Out (PRO)
1127 University, NE
Albuquerque, NM 87102
(505) 842–9045; (800) 542–5176 (in NM)
Contact: Director

ARC of New Mexico
3500–G Commanche, NE
Albuquerque, NM 87107
(505) 883–4630
Contact: John Foley, Exec. Dir.

New York

TSA—Central New York Chapter
(serves Elmira, Binghampton, Syracuse, Utica,
and Watertown)
For current phone number,
contact national TSA

TSA—Long Island Chapter
(serves Nassau and Suffolk Counties, Queens,
and the Bronx)
For current phone number,
contact national TSA

TSA—Mid-Western NY Chapter
(serves Rochester)
For current phone number,
contact national TSA

TSA—New York City West Chapter
(serves Brooklyn, Manhattan, and Staten Island)
For current phone number,
contact national TSA

TSA—Westchester/Rockland County Chapter
(serves Westchester and Rockland Counties)
For current phone number,
contact national TSA

TSA—Western New York Chapter
(serves Buffalo and Jamestown)
For current phone number,
contact national TSA

New York ALD
8 Weiser St.
Glenmont, NY 12077
(518) 463–6225 (H)
(518) 783–1644 (W)
Contact: Virginia Rossuck, President

ALD State Office
90 South Swan St.
Albany, NY 12210
(518) 436–4633

Office for Education of Children with Handicapping Conditions
Department of Education
1073 Education Building Annex

Albany, NY 12234–0001
(518) 474–5548
Contact: Tom Neveldine

Office for Education of Children with Handicapping Conditions (Ages 3–5)
Department of Education
1073 Education Building Annex
Albany, NY 12234–0001
(518) 474–8917
Contact: Bureau Chief

Office of Vocational Rehab.
Department of Education
One Commerce Plaza, 16th Fl.
Albany NY 12234
(518) 474–2714
Contact: Larry Gloeckler

Office of Mental Retardation and Developmental Disabilities
44 Holland Ave.
Albany, NY 12229
(518) 473–1997
Contact: Elin Howe, Commissioner

Bureau of Children and Families
Office of Mental Health
44 Holland Ave.
Albany, NY 12229
(518) 474–6902
Contact: Gloria Newton-Logsdon, Assoc. Commissioner

New York State Developmental DIsabilities
Planning Council
155 Washington Ave., 2nd Fl.
Albany NY 12210
(518) 432–8233
Contact: Isabel Mills, Exec. Director

University Affiliated Facility
Rose F. Kennedy Center
Albert Einstein College of Medicine
Yeshiva Univrsity
1410 Pelham Parkway
South Bronx, NY 10461
(212) 430–2325
Contact: Dr. Herbert Cohen, Director

University Affiliated Program for Dev. Dis.
University of Rochester Medical Center
601 Elmwood Ave.
Rochester, NY 14642
(716) 275–2986
Contact: Phillip Davidson, Director

NY Comm. on Quality of Care for the
Mentally Disabled
99 Washington Ave.
Albany, NY 12210

518/473–4057
Contact: Clarence Sundram, Commissioner

Advocates for Children of New York, Inc.
24–16 Bridge Plaza South
Long Island, NY 11101
(718) 729–8866
Contact: Norma Rollins, Director

Parent Network Center
1443 Main St.
Buffalo, NY 14209
(716) 885–1004
Contact: Joan Watkins, Director

Parent-to-Parent
Senate Select Committee on the Disabled
Legislative Office Building
Albany, NY 12247
(518) 455–2096
Contact: Marilyn Wessels, Director

Parent-to-Parent
Family Support Project for the Developmentally Disabled
North Central Bronx Hospital
3424 Kossuth Ave.
Bronx, NY 10467
(212) 519–4796

New York State ARC, Inc.
393 Delaware Ave.
Delmar, NY 12054
(518) 439–8311
Contact: Director

North Carolina

TSA—North Carolina Chapter
(serves entire state)
For current phone number,
contact national TSA

LDA of North Carolina
510 Colony Woods Dr.
Chapel Hills, NC 27514
(919) 966–4041 (W)
(919) 942–1352 (H)
Contact: Laura Thomas, President

LDA State Office
Box 3542
Chapel Hill, NC 27514
(919) 967–9537

Division for Exceptional Children
Department of Public Instruction
Education Building, Room 442
116 W. Edenton
Raleigh, NC 27603
(919) 733–3921
Contact: Lowell Harris, Director

Div. of Vocational Rehab.
Dept. of Human Resources
620 North West St.
P.O. Box 26053
Raleigh, NC 27611
(919) 733–3364
Contact: Claude Myer, Director

North Carolina Council on Dev. Disabilities
1508 Western Blvd.
Raleigh, NC 27606
(919) 733–6566
Contact: Director

Governor's Advocacy Council for Persons with
Disbilities
1318 Dale St., Suite 100
Raleigh, NC 27605
(919) 733–9250
Contact: Lockhart Fallin-Mace, Director

Exceptional Children's Assistance Center
P.O. Box 16
Davidson, NC 28036
(704) 892–1321
Contact: Connie Hawkins, Director

Family Support Network
CB #7340 Trailer 31, Daniels Rd.
University of NC at Chapel Hill
Chapel Hill, NC 27599–7340
(919) 966–2841
Contact: Michael Sharp

ARC of North Carolina
16 Rowan St., P.O. Box 20545
Raleigh, NC 27619
(919) 782–4632
Contact: Director

North Dakota

North Dakota Tourette Syndrome Association
3004 Chestnut St.
Grand Forks, ND 58201
(701) 746–7182
Contact: Peggy Chisholm, President

Tourette Syndrome Clinic
The Child Evaluation and Treatment Center
Medical Center Rehabilitation Hospital and
Clinics
Box 8202
Grand Forks, ND 58202

North Dakota Association for Children and
Adults with Learning Disabilities (ACLD)
Box 814
Fargo, ND 58107
(701) 293–7914
Contact: Deb Dawson

Special Education Division
Department of Public Instruction
600 East Blvd.
Bismarck, ND 58505
(701) 224–2277
Contact: Gary Gronberg, Director

Special Education Division (Ages 3–5)
Department of Public Instruction
State Capital
Bismarck, ND 58505–6440
(701) 224–2277
Contact: Coordinator

Dept. of Vocational Rehab.
State Board of Social Services
State Capitol Building
Bismarck, ND 58505
(701) 224–2907
Contact: Gene Hysjulien, Exec. Director

Developmental Disabilities Division
Department of Human Services
State Capitol Building
600 East Blvd.
Bismarck, ND 58505
(701) 224–2907
Contact: Acting Director

North Dakota Developmental Disabilities
    Council
Department of Human Services
State Capitol Building
Bismarck, ND 58505
(701) 224–2970
Contact: Tom Wallner, Director

Protection and Advocacy Project
400 E. Broadway, No. 515
Bismarck, ND 58501
(701) 224–2972; (800) 472–2670 (in ND)
Contact: Barbara Braun, Director

Pathfinder Parent Ctr.
16th St. & 2nd Ave., SW
Arrowhead Shopping Center
Minot, ND 58701
(701) 852–9426
Contact: Kathryn Erickson, Dir.

ARC of North Dakota
417½ E. Broadway, No. 9
P.O. Box 2776
Bismarck, ND 58502
(701) 223–5349
Contact: Exec. Director

Ohio

TSA of Ohio, Inc.
Park 50 Techne Center
100 Techne Center Dr., Suite 118

Milford, OH 45150
(513) 831–2976; (800) 543–2675 (in OH)
Contact: Judy King

Tourette and Tic Clinic
Ohio State University
Department of Psychiatry
Upham Hall
473 W. 12th Ave.
Columbus, OH 43210

Ohio Association for Children and Adults with
    Learning Disabilities (ACLD)
2874 Castlewood Road
Columbus, OH 43209
(614) 231–3321
Contact: Bernice Stewart, President

ACLD State Office
1480 Pearl Road, #5
Brunswick, OH 44212
(216) 273–7388

Division of Special Education
Department of Education
933 High St.
Worthington OH 43085–4017
(614) 466–2650
Contact: Frank E. New, Director

Early Childhood Section (Ages 3–5)
Department of Education
65 S. Front St., Room 202
Columbus, OH 43266
(614) 466–0224
Contact: Jane Wiechel, Assistant Director

Rehabilitation Services Commission
400 E. Campus View Blvd.
Columbus, OH 43235
(614) 438–1210
Contact: Robert Rabe, Administrator

Department of Mental Retardation and
    Developmental Disabilities
State Office Tower
30 E. Broad St., Room 1280
Columbus, OH 43224
(614) 466–5214
Contact: Robert Brown, Director

Ohio DD Planning Council
Dept. of MR/DD
8 E. Long St.
Atlas Bldg., 6th Fl.
Columbus, OH 43215
(614) 466–5205
Contact: Ken Campbell, Exec. Dir.

Ohio Legal Rights Service
8 E. Long St., 6th Floor
Columbus, OH 43215

(614) 466–7264; (800) 282–9181 (in OH)
Contact: Carolyn Knight, Exec. Director

Affiliated Cincinnati Center for Devel. Disabilities
Pavilion Building
Elland and Bethesda Ave.
Cincinnati, OH 45229
(513) 559–4623
Contact: Dr. Jack Rubenstein, Director

The Nisonger Center
Ohio State University
McCambell Hall
1581 Dodd Dr.
Columbus OH 43210–1205
(614) 292–8365
Contact: Stephen Schroeder, Director

Tri-State Organized Coalition for Persons with Disabilities
SOC Information Center
106 Wellington Place, Lower Level
Cincinnati, OH 45219
(513) 381–2400
Contact: Cathy Heizman, Director

Ohio Coalition for the Education of Handicapped Children
933 High St., Suite 106
Worthington, OH 43085
(614) 431–1307
Contact: Margaret Burley, Director

ARC of Ohio
360 3rd St., Suite 101
Columbus, OH 43215
(614) 228–4412
Contact: Carolyn Sidwell, Exec. Director

Oklahoma

TSA—Oklahoma Chapter
(serves entire state)
For current phone number,
contact national TSA

Oklahoma Association for Children and Adults with Learning Disabilities (ACLD)
1701 Leawood Dr.
Eadmond, OK 73034
(405) 341–2980, ext. 2236 (W)
(405) 348–4080 (H)

ACLD State Office
3701 NW 62nd St.
Oklahoma City, OK 73112
(405) 943–9434
Contact: Jeanne Asher

Special Education Division
Department of Education
Oliver Hodge Memorial Building, Room 215

Oklahoma City, OK 73105–4599
(405) 521–3351
Contact: Director

Section for Exceptional Children (Ages 3–5)
Department of Education
2500 N. Lincoln Blvd., Ste. 263
Oklahoma City, OK 73105
(405) 521–3351
Contact: Coordinator

Rehabilitation Services Division
2409 N. Kelley
Oklahoma City, OK 73125
(405) 424–6006, ext. 2840
Contact: Jerry Dunlap

Developmental Disability Services
Department of Human Services
P.O. Box 25352
Oklahoma City, OK 73125
(405) 521–3571
Contact: Eranell McIntosh-Wilson, Administrator

Oklahoma Developmental Disability Planning Council
Box 25352
Oklahoma City, OK 73125
(405) 521–4984
Contact: Director

Protection and Advocacy Agency
Osage Building, Room 133
9726 E. 42nd St.
Tulsa, OK 74146
(918) 664–5883
Contact: Dr. Bob VanOsdol, Director

Parents Reaching Out in Oklahoma (PRO—Oklahoma)
1917 S. Harvard Ave.
Oklahoma City, OK 73128
(800) 959–4142; (405) 681–9710
Contact: Connie Motsinger, Director

Positive Reflections, Inc.
6141 NW Grand, Suite 103
Oklahoma City, OK 73116
(405) 843–9114
Contact: Dana Baldridge or Nancy Thompson

Oregon

TSA—Southern Oregon Chapter
(serves Eugene, Klamath Falls, and Medford)
For current phone number,
contact national TSA

Special Education and Student Services Division
Department of Education
700 Pringle Parkway, S.E.

Salem, OR 97310
(503) 378–3591
Contact: Karen Brazeau, Assoc. Superintendant

Division of Special Education (Ages 3–5)
Department of Education
700 Pringle Parkway, S.E.
Salem, OR 97301
(503) 373–1484
Contact: Mike Barker, Coordinator

Vocational Rehabilitation Division
Department of Human Resources
2045 Silverton Rd., N.E.
Salem, OR 97310
(503) 378–3830
Contact: Joil Southwell, Administrator

Program for Mental Retardaton and Developmental Disabilities
Department of Human Resoruces
2575 Bittern St., N.W.
Salem, OR 97310
(503) 378–2429
Contact: James Toews, Asst. Administrator

Oregon Dev. Disabilities Planning Council
540 24th Place, NE
Salem, OR 97301
(503) 373–7555
Contact: Russ Gurley, Dir.

Oregon Advocacy Center
Board of Trade Bldg.
310 SW 4th Ave., Ste. 625
Portland, OR 97204–2309
Contact: Elam Lantz, Jr., Exec. Director

Center on Human Development
Clinical Services Building
College of Education
University of Oregon—Eugene
Eugene, OR 97403
(503) 686–3591
Contact: Dr. Hill Walker, Director

Crippled Children's Division
Child Development and Rehabilitation Center
Oregon Health Sciences University
P.O. Box 574
Portland, OR 97207
(503) 279–8362
Contact: Director

Oregon COPE Project (Coalition in Oregon for
Parent Education)
999 Locust St., NE, Box B
Salem, OR 97303
(503) 373–7477
Contact: Cheron Mayhall, Director

Parent-to-Parent
Oregon COPE Project
999 Locust St., NE, Box B
Salem, OR 97303
(503) 373–7477

ARC of Oregon
1745 State St.
Salem, OR 97301
(503) 581–2726
Contact: Janna Starr, Exec. Director

Pennsylvania

TSA—South Central Penn. Chapter
(serves Altoona, Harrisburg, Lancaster, Lehigh
Valley, Philadelphia, Reading, and Williamsport)
For current phone number,
contact national TSA

TSA—Northeast Penn. Chapter
(serves Scranton and Wilksbarre)
For current phone number,
contact national TSA

TSA—Western Penn. Chapter
(serves Greensburg, Johnstown, and Pittsburgh)
For current phone number,
contact national TSA

TSA—Erie Penn. Chapter
(serves Bradford, DuBois, Erie, New Castle,
and Oil City)
For current phone number,
contact national TSA

Philadelphia O.C.D.
1062 Lancaster Ave., Suite 9
Rosemont, PA 19010
Contact: Gail Franklin

Pennsylvania ACLD
2551 W. 8th St.
Erie, PA 16505
(814) 838–1966, ext. 303
Contact: Sr. Joyce Lowry, President

ACLD State Office
Toomey Building, Suite 23
Eagle, Box 308
Uwichland, PA 19408
(215) 458–8193; (800) 692–6200
Contact: Mary Rita Hanley

Bureau of Special Education
Dept. of Education
333 Market St.
Harrisburg, PA 17126–0333
(717) 783–6913
Contact: James Tucker, State Dir.

Bureau of Special Education (Ages 3–5)
Department of Education
333 Market Street
Harrisburg, PA 17126–0333
(717) 783–6913
Contact: Special Education Advisor

Bureau of Vocational Rehabilitation
Department of Labor and Industry
Labor and Industry Building, Room 1300
7th and Forster Streets
Harrisburg, PA 17120
(717) 787–5244
Contact: Director

Developmental Disabilities Planning Council
Forum Building, Room 569
Commonwealth Ave.
Harrisburg, PA 17120
(717) 787–6057
Contact: David Schwartz, Executive Director

Protection and Advocacy, Inc.
116 Pine St.
Harrisburg, PA 17101
(717) 323–8110; (800) 692–7443
Contact: Kevin Casey, Executive Director

Developmental Disabilities Program
Temple University
9th Floor, Ritter Annex
13th St. and Cecil Moore Ave.
Philadelphia, PA 19122
(215) 787–1356
Contact: Dr. Edward Newman, Director

Parents Union for Public Schools
311 S. Juniper St., Ste. 602
Philadelphia, PA 19107
(215) 546–1212
Contact: Christine Davis, Dir.

Parent Education Network
240 Haymeadow Dr.
York, PA 17402
(717) 845–9722
Contact: Louise Thieme, Director

Mentor Parent Program
Rte. 257, Salina Rd.
P.O. Box 718
Seneca, PA 16346
814/676–8615; 800/447–1431
Contact: Gail Walker, Dir.

Parent-to-Parent
Parent Education Network
240 Haymeadow Dr.
York, PA 17402
(717) 845–9722

ARC of Pennsylvania
123 Forester Place
Harrisburg, PA 17102
(717) 234–2621
Contact: W.A. West, Exec. Director

Puerto Rico

Puerto Rico ACLD
GPO Box 1905
Sam Juan, PR 00936
(809) 761–0816; (809)788–6252
Contact: Mildred De Velazuez, President

Special Education Programs
Department of Education
Box 759
Hato Rey, PR 00919
(809) 764–8059
Contact: Lucila Torres Martinez, Assistant
Secretary of Special Education

Early Childhood Education (Ages 3–5)
Department of Education
Box 759
Hato Rey, PR 00919
(809) 759–7228
Contact: Awilda Torres

Division de Rehabilitation Vocational Depart-
ment de Servcios Sociales
Apartado 1118
Hato Rey, PR 00919
(809) 725–1792
Contact: Angel Jimenez

Developmental Disabilities Council
Box 9543
Santurce, PR 00908
(809) 722–0590
Contact: Maria Luisa Mendia, Director

Ombudsman for the Disabled
Box 5163
Hato Rey, PR 00919
(809) 766–2333
Contact: Director

Associate de Padres Pro Bienestar/Ninos In-
pedios de PR, Inc.
Box 21301
Rio Piedras, PR 00928
(809) 765–0345; (809) 763–4665
Contact: Carmen Selles Vila, Director

Rhode Island

Rhode Island Chapter—OC Foundation
Butler Hospital
345 Blackstone Blvd.
Providence, RI 02906

Rhode Island Association for Children and
Adults with Learning Disabilities (ACLD)
103 Harris Ave.
Johnston, RI 02919
(401) 231–0914 (H)
(401) 461–0820, ext. 539 (W)
Contact: Norma Veresko, President

Special Education Program
Department of Education
Roger Williams Building, Room 209
22 Hayes St.
Providence, RI 02908
(401) 277–3505
Contact: Robert Pryhoda, Director

Special Education Program Services Unit
(Ages 3–5)
Department of Elementary and Secondary
Education
Roger Williams Building, Room 209
22 Hayes St.
Providence, RI 02908
(401) 277–3505
Contact: Amy Cohen, Preschool ECSE Consultant

Vocational Rehabilitation
Department of Human Services
40 Fountain St.
Providence, RI 02903
(401) 421–7005
Contact: Sherri Campanelli, Administrator

Rhode Island Developmental Disabilities
Council
600 New London Ave.
Cranston, RI 02920
(401) 464–3191
Contact: Director

Rhode Island Protection and Advocacy System, Inc.
55 Bradford St., 2nd Floor
Providence, RI 02903
(401) 831–3150
Contact: Linda Katz, Exec. Director

Child Development Center
Rhode Island Hospital
593 Eddy St.
Providence, RI 02920
(401) 277–5681
Contact: Dr. Siegfried Pueschel, Director

Parent-to-Parent
R.I. Department of Education
22 Hayes St., Room 209
Providence, RI 02908

(401) 277–3505
Contact: Connie Susa, Parent Training
Specialist

ARC of Rhode Island
99 Bald Hill Rd.
Cranston, RI 02920
(401) 436–9191
Contact: James Healey, Exec. Director

South Carolina

Tourette Syndrome Association
South Carolina Contact
Marilyn Eskew
2603 Warren Dr.
Anderson, SC 29621
(803) 224–0683

South Carolina Association for Children and
Adults with Learning Disabilities (ACLD)
1792 Sharonwood Lane
Rock Hill, SC 29730
(803) 366–4141 (W)
(803) 366–5042 (H)
Contact: Ellen Mayes

Office of Programs for the Handicapped
Department of Education
Santee Building, A–24
100 Executive Center Dr.
Columbia, SC 29201
(803) 737–7810
Contact: Dr. Robert Black, Director

Programs for the Handicapped (Ages 3–5)
Department of Education
100 Executive Center Dr.
Santee Buildign, Suite 210
Columbia, SC 29210
(803) 737–8710
Contact: Mary Ginn, State Plan Coordinator

Vocational Rehabilitation Department
1410 Boston Ave
P.O. Box 15
West Columbia, SC 29171
(803) 734–4300
Contact: Joseph Dusenbury, Commissioner

South Carolina Developmental Disability Planning Council
1205 Pendleton Street, Room 372
Columbia, SC 29201
(803) 734–0465
Contact: LaNelle DuRant, Exec. Director

South Carolina Protection and Advocacy System for the Handicapped, Inc.
3710 Landmark Dr., Suite 208
Columbia, SC 29204

(803) 782–0639; (800) 922–5225
Contact: Louise Ravenel, Exec. Director

University Affiliated Facility of South Carolina
Center for Developmental Disabilities
Benson Building, Pickens St.
University of South Carolina
Columbia, SC 29208
(803) 777–4839
Contact: Director

Parents Reaching Out to Parents
220 Great North Road
Columbia, SC 29223
(803) 737–4048
Contact: Sue Slater, Director

ARC of South Carolina
Box 21983
Columbia, SC 29221
(803) 754–4763
Contact: John Beckley, Exec. Director

South Dakota

Tourette Syndrome Association
South Dakota Contact
Ron Wentzel
RR2, Box 93
Parker, SD 57053
(605) 297–4291

LDA of South Dakota
4022 Helen Court
Rapid City, SD 57701
(605) 342–4320
Contact: Dixie Davis, President

Section for Special Education
Department of Education
Kneip Office Building
700 N. Illinois St.
Pierre, SD 57501
(605) 773–3315
Contact: Dean Myers, Director

Section for Special Education (Ages 0–5)
Department of Education and Cultural Affairs
700 Governors Dr.
Pierre, SD 57501
(605) 773–4329
Contact: Paulette Levisen

Division of Rehabilitation Services
700 N. Governors Dr.
Pierre, SD 57501
(605) 773–3195
Contact: David Miller, Director

Developmental Disabilities and Mental Health
700 N. Illinois St.
Pierre, SD 57501

(605) 733–3438
Contact: Dianne Weyer

South Dakota Advocacy Project
221 S. Central Ave.
Pierre, SD 57501
(605) 224–8294; (800) 742–8108
Contact: Robert Kean, Exec. Director

South Dakota University Affiliated Facility
Center for Developmental Disabilities
U.S.D. School of Medicine
Vermillion, SD 57069
(605) 677–5311
Contact: Cecilia Rokusek, Acting Director

Parent-to-Parent
Center for Developmental Disabilities
USD School of Medicine
414 E. Clark
Vermillion, SD 57069
(605) 677–5311

ARC of South Dakota
P.O. Box 502
Pierre, SD 57501
(605) 224–8211
Contact: John Stengle, Exec. Director

Tennessee

TSA—Tennessee State
(serves entire state)
For current phone number,
contact national TSA

Tennessee Association for Children and
Adults with Learning Disabilities (ACLD)
P.O. Box 114
Pocahontas, TN 38061
(901) 528–6159 (W)
(901) 525–2206 (H)
Contact: William Burne, President

Special Education Programs
Department of Education
132 Cordell Hull Building
Nashville, TN 37219
(615) 741–2851
Contact: Assoc. Commissioner

Division of Vocational Rehabilitation
Department of Human Services
400 Deaderick St., 15th Floor
Nashville, TN 37219
(615) 741–2521
Contact: Patsy Mathews, Assistant Commissioner

Office of Children and Adolescent Services
Doctors Building
706 Church Street
Nashville, TN 37219

(615) 741–3708
Contact: Director

Developmental Disability Planning Council
Doctors Building, 3rd Floor
706 Church St.
Nashville, TN 37219
(615) 741–3807
Contact: Wanda Willis, Director

Effective Advocacy for Citizens with Handicaps (EACH)
P.O. Box 121257
Nashville, TN 37212
(615) 298–1080; (800) 342–1660
Contact: Harriette Derryberry, Director

Center for Developmental Disabilities
University of Tennessee, Memphis
711 Jefferson Ave.
Memphis, TN 38105
(901) 528–6511
Contact: Dr. Gerald Golden, Director

Parents Offering Support to Other Parents (POSTOP)
801–A Teaberry Lane
Knoxville, TN 37919
(615) 691–2418
Contact: Ann Farr

Support and Training for Exceptional Parents (STEP)
1805 Hayes St., Ste. 100
Nashville, TN 37203
(615) 327–0294
Contact: Carol Westlake, Dir.

ARC of Tennessee
1805 Hayes, Suite 100
Nashville, TN 37203
(615) 327–0294
Contact: Roger Blue, Exec. Director

Texas

TSA—Dallas/Ft. Worth Chapter
(serves Dallas, Ft. Worth, Greenville, Longview, Lufkin, Texarkana, Tyler, and Wichita Falls)
For current phone number, contact national TSA

TSA—Houston Chapter
(serves Beaumont, Bryan, Conroe, Houston, Palestine, Pasadena, and Victoria)
For current phone number, contact national TSA

TSA—South Central Texas
(serves Austin, Corpus Christi, McAllen, San Antonio, Temple, and Waco)
For current phone number, contact national TSA

TSA—South Plains Chapter
(serves Abilene, Amarillo, Childress, and Lubbock)
For current phone number, contact national TSA

Texas Association for Children and Adults with Learning Disabilities (ACLD)
2909 Wildflower
Bryan TX 77802
(409) 776–2807
Jean Kueker, President

ACLD State Office
1011 W. 31st Street
Austin, TX 78705
(512) 458–8234

Special Eduation Programs
Texas Education Agency
Wm. B. Travis Bldg., Room 5–120
1701 N. Congress Ave.
Austin, TX 78701–2486
(512) 463–9414
Contact: Jill Gray, Director

Special Education Programs (Ages 3–5)
Texas Education Agency
Wm. B. Travis Bldg.
1701 N. Congress Ave.
Austin, TX 78701
(512) 463–9414
Contact: Coordinator

Texas Rehab. Commission
4900 N. Lamar
Austin, TX 78751
(512) 483–4001
Contact: Vernon M. Arrell, Commissioner

Children and Youth Mental Health Services
Department of Mental Health and Mental Retardation
Box 12668, Capitol Station
Austin, TX 78711
(512) 465–4657
Contact: Regenia Hicks

Texas Planning Council for Dev. Disabilities
4900 N. Lamar Blvd.
Austin, TX 78751–2316
(512) 483–4080
Contact: Roger Webb, Exec. Dir.

Advocacy, Inc.
7800 Shoal Creek Blvd.
Suite 171–E
Austin, TX 78757

(512) 454–4816; (800) 252–9108
Contact: Exec. Director

University Affiliated Center
200 Treadway Plaza
6400 Harry Hines Blvd.
Dallas, TX 75235
(214) 688–7117
Contact: Dr. Mark Swanson, Director

Partnerships for Assisting Texans with Handicaps (PATH)
6465 Calder Ave., Suite 202
Beaumont, TX 77707
(409) 866–4726
Contact: Janice Foreman, Director

ARC of Texas
833 Houston St.
Austin, TX 78756
(512) 454–6694
Contact: Director

Utah

TSA—Utah Chapter
(serves entire state)
For current phone number,
contact national TSA

LDA of Utah
2030 E. 9100 St.
Sandy, UT 84093
(801) 943–4425
Contact: Linda Smity, President

LDA State Office
P.O. Box 112
Salt Lake City, UT 84110
(801) 364–0126

Special Education Section
State Office of Education
250 E. 500 South
Salt Lake City, UT 84111–3204
(801) 538–7706
Contact: Steve Kukic, Director

Special Education Section (Ages 3–5)
State Office of Education
250 E. 500 South
Salt Lake City, UT 84111
(801) 538–7700
Contact: John Killoran

Office of Rehab.
State Board of Education
250 E. 500 South
Salt Lake City, UT 84111
(801) 538–7530
Contact: Judy Ann Buffmire, Exec. Director

Division of Mental Health
Department of Social Services
120 N. 200 West, 4th Floor
P.O. Box 45500
Salt Lake City, UT 84145–0500
(801) 538–4270
Contact: Children and Adolescents Program
Specialist

Utah Council for People with Disabilities
120 N. 200 West
P.O. Box 1958
Salt Lake City, UT 84110
(801) 538–4184
Contact: Director

Legal Center for the Handicapped
455 E. 400 South, Ste. 201
Salt Lake City, UT 84111
(801) 363–1347; (800) 662–9080
Contact: Phyliss Geldzahler, Exec. Director

Developmental Center for Handicapped Per-
sons
Utah State University
Logan, UT 84322–6800
(801) 750–1981
Contact: Dr. Marvin Fifield, Director

Utah Parent Center
2290 E. 4500 South, No. 110
Salt Lake City, UT 84117
(801) 272–1051; (800) 468–1160 (in UT)
Contact: Helen Post

Parent-to-Parent
455 E. 400, South, Ste. 300
Salt Lake City, UT 84111
(801) 364–5060; (800) 662–4058

ARC of Utah
455 E. 400, South, Ste. 300
Salt Lake City, UT 84111
(801) 364–5060
Contact: Ray Behle, Exec. Director

Vermont

Tourette Syndrome Association Contact
Thelma Mason
P.O. Box 118
Newfane, VT 05345
(802) 365–4481

TSA Contact
Jan Farrell
34 Woodlane Apartments
Bristol, VT 05443
(802) 453–3266

TSA Contact
59 Terrill St.
Unit #4

Rutland, VT 05701
(802) 747–4436
Contact: Joan Canney

Division of Special Education
Department of Education
120 State Street
Montpelier, VT 05602–3403
(802) 828–3141
Contact: Marc E. Hull, Director

Special Education Unit (Ages 3–5)
Department of Education
120 State Street
Montpelier, VT 05602–2703
(802) 828–3141
Contact: Preschool Coordinator

Vocational Rehabilitation Division
Dept. of Social and Rehabilitation Services
103 S. Main St.
Waterbury, VT 05676
(802) 241–2189
Contact: Richard Douglas, Director

Vermont Developmental Disability Council
103 S. Main St.
Waterbury, VT 05676
Contact: Thomas Pombar, Director

Citizen Advocacy, Inc.
Champlain Mill, Box 37
Winooski, VT 05404
(802) 655–0329
Contact: Katherine Lenk, Dir.

Vermont Developmental Disability Law
Project
12 North St.
Burlington, VT 05401
(802) 863–2881
Contact: Judy Dickson, Director

Vermont Information and Training Network
(VITN)
Vermont/ARC
Champlain Mill, No. 37
Winooski, VT 05404
(802) 655–4016
Contact: Connie Curtain, Director

Vermont ARC
Champlain Mill, No. 37
Winooski, VT 05404
(802) 655–4014
Contact: Joan Sylvester, Exec. Director

Virginia

TSA—Greater Washington Chapter
(serves Maryland, Virgina, and D.C.)
For current phone number,
contact national TSA

LDA of Virginia
P.O. Box 717
Woodstock, VA 22664
(703) 459-8804
Contact: Attracta Owens, President

Special and Compensatory Education
Department of Education
P.O. Box 6Q
Richmond, VA 23216–2060
(804) 225–2402
Contact: Wm. Helton, Director

Division of Special Education Programs (Ages
3–5)
Department of Education
P.O. Box 6Q
Richmond VA 23216–2060
(804) 225–2873
Contact: Coordinator

Dept. of Rehabilitation Services
State Board of Vocational Rehabilitation
P.O. Box 11045
Richmond, VA 23230
Contact: Susan Urofsky, Commissioner

Developmental Disability Planning Council
Monroe Building, 17th Floor
101 N. 14th St.
Richmond, VA 23219
(804) 225–2042
Contact: Administrator

Department for Rights of the Disabled
James Monroe Building, 17th Floor
101 N. 14th St.
Richmond, VA 23219
(804) 225–2042; (800) 553–3962 (TDD and
Voice)
Contact: James Rothrock, Director

Virginia Institute for Devel. Dis.
Virginia Commonwealth University
301 W. Franklin St., Box 3020
Richmond, VA 23284–3020
(804) 224–3876
Contact: Dr. Howard Garner, Director

Parent Education Advocacy Training Center
(PEATC)
228 S. Pitt St., Room 300
Alexandria, VA 22314
(703) 836–2953
Contact: Winifred Anderson, Director

Parent-to-Parent of Virginia
1518 Willow Lawn Dr.
Richmond, VA 23230
(804) 282–4255
Contact: Mary Cunningham, Coordinator

ARC of Virginia
6 N. 6th St.
Richmond, VA 23219
(804) 649–8481
Contact: Chris Rowe, Exec. Director

Washington

TSA—Washington State Chapter
(serves entire state)
For current phone number,
contact national TSA

LDA of Washington
18921 27th Dr., SE
Bothell, WA 98012
(206) 481–8918
Contact: Carol Schneider

LDA State Office
17530 NW Union Hill, Suite 100
Redmond, WA 98052
(206) 882–0792
Special Education Section

Superintendent of Public Instruction
FG–11 Old Capitol Building
Olympia, WA 98504–0001
(206) 753–6733
Contact: John Pearson, Director

Superintendent of Public Instruction (Ages 3–5)
FG–11 Old Capitol Building
Olympia, WA 98504
(206) 753–0317
Contact: Michael Conn-Powers, ECSE Coordinator

Division of Vocational Rehab.
Dept. of Social and Health Services
MS: OB–21C
Olympia, WA 98504
(206) 753–2544
Contact: Sharon Stewart-Johnson, Director

Division of Developmental Disabilities
Dept. of Social and Health Services
P.O. Box 1788, OB–42C
Olympia, WA 98504
(206) 753–3900
Contact: Susan Elliott, Director

Child and Adolescent Services
Mental Health Division
MS: OB–42F
Olympia, WA 98504
(206) 753–5414
Contact: Jann Hoppler, Administrator

Developmental Disability Planning Council
Ninth and Columbia Building
MS: GH–52

Olympia, WA 98504–4151
(206) 753–3908
Contact: Sharon Hansen, Exec. Director

WA Protection & Advocacy System
1401 E. Jefferson
Seattle, WA 98122
(206) 324–1521
Contact: Mark Stroh, Exec. Dir.

Child Development and Mental Retardation Center
University of Washington
Seattle, WA 98195
(206) 543–2832
Contact: Dr. Michael Guralnick, Director

Parents Advocating Vocational Educational (PAVE)
6316 S. 12th St.
Tacoma, WA 98645
(206) 565–2266; (800) 5–Parent (In WA)
Contact: Kathy Babel, Coordinator

Pierce County Parent-to-Parent
12208 Pacific Highway, SW
Tacoma, WA 98499
(206) 588–1741
Contact: Betty Johnston, Coordinator

ARC of Washington
1703 E. State St.
Olympia, WA 98506
(206) 357–5596

West Virginia

TSA—West Virginia Chapter
(serves entire state)
For current phone number,
contact national TSA

West Virginia Association for Children and Adults with Learning Disabilities (ACLD)
Rt. 3, Box 70
Mineral Wells, WV 26150
(304) 489–9621
Contact: James Freeman, President

Office of Special Education
Department of Education
B–304, Building 6
Capitol Complex
Charleston, WV 25305
(304) 348–2696
Contact: Nancy Thabet, Director

Preschool Handicapped (Ages 3–5)
Office of Special Education
Department of Education
B–304, Building 6
Capitol Complex
Charleston, WV 25305

(304) 348–2696
Contact: Pam George, Coordinator

Division of Rehabilitation Services
State Board of Rehabilitation
State Capitol
Charleston, WV 25305
(304) 766–4601
Contact: John Panza, Director

Office of Behavioral Health
Dept. of Health and Human Resources
1800 Washington St., East
Charleston, WV 25305
(304) 348–0627
Contact: George Lilley, Director

Developmental Disaility Planning Council
1601 Kanawha Blvd., West
Charleston, WV 25312
(304) 348–0416
Contact: Richard Kelly, Director

West Virginia Advocates
1524 Kanawha Blvd., East
Charleston, WV 25311
(304) 346–0847; (800) 950–5250 (in WV)
Contact: Vicki Smith, Exec. Dir.

University Affiliated Center for Devel. Disab.
West Virginia University
509 Allen Hall/P.O. Box 6122
Morgantown, WV 26506–6122
(304) 293–4692
Contact: Ashok Dey, Director

Project STEP
116 E. King St.
Martinsburg, WV 25401
(304) 263–HELP
Contact: Carol Tamara, Director

ARC of West Virginia
16 Echo Terrace
Wheeling, WV 26003
(304) 485–5283
Contact: President

Wisconsin

TSA—Wisconsin Chapter
(serves entire state)
For current phone number,
contact national TSA

Wisconsin Association for Children and Adults
    with Learning Disabilities (ACLD)
2622 Oak Crest Dr.
Neenah, WI 54956
(414) 722–4977
Contact: Carolyn Tietje, President

Obsessive Compulsive Information Center
University of Wisconsin
Department of Psychiatry
600 Highland Ave.
Madison, WI 53792

Division of Handicapped Children and Pupil
    Services
Department of Public Instruction
125 S. Webster St.
P.O. Box 7841
Madison, WI 53707–7841
(608) 266–1649
Contact: Victor J. Contrucci, Director

Early Childhood Handicapped Programs (Ages
    3–5)
Department of Public Instruction
P.O. Box 7841
Madison, WI 53707
(608) 266–6981
Contact: Jenny Lange, Supervisor

Division of Vocational Rehab.
Department of Health and Social Services
1 W. Wilson St., Room 830
Madison, WI 53702
(608) 266–2168
Contact: Judy Norman-Nunnery, Administrator

Developmental Disabilities Office
Department of Health and Human Services
P.O. Box 7851
Madison, WI 53707
(608) 266–9329
Contact: Dennis Harkins, Director

Wisconsin Council on Developmental Dis-
    abilities
722 Williamson St., 2nd Fl.
Madison, WI 53707
(608) 266–7826
Contact: Jayn Wittenmyer, Exec. Director

Wisconsin Coalition for Advocacy, Inc.
16 N. Carroll St., Suite 400
Madison, WI 53703
(608) 267–0214
Contact: Lynn Breedlove, Executive Director

Waisman Center University Affiliated Facility
1500 Highland Ave.
Madison, WI 53705–2280
(608) 263–5940
Contact: Terrence Dolan, Director

Parent Education Project
United Cerebral Palsy of SE Wisconsin
230 W. Wells St., No. 502
Milwaukee, WI 53203
(414) 272–4500
Contact: Liz Irwin, Director

Parent-to-Parent
121 S. Hancock St.
Madison, WI 53703
(608) 251–9272
Contact: Coordinator

ARC of Wisconsin
121 S. Hancock St.
Madison, WI 53703
(608) 251–9272
Contact: Jon Nelson, Exec. Director

Wyoming

TSA Contact
Phyliss Henley
Box 412
Thermapolis, WY 82443
(307) 864–3603

TSA Contact
Jaime Eager
P.O. Box 14
Glen Rock, WY 82637
(307) 436–8533

Special Programs Unit
Department of Education
Hathaway Building, 2nd Fl.
Cheyenne, WY 82002–0050
(307) 777–7414
Contact: Ken Blackburn, Director

Division of Vocational Rehab.
Department of Employment
1100 Herschler Bldg.
Cheyenne, WY 82002
(307) 777–7385

Division of Community Programs
356 Hathaway Bldg.
Cheyenne, WY 82002
(307) 777–7115
Contact: Darrell Farris

Wyoming Protection and Advocacy System, Inc.
2424 Pioneer Ave., No. 101
Cheyenne, WY 82001
(307) 638–7668
Contact: Jeanne Kawcak, Exec. Director

Parent-to-Parent
Council on Developmental Disabilities
Barrett Building, Room 408
301 Central Ave.
Cheyenne, WY 82002
(307) 777–7230
Contact: Brett Wilson, Program Manager

ARC of Wyoming
P.O. Box 2161
Casper, WY 82601

(307) 265–6627
Contact: Lorinda Vetter, Exec. Director

Canadian TSA Chapters and TS Clinics

Alberta

TS Foundation of Alberta
Valerie Korman
7639–22 St. S.E.
Calgary, Alta. T2C 0W9
(403) 279–8792

Movement Disorder Clinic
University of Calgary Medical Unit
3350 Hospital Dr., NW
Calgary, Alta. T2N 4N1
(403) 270–1110

TSA
Calgary Chapter
c/o Valerie Korman,
7639 22 St. SE
Calgary, Alta. T2C 0W9
(403)279–8792

TSA
Edmonton Chapter
c/o Janet Smart
8215 185 St.
Edmonton, Alta. T5T 1G9

British Columbia

Tourette Syndrome Clinic
Jack Ledger House
Arbutus Road
Victoria, BC
(604) 479–6913

Movement Disorder Clinic
University Hospital, UBC Site
2211 Wesbrook Mall
Vancouver, BC V6T 1W5
(604) 228–7660

TSA
Vancouver Island Chapter
c/o Judy Rogers
4056 Valerie Place,
Victoria, BC V8X 2K9
(604) 479–6913

TSA
Greater Vancouver Chapter,
c/o P. Seidelman
4371 Coventry Dr.
Richmond, BC V7C 4R7
(604) 271–0492

TSA Representatives
Myrtice & Doug Alpen
1733 Sloan Ave.
Prince Rupert, BC V8J 2B5
(604) 627–8129

TSA Representatives
Ken & Mary-Ann Armstong
411–6716 Dover Road
Nanaimo, BC V9V 1L8
(604) 390–3813

Manitoba

Tourette Syndrome Clinic
St. Boniface General Hospital
409 Tache Ave.
Winnepeg, Man. R2N 2A6
(204) 237–2690

Manitoba Society for TS
Murray McKnight
1650 Main St.
Box 25064
Winnipeg, Man. R2V 4C7
(204) 889–4463

New Brunswick

TSA
New Brunswick Chapter
c/o Hope Green
RR 2
Sackville, N.B. E0A 3C0
(506) 536–0912

TSA Representative
Claudett Vinneau
660 Vanier Blvd.
Barthurst, N.B. E2A 3N9

Newfoundland

Newfoundland Chapter TSA
c/o Rosalind M. Foley
P.O. Box 14072
St. John's, Nfld. A1N 2P5
(709) 834–9443

Nova Scotia

Isaak Walton Killam Hospital for Children
Dr. Aiden Stokes
Tourette Diagnostic Center
5850 University Ave.
Halifax, B.C. B3H 1V7
(902) 428–1875

TSA
Nova Scotia Chapter
c/o Norma McNamara
P.O. Box 3256 East

Dartmouth, N.S.B2W 5G2
(902) 462–8066

Cape Breton Chapter
c/o Mary Lou Setchell
26 Carmichael
Sydney River, N.S. B1S 3H9
(902) 564–4694

Ontario

Children's Hospital of Eastern Ontario
401 Smyth
Ottawa, Ont. K0H 8L1
(613) 737–7600

Psychobiological Medicine Unit
Toronto Hospital, Western Division
399 Bathurst St.
Toronto, Ont. M5T 2R2
(416) 369–5794

Movement Disorder Clinic
25 Leonard St., Suite 3
Toronto, Ont. M5T 2R2
(416) 363–3063

TS Foundation of Ontario
Sam Waye, President
100 College St.
Toronto, Ont. P0A A1A
(416) 449–4842

TSA
Greater Metro Toronto Chapter
c/o Diane Robertson
P.O. Box 407, Station S
Toronto, Ont. M5M 4M9
(416) 782–9406

TSA
Brantford Area Chapter
c/o Elfrieda Neumann
290 Erie Ave.
Brantford, Ont. N3S 2H6
(519) 759–7885

TSA
Natonal Capital Region Chapter
c/o Marcia Zuker
51 St. Remy Dr.
Nepean, Ont. K2J 1H5
(613) 825–2561

Wellington-Waterloo Chapter
c/o Sheila Montyro
Box 1312
Guelph, Ont. N1H 6N6
(519) 822–8192

TSA Representative
Margo Liaw
70 Appleton Trail

Brampton, Ont. L6W 4L3
(416) 455–1806

TSA Representative
Mary Jo Chartrand
20 Rexway Road
London, Ont. N6G 3C3
(519) 473–1746

TSA Representative
Bob Atack
120 Brookside Cres.
Kitchner, Ont. N2N 1H1
(519) 576–6825 (evenings only)

TSA Representative
Mrs. J. Albo
340 Toledo St.
Thunder Bay, Ont. P7A 2R6
(807) 344–8207

TSA Representative
R.K. Bradey
5 Waubuno Cres.
Parry Sound, Ont. P2A 2R6
(705) 746–5660

TSA Representative
Mrs. Jeannine Delorme
1245 Voyageur St.
Sudbury, Ont. P3A 3Z5
(705) 566–0888

Prince Edward Island

TSA
P.E.I. Chapter
c/o Susan Lambe
RR 2
Albany, PEI, C0B 1A0
(902) 855–2221

Quebec

Clinical Psychophamacology Unit
Allen Memorial Institute
1025 Pine Ave. West
Montreal, PQ H3A 1A1
(514) 842–1231, ext. 5519

Hopital Sainte-Justine
3175 Cote Sainte-Catherine
Montreal, PQ H3T 1C5
(514) 345–4931

Association Quebecoise du Syndrome de la
Tourette
c/o Evelyne Paiement
3791 Kent
Montreal, PQ H3S 1N4
(514) 345–0251

TSA Representatives
Carmen & France Bellemare
2105 rue Lemieux
Duberger, PQ G1P 2T8
(418) 688–8284 (6–8 p.m.)

Saskatchewan

TSA Representative
Dr. Carlos Maningas
University Hospital (Paed.)
Saskatoon, Sask. S7N 0W8
(306) 966–8108

TSA Representative
Debbie Stewart
3499 Olive Grove
Regina, Sask. S4V 2P4
(306) 751–0041

INDEX